COLONIALISM & THE MEDICAL EXPERIENCES IN THE SUDAN 1504-1956

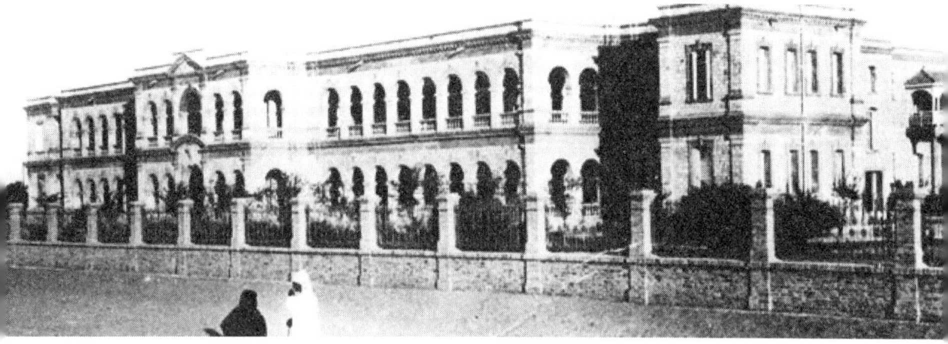

COLONIALISM & THE MEDICAL EXPERIENCES IN THE SUDAN 1504-1956

Volume I

The Roots of Medicine, Medical Research & Education (1504-1924)

Tarik Elhadd

THE RED SEA PRESS
TRENTON | LONDON | NEW DELHI | CAPE TOWN | NAIROBI | ADDIS ABABA | ASMARA | IBADAN

THE RED SEA PRESS
541 West Ingham Avenue | Suite B
Trenton, New Jersey 08638

Book design: Dawid Kahts
Cover design: Asharful Haq

Cataloging-in-Publication Data may be obtained from the Library of Congress.

ISBNs: 978-1-56902-653-3 (HB)
978-1-56902-654-0 (PB)

This book is dedicated to the soul of my late father,

Abdelkariem Elhadd,

a very fine man in every sense.

'One should write books as one writes letters, with [a] vivid sense of whom is addressing.'

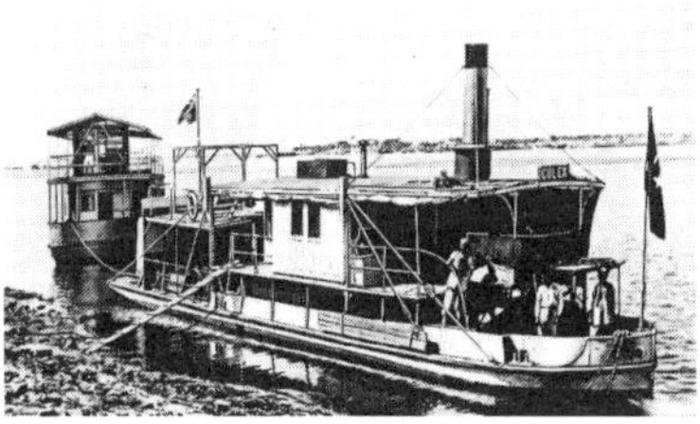

Table of Contents

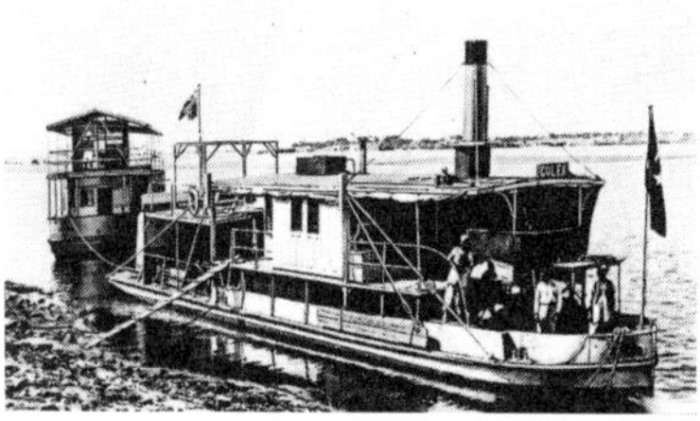

Illustrations

Maps

Abbreviations

AMO:	Assistant Medical Officer
EA:	Egyptian Army
EAMC:	Egyptian Army Medical Corps
GMC:	Gordon Memorial College
Eff.:	Effendi
KSM:	Kitchener School of Medicine
PMO:	Principal Medical Officer
MO:	Medical Officer
MD:	Medical Department
MTS:	Midwifery Training School
RAMC:	Royal Army Medical Corps
SMD:	Sudan Medical Department
SMS:	Sudan Medical Service
SPS:	Sudan Political Service
SSC:	Sleeping Sickness Commission
WTRL:	Wellcome Tropical Research Laboratory

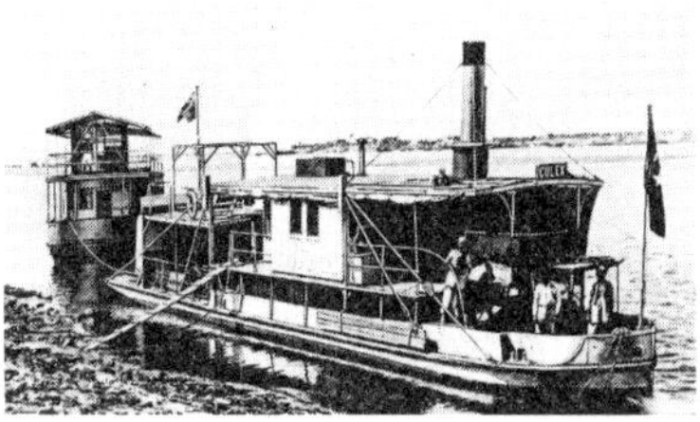

Acknowledgements

This book is the by-product of hard and painstaking work which was carried out over several years. It would not have become the work as it is, if I didn't have the help and support of many, including family, colleagues, and friends as well as many of those who have shaped the history of the Sudan health. I would like to pay special tribute to Professor Ali Khogali Ismail, the first Sudanese medical physiologist, and first Sudanese professor of physiology and later WHO envoy to the East Mediterranean Region. He has provided invaluable evidence of an important era in the evolution of the medical education in the Sudan. The seeds of the many trees of this book were sowed during many trips to the Sudan Archives at Durham and to the Cambridge University Library. I would like to acknowledge the help of Mrs Jane Hogan, Francis Gotto and Mr Mark Harkness at the Palace Green Library at Durham University, and the librarians at the Rare Manuscript reading Room at Cambridge. Bill and Mandy Kelly were so ever generous to make those trips comfortable by hosting me at 'Gill House', enjoying their lovely company and kind hospitality. I also spent some time at the main library of Wellcome Foundation Trust in Euston Road, London. My trips to Cambridge University Library and the help and support I got from the staff at the Manuscript Reading Room, the Royal Commonwealth Society Archive Centre and the Rare Books Reading Room very much helped to bridge the gap in the documentation in various sections. During my trips to Cambridge I was blessed and honoured to have stumbled on Mr. Moses Anafu, a retired Ghanaian diplomat, whose help and advise were useful to direct my attention to other areas which proved to be helpful in writing this treatise. Several friends and colleagues have made very useful suggestions and comments when read some of the chapters. Special thanks go to Dr. Paul Rafferty, Dr. James Walker, Dr. Bill Kelly, Dr. Ghazi Salah al-Din al-Atabani, Dr. Andy Collier, Dr. Peter Newman and Anne Crichton Harris. Others helped by guiding me to certain references and books, others by even providing some rare copies. Special thanks to Hadi Stamboli (Great grandson of Georgeos Stamboli, the famous Sudanese Syrian who was assigned by the Mahdi to be the guardian of the Christian community at el-Obeid, following the fall of the city in 1883. I would like also to thank Dr. Catherine Greer, a medical missionary whom I met at Elgin, in the Scottish Highlands in 2010, for furnishing me with the rare book of Dr. Kenneth Fraser, 'The Doctor Comes to Lui'. Also I would like to pass special thanks to Dr. Mervyn Humphreys, son of the late Dr. Roy Mervyn Humphreys, of the Sudan Medical Service (SMS), and to his daughter, Mrs Miranda Waller. I would like also to thank Dr. David Clarke, son of Dr. Patrick Clarke, a veteran of the SMS and later an eminent neurosurgeon in the northeast of England. Special tribute is paid to the memory of Dr. Kenneth Owen, one of the last SMS doctors, and later a very distinguished urologist at St Mary Hospital, London. Dr. Owen, sadly, passed away in June 2013. Both Drs Owen and Clarke provided me with first hand memoirs of their lives and times in Sudan as doctors in the SMS in the 1940s and 1950s respectively. Lastly, I would like to thank Mrs Sirloin Streeten, daughter of the late professor John Mynors who helped me greatly during my interview of her mother Una Mynors. Special thanks go to Professor Ahmed Ibrahim Abu Shouk, Professor of Modern and Contemporary History at Qatar University, Qatar, for his very useful and expert comments, and to Rogaia Mustafa Abu Sharaf for her help and guidance. A special note is a word of tribute to the memory of the late Ahmed Yusif Mustafa Altenie, former Sudanese ambassador and a well beloved and a cultural man, who has been following the final stages of this work. Special thanks to Dr. Eric Kirpatrick, Dr. Kariem Elhadd, Mrs. Aiza Mahmoud and Dr. Richard Quinton for their invaluable help and efforts reading and making corrections in the galley proof of the manuscript

Finally I would like to express my extreme gratitude to my wife Sarah Elarabi and my kids, Kariem, Ahmed, Amr and Shaza Elhadd, and my son-in-law, Khaled Gabra, as without their patience and support during the long and painstaking process of writing this book, this wouldn't have been possible so they have all my love and gratitude.

To Ahmed Ibrahim Abu Shouk, Ann Crichton-Harris, Richard Quinton and Ali B. Ali Dinar special thanks for writing blurbs for the work. Finally, to Professor Heather Sharkey, Professor of History, Pennsylvania University, my deep gratitude for taking the time and efforts to read the manuscript and writing a foreword for the book. I have been honoured and touched by her contribution. At the end, without the help and support of my family, my wife Sarah Ahmed Elarabi, and my kids, Kariem, Shaza, Ahmed and Amr, this work wouldn't have been possible to see light, so they have my love and gratitude.

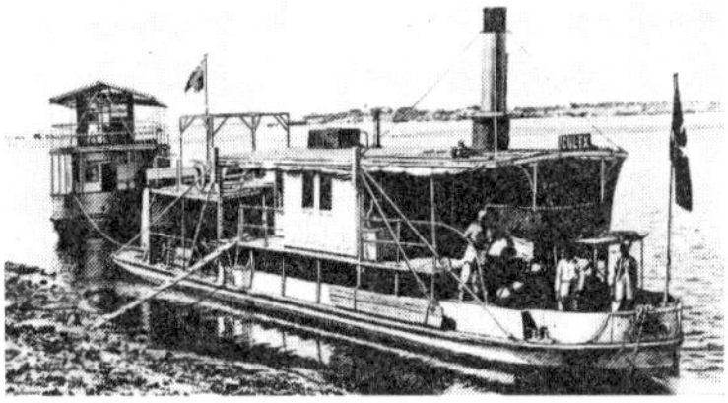

Foreword

Heather J. Sharkey
University of Pennsylvania

This sweeping history of Sudanese medicine comes to us from Tarik Elhadd, a distinguished endocrinologist who studied medicine at the University of Khartoum before pursuing a successful career in England, Scotland, Sudan, Saudi Arabia, and now Qatar. Having dedicated his life's work to promoting good health, with a specialty in treating diabetes, Dr. Elhadd pays tribute here to the generations of men and women who established and maintained medical practices and institutions, or who left records that help us to appreciate the history of sickness, healing, and health in Sudan. Today, when the world is coping with the COVID-19 pandemic, Dr. Elhadd's narrative feels more relevant than ever as a testament to humankind's long-running and ongoing quest for survival and well-being.

Readers will see that this account is wide-ranging and inclusive. Dr. Elhadd describes the efforts of many kinds of medical practitioners, among them doctors, midwives, sanitation engineers, researchers, traditional barbers (who historically in Sudan, as in Europe, functioned as surgeons, dentists, and bloodletters), and others. He surveys sites of organized care and training: not only hospitals, but also quarantine stations and laboratories. He considers recurrent diseases that afflicted Sudanese populations – everything from guinea worm, malaria, and cholera to bilharzia and plague. He cites practices and treatments, including some based on local knowledge about the restorative powers of herbs and foods. He tells us (to cite just a few examples) that some Sudanese people once used an infusion of *hilba* (fenugreek) to treat dysentery, advised people recovering from fractures to eat dates, and treated wounds by wrapping them in bandages which they then coated with butter. Moving into the twentieth century, he describes how a generation of British tropical disease specialists, armed with microscopes, advanced the frontiers of knowledge by identifying and studying parasites, such as those that cause leishmaniasis (kala azar). He also notes cumulative efforts to promote public health, for example, by vaccinating against smallpox in the nineteenth century and, later, in the early twentieth, by promoting mosquito-eradication programs to reduce the spread of malaria.

As title of the volume makes clear, Dr. Elhadd envisions the book as stretching from the Funj era (circa 1500-1800) to the end of the Anglo-Egyptian period (1898-1956). Alas, sources for the Funj period are slim, making written accounts by early European travelers, such as James Bruce and John Lewis Burckhardt, critical for what they say about local ailments, epidemics, and people's responses to them. Sometimes travelers dabbled in healthcare themselves, with mixed results. Consider the English explorer W.G. Browne, who visited Sudan in the 1790s: he described inoculating five slave children of Fertit origin against smallpox, but noted that one of them died from the consequences.

For the nineteenth century, European travel accounts remain Dr. Elhadd's major source; for the twentieth century, he relies heavily on the memoirs and other papers of British officials and medics, many of which are now stored in archives. One consequence of this source base is that the actions of Europeans – and of Britons above all – loom large in this history of medicine. Dr. Elhadd acknowledges that Egyptian doctors and later, in the twentieth century, Syrian and Lebanese doctors (many of them graduates of the American University of Beirut) were central players in Sudanese medicine, too, although information about them is scarce.

Of course, the reliance on European and especially British written sources, and the lack of comparable sources in Arabic, makes it hard to see what Sudanese people did or achieved in medical history. Indeed, Sudanese people remain largely nameless in medical sources before the mid-twentieth century. Studies in folklore and ethnography help to some degree, by giving a sense of popular customs and practices, but do so, again, without citing individuals in action. This challenge of sources is one that faces all historians of Sudan.

The institutional development of medicine in Sudan bears an intimate relationship to the two waves of colonialism that rolled through the country, during the Turco-Egyptian era (circa 1820-1885) and later in the Anglo-Egyptian period. Not surprisingly, the health of soldiers – on whose coercive powers colonial powers depended – remained a top concern for Egyptian and British authorities. Indeed, both regimes established hospitals – the first of their kind in the region – which prioritized the care of men, and of diseases or injuries from which soldiers were likely to suffer, such as syphilis, gonorrhea, dysentery, and battle wounds.

After the conquest of 1820, Turco-Egyptian authorities realized that the stability of their regime – and of the local society and economy that anchored it – required a broad and stable base of public well-being; they could not focus efforts on soldiers alone. After all, epidemics paid no heed to social rank, and struck Turco-Egyptian leaders, too. Consider Mahu Bey Urfali, the Kurd who became governor of Sinnar: he perished during the smallpox outbreak that struck the wider Sudanese population in 1826. Cholera was particularly devastating, and often came with pilgrims returning from Mecca. Eager to monitor cholera and to stop it from spreading, Turco-Egyptian authorities opened quarantine stations on Sudan's Red Sea coast, at Massawa and Suakin, and from the 1860s expanded efforts to vaccinate travelers against smallpox. We can see with such practices the beginnings of concerted state-led programs of public health.

The Mahdist period (c. 1881-1898) was an interlude in the history of colonialism and its medical programs. Nevertheless, the Mahdi and later the Khalifa pursued their own public health agendas. For example, they issued proclamations ordering residents of Omdurman, their capital, to keep the streets clean of garbage, while banning public urination and defecation. They made urban sanitation a priority. They ordered the continuation of smallpox vaccination campaigns, since epidemics worried them, too. And with good reason: the Mahdi himself died, on the heels of his victory at Khartoum in 1885, during an outbreak of what may have been either cerebrospinal meningitis or typhus.

Following the 1898 conquest, British authorities wanted to cultivate a robust force of laborers as part of their strategy for economic development. To this end, they expanded the Sudanese medical and public health systems, while developing feeder schools and programs. They also elaborated systems of urban sanitation, waste management (including sewage systems), and quarantine. In 1902, for example, they opened a new quarantine station at Wadi Halfa to monitor travelers coming from Egypt, where cholera was, again, a major concern. At the same time, new institutions emerged that offered formal healthcare to a broader array of the populace. An important step in this direction occurred in 1921 when the British sisters Mabel and Gertrude Wolff established the Midwifery Training School in Omdurman, focused on the care of pregnant women, new mothers, and their babies.

Dr. Elhadd features many colourful characters in his account. Among them is the Egyptian, Hasan Effendi Zaki. Taken as a prisoner of war during the Mahdist revolution, when he was serving as a military doctor in the Egyptian Army, Hasan Effendi Zaki became personal physician to the Mahdi and the Khalifa, and led the Mahdist state's vaccination campaigns; after 1898, he transitioned to serve the Anglo-Egyptian regime as well. He wrote an Arabic account of Mahdist-era medicine, which Rudolf van Slatin (a fellow prisoner of the Mahdi, and later Inspector-General of the Anglo-Egyptian Sudan) translated into English and helped to publish in 1908. Hasan Effendi Zaki described the work of surgeons and barbers in setting bones and treating wounds, and in circumcising boys. He also recorded popular treatments for injuries, describing how, for example, Sudanese would cover wounds with a paste made from ground coffee and water, or apply a mixture of sesame oil and beeswax.

Dr. Elhadd obviously admires many of the figures he profiles. He lavishes praise, for instance, on Henry Wellcome, the pharmaceutical entrepreneur, whose philanthropy initiated and sustained the Wellcome Tropical Research Laboratory. He describes the cutting-edge research that this laboratory sponsored in the study of diseases like sleeping sickness (trypanosomiasis). He examines the contributions that individual researchers made, even while noting their achievements beyond medicine. William Byam, for instance, who helped to lead the Anglo-Egyptian state's fight against malaria, was a serious philatelist who wrote studies on postage stamps and won international accolades in this field. Sheffield Neave not only became a world expert in sleeping sickness and the tse-tse fly which spread it; he also studied the Bari people and their use of medicinal plants, and collected insect and botanical specimens which he gave to museums. Dr. Elhadd presents Andrew Balfour as "a genius" in the field of tropical medicine whose "protean and diverse interests place him undoubtedly as a polymath of science." Amid the fight against malaria, Balfour researched mosquitoes so extensively that his colleagues named a Sudanese species, which they discovered, in his honor: they called it *Uranotaenia balfouri*.

Dr. Elhadd opens his narrative by explaining the epiphany which led him to write this book. One day, while living in Ayr, a historic market town south of Glasgow in Scotland (where he was working as a staff endocrinologist in the local hospital), he was driving his son to a friend's house when he saw that the street leading up to it was called Dongola Road – named, as it turns out, after Kitchener's Dongola Expedition of 1896, which preceded the Anglo-Egyptian overthrow of the Mahdist state two years later. Finding a reference to the Sudanese Nile town of Dongola in that corner of Ayr inspired him to trace the arcs that have linked Sudanese specialists like himself to the British and other medical practitioners who came before him.

Dr. Elhadd's interest in the history of Sudanese medicine springs from his experiences as someone who is proud to be Sudanese, and also proud of his advanced training and professional service in the United Kingdom. His account on these pages testifies to strong and historic Anglo-Sudanese connections, as well as to the links that have bound Sudan and its peoples to others on the world stage. In short, Dr. Elhadd provides a panoramic sweep of Sudanese history which brings local, regional, and international perspectives to bear on this lively study of medicine, sickness, and public health.

Heather J Sharkey,
Professor,
Department of Near Eastern Languages & Civilization
University of Pennsylvania

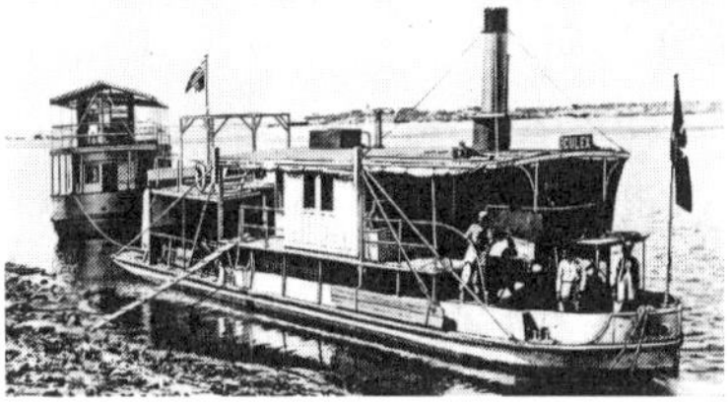

Prologue

From the Dongola Expedition to Dongola Road, Ayr

Time and destiny took me from eastern Sudan, where I passed the first educational milestones that shaped my early life, to central Sudan and Egypt, before completing my medical training in Khartoum and graduating in medicine in the early 1980s. Then ambition and a zeal for knowledge took me to Great Britain, a country destined to greatly influence my adult years and the whole of my professional life. The writing of this book is a mixture of nostalgia, love of narration and history, and an expression of deep gratitude to my home country, Sudan, and my adopted country, Britain. I am not a historian and I won't claim to be one, nor do I have a wide knowledge of history, but I felt that my lifelong love and passion for history since I was a child has very much helped me in writing this book. That love evolved since I was a young child of six sitting with my paternal grandmother, attentively listening to stories from old Sudanese and Arabic folklore. That early childhood experience captured my imagination and possibly sowed the first seeds of my love of history. It was during my first year in secondary education, in 1974/5, that I became fascinated with yet another character who had an impact on my ongoing love of and passion for history. That was the history teacher at el-Gedaref High Secondary School, 'Uztaz'[1]

Gubarah Mohamed Ahmed, from the Singa region, a prolific history teacher, with glowing bright eyes and a gallant character.

Many years later, well into the second millennium and in a friendly and quiet suburb of Ayr, a historical market town in south-west Scotland, the writing of this book had its beginnings. It was an irony that one day, while I was dropping my youngest son, *Amr,* to the house of one of his friends and school-mates, that I noticed that the road leading to that house is called *'Dongola Road'*. What a coincidence! The famous Nile Expedition led by Lord Kitchener during the Reconquest of the Sudan in the 1890s, took a decisive turn with the '*Dongola Expedition*'; the subsequent fall of the town of Dongola[2] indeed paved the way to the eventual capture of Omdurman in 1898 and the creation of the Anglo-Egyptian Sudan. That marked the beginning of an important chapter in the history of the Sudan, and it proved to be crucial to the beginnings of modern medicine there. Hence, the choice of the title of this prologue, comes from the amazing coincidence of the name of the northern Sudan town of Dongola occurring in the Scottish town where I first began writing this treatise.

This book is an attempt to write a comprehensive account of Sudan's medical history. I have to pay special tribute to the memory of the late Professor Richard Leslie Hill, whose selflessness devotion in documenting the history of Sudan has enabled many, including myself, to know much about Sudan. Professor Hill's immense contribution to creating a repository for modern Sudanese history was unsurpassed, and he deserves to be acknowledged and appreciated by the Sudanese. Hill, an Englishman who was brought up in New Zealand and studied history at Oxford, was recruited to work for the Sudan Political Service, where he was employed by Sudan Government Railways (SGR). One day, Richard Hill went in search of a biographical dictionary of the Sudan and, when told that there was none, authored the first biographical dictionary of the Sudan. It was through the orchestrating efforts of Richard Hill that the core of the Sudan Archives at Durham was created. This repository has enabled many researchers to have access to rare documents about the Sudan. Here, I would like to pay tribute to the many men and women who have contributed to the common history of the Sudan and Britain and to its legacy. There were some English, a good score of the Welsh, some Irish, and many Scots. There were also many Syrians[3] and a good number of Egyptians. Those men and women were a 'special breed', as Elliot Balfour, son of Sir Andrew Balfour, and later Governor of Northern Province in Sudan, wrote: 'We are a dying breed, they are not making new of us any more'. Doctors, who worked in the Sudan, were mostly distinguished during their career in their medical schools before joining. Many made outstanding contributions to the service in Sudan, and went on to excel following their relocation back to Britain. Of these, I mention Andrew Balfour, William Byam, Robert Archibald, Eric Pridie, Kenneth Owen, Patrick Clarke, Bill MacGowan, Patrick D'Arcy, and the list goes on. On the other hand, most of the Sudanese doctors who came and worked in Britain through the amazing decades of evolving relations were also a 'special breed'.

I have done my best to compile some biographical details of many doctors, British, Syrian, Egyptian, and Sudanese, who represent the common legacy of the relationship between Britain and the Sudan. The details of many of those I have included, narrating their stories and mapping their legacy, are sketchy or limited. It was a painstaking task to gather the scattered information from various places. Some had left a rich saga of their 'days & ways' in the Sudan, others left very little trace, and many left none. Those who left a wealth of published or other written material have received more detailed inclusion in this text. These include Andrew Balfour, Albert Chalmers, Robert Archibald, John Bloss, William Byam, Leonard Bousfield, Patrick D'Arcy, Mabel Wolff, and Alexander Cruickshank, to mention but a few. Others were still alive at the time of writing this thesis, such as Dr. Kenneth Owen, whom I had the opportunity of meeting and interviewing. Others, like Patrick Clarke, who, although frail and feeble, nonetheless permitted a visit, was ever so kind in writing some of his reminisces in his own handwriting, which was a joy to read and 'try to figure out'. So, when reading this book, these points should be borne in mind and this will readily explain why my accounts of some characters like Bousfiled, Byam & Balfour, Kenneth Owen and Patrick Clarke, and others are rich and in depth. Others about whom the information and details were rather patchy and scarce were mentioned only in passing. Some could not even be traced.

I started this project well into 2007 with various trips to the Sudan Archives at Durham. Later, I made several trips to the Wellcome Library and to the University of Cambridge Library. I strove to meet descendants or relatives of the staff of the Sudan Medical Service, and I was blessed to have met a few. One touching experience was when I met Dr. Kenneth Owen, a veteran, who worked in the Sudan in the 1940s. Meeting him and interviewing him was a special and memorable experience. I have to pay tribute to his kind help. Despite his many ripe years, Ken was happy to meet me at his farmhouse, 'Hillside Farm', in Gloucestershire in the spring of 2009. The way I stumbled on him is narrated in volume 2 (forthcoming). I also have to pay great tribute to Patrick Clarke, an eminent northeast of England neurosurgeon who worked in the Sudan in 1950s (and like Ken Owen also at Wad Medani). Although I could not meet him personally, he was very kind to exchange letters with me, in which he poured forth his 'Sudan Reminisces'. I also would like to thank his son, Dr. David Clarke, a former Convenor of the Scottish Museum. It was courtesy of Professor Ali Khogali's wife, Friyal, that I managed to meet Una Mynors and Sirloin Streeten, wife and daughter, respectively, of the late Professor Mynors, one of the eminent surgeons in the SMS. Finally, I was also privileged to have met Dr. Mervyn Humphreys, son of Dr. Roy Humphreys at his house in Farendon, Oxfordshire, in summer of 2009. Roy Humphreys was among the first waves of British doctors to flock to the Sudan in the early 1920s. He went on to stay in Sudan till 1944. He was the second lecturer of medicine at Kitchener School of Medicine and the first to hold the post of Senior Physician at Khartoum. His story with the sword of Darfur Sultan, Ibrahim Garrad, is narrated elsewhere.[4]

Endnotes

1 Ustaz: an Arabic name for teacher.

2 Dongola, an ancient market town in Northern Sudan.

3 The name Syrian applies to both Syrian and Lebanese prior to the appearance of Greater Lebanon in 1920 and declaration of Independence of Lebanon in 1943.

4 *Sudanese Studies Association Bulletin*, Vol. 28, No. 2, Fall 2010.

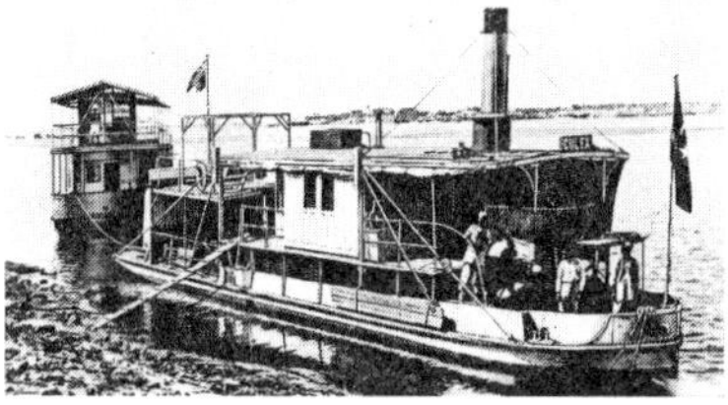

Introduction

This book attempts to bridge the existing gap in the documentation of Sudan's medical heritage. Despite the fact that that the medical history the Sudan is quite rich compared to other countries in Africa and the Middle East, there is a dearth of documentation, as most of the pertinent records are scattered piecemeal. There is a perceived need for a treatise that will trace the evolution of medicine in the Sudan. Thus, the present work attempts to set forth a rather comprehensive account of the history of medicine in the Sudan, pieced together from primary source material that I have compiled over the course of years. The idea originated in my special interest in medical biography. Indeed, the initial exercise was an attempt to compile some biographical details of the prominent British medical staff who laid the groundwork for the establishment of the modern Sudanese medical services. The deeper my research into the theme went, the more I came to realize just how deficient our knowledge of the history of Sudan's medical heritage is. Earlier attempts to write on the medical history of Sudan—e.g., those of Dr. Paul Squires (a pioneer of the medical services in modern Sudan)[1], the academic theses of Dr. Ahmed Bayoumi (1972) and Dr. Heather Bell (1999), and the late Professor Patrick D'Arcy's documentary on the Wellcome Laboratory at Khartoum—present but a sketchy picture of the evolution of modern medicine in the region. Seeing the need for a more comprehensive treatment of the subject, I have tried to present a more panoramic and global picture of this history. The works of Bayoumi and Bell were both primarily academic theses focusing on specific themes. The earlier work by Paul Squires, who was in close touch with the medical service for nearly forty years, had the advantage of being first-hand documentation, but it lacked depth. Indeed, when it was first published in 1958 (the year I was born), it was criticized as having no scientific depth. C. A. Bozman concluded his review by stating that 'Dr. Squires certainly succeeds in whetting one's appetite for the full-scale history yet to come from some other source, of a service and a period so important in the development of medical knowledge in regard to some of the major problems of health in hot climates'[2]. Modern pioneers of Sudan history, such as Richard Hill, Peter Malcolm Holt, and Martin Daly, mentioned a few scattered notes about the medical services during the Anglo-Egyptian era. At the national level in the Sudan, Dr. Ahmed Alsafi, a renowned expert on Sudanese complementary and traditional medicine, has established a way to document and preserve the Sudanese medical heritage. Through his Sudan Medical Heritage Foundation, he has made a major contribution by documenting biographies of some contemporary Sudanese pioneers of medicine.

Evidence of medical practices in the Sudan prior to the early nineteenth century surfaced in the writings of some European explorers/travellers. The first European physician to have come to 'Nubia & Sennar' was the French doctor and apothecary, Charles Jacques Poncet, who traversed the Sudanese frontiers on his way to treat the Abyssinian monarch, Iyasu ('The Great') in 1699. Poncet was sent by the French King as a diplomatic envoy and as a physician to treat Iyasu. He was accompanied by a Jesuit priest named Charles Francis Xavier De Brevedent. Their mission was followed in 1705 by a group of Jesuit priests, including the German Theodoro Krump. Father Krump left a rich legacy of medical enterprises. Krump also wrote some accounts of the traditional Sudanese medical practices and superstitions as he witnessed them. The first British explorer documented to have visited Sudan was the Scottish 'Laird', James Bruce. Bruce and his fellow Briton, George William Browne, and the Anglo-Swiss John Lewis (Johann Ludwig) Burckhardt wrote extensively about their observations on the health of the Sudanese, and the various diseases they witnessed during their stay in the Sudan.

Many European travellers in those days used to adopt the persona of a physician to impress, to gain easy access, and to ensure safety during travels in those rough times. The aforementioned travellers were no exception.

The introduction of modern European medicine to the Sudan in the nineteenth century took place following the incorporation of the Sudanese hinterland into the domain of the empire of Muhammad Ali Pasha, the prolific Albanian/Macedonian Viceroy of Egypt, when he reigned supreme in Egypt following the defeat of Napoleon Bonaparte. Muhammad Ali and his successor in the dynasty he established in Egypt, Abbas I, were not interested in setting up sound public services in the southern frontiers they acquired following the invasion of 'Nubia and Sennar' in 1820. The medical services established in what came to be known as the Turco-Egyptian Sudan (1821-1885) were rudimentary and backward compared with the services established in the remaining part of his expanding empire. The first modern hospital was built at Khartoum circa 1826, but treatment was restricted to the ruling Turkish and Egyptian elite and the military. Despite significant reforms that were carried out by Mohamed Sa'ied Pasha (r. 1853-1863), the services remained poor and very limited. It was only during the reign of Ismail Pasha ('The Magnificent') that the public services of the Turco-Egyptian Sudan saw some improvement, especially during the tenure of Charles Gordon (1877-1880). The medical staff consisted mainly of French, Italians, Egyptians, Turkish, and a few Germans, Greeks, and only a handful from Britain. At the time of the rise of the Mahdi in 1881, there was a military hospital in each 'Mudeiryyia' in the country. Following the establishment of the Mahdist State on the ruins of the Turco-Egyptian Sudan, the medical establishment created by 'The Turks' was swept away. From the medical and dispensary staff during the Turco-Egyptian regime, only one Egyptian doctor, Dr. Hassan Effendi Zaki, survived the revolution and was taken as the private physician of the Mahdi and then of his successor, the Khalifa Abdullahi. The medical services that had been in place during the Mahdiyya went into oblivion, but for the sole practice of Dr. Zaki, who survived the years of turmoil and was appointed to the Egyptian Army Medical Corps following the Nile Expedition and the Reconquest of 1898. With the success of the Reconquest, led by Lord Kitchener, the fate of the Mahdist State was sealed at Omdurman on September 2nd, 1898. It is worth noting here that two regions in the old Turco-Egyptian Sudan remained under Anglo-Egyptian control throughout the Mahdiyya. Those included Mahdiyya: Wadi Halfa and Suakin. Evidence of some medical services by military doctors could be traced and are included in the early chapters of this work. The memoirs of Dr. William Thornton of the Indian Medical Services and Sir Arthur Slogget give some idea of the health and medical problems of Wadi Halfa and Suakin during the Mahdiyya. Slogget, a distinguished physician, is credited with having set important milestones in military medicine and the discovery of a particular strain of staphylococcus, will be examined.

It was to the credit of the new British administration that it established a basis for modern medicine in the Sudan at the turn of the twentieth century. It is important to note that the establishment began in a hybrid way. At the beginning, the health services were more or less centred on delivering health care for the invading British troops and their families, thus, the military medical personnel were the spearhead. However, this was shortly extended to the natives when a policy of 'pacification' was adopted to try to contain any resistance to the new order. The entwining of health and education was at the heart of that policy of pacification. Soon after the Reconquest, Lord Kitchener made his famous appeal to establish a school in memory of Charles Gordon, to educate the Sudanese. The Gordon Memorial College (GMC) was inaugurated in 1902, accompanied shortly thereafter by the hosting of the Wellcome Tropical Research Laboratory (WTRL) in the eastern wing of the college. That enterprise was a benevolent act of the Anglo-American pharmaceutical tycoon, Henry Solomon Wellcome. Wellcome was among the first notables to visit Sudan immediately after the Reconquest. That laboratory and its first director, Dr. Andrew Balfour, added a new dimension to GMC by making it the hub of medical research into tropical medicine in the first school of modern education. Further, Dr. Balfour was the one chosen to guide and deliver the first milestones of modern public health in Khartoum. His first task was to focus on the eradication of mosquitoes, curbing the menace of malaria, and then, secondarily, tackling the issue of improving sanitation—a mission deemed to be impossible, but accomplished with vigour and perfection. He went on to set up a strong program of public health services for the capital of the Anglo-Egyptian Sudan (with the possible exclusion of Omdurman, the Mahdists' capital). A Central Sanitary Board was established in 1905, with Balfour as one of its key members. This board was tasked with delivering public health services under the continuing auspices of the Wellcome Laboratory for the duration of Dr. Balfour's service (1903-1913). The indefatiguable energies of Balfour and his laboratory staff transformed the capital of the new regime into a healthy city, probably second to none in the British colonial mosaic. When he left, the task was handed over to Dr. Leonard Bousfield, who became the second Khartoum Medical Officer of Health, until his retirement in 1922. Beyond this date, the public health domain became the heart of the new service, the Sudan Medical Service (SMS), which succeeded the Sudan Medical Department (SMD) in 1924. The position of Assistant Director of Public Health became a key senior post of the service, representing the demand for expansion of the service and the central role it played in public health efforts in the vast country of Anglo-Egyptian Sudan.

For the first few, years the health services were carried out by military doctors; the members of the Royal Army Medical Corps (RAMC), who, on appointment, would be seconded to the Egyptian Army Medical Corps and then employed by the Government of the Anglo-Egyptian Sudan. It took nearly six years to establish the first civil health department, the SMD. Allocation of resources was meagre. The civilian staff that were recruited were only a handful in number and conflict between them and the ruling military hierarchy greatly complicated things at the outset, and probably slowed down the evolution of the service in the first two decades. However, with more stability in the country and more resources becoming available, especially after the First World War, the SMD took its first major steps forward at the beginning of the 1920s. As the number of military doctors was very small, the service in its early years relied heavily on recruiting doctors from Syria. Those were primarily graduates of two medical schools in Beirut (prior to 1932, Lebanon did not exist as a separate political entity). By 1909, there were about thirty Syrian doctors in the SMD, while the British doctors numbered no more than six. As the service was still under military control, like their British counterparts, they were employed initially by the Egyptian Army and then seconded to the Sudan Government. Despite its difficult beginnings, pioneering work in public health and research into endemic and tropical diseases at SMD made huge strides. In the pre-war years and despite the allocation of little funds, more hospitals were built in cities and towns and old ones were replaced. Novel ideas, such as better use of limited resources, enabled the health service to flourish; and, with more British and Syrian medical staff flocking to the country, training initiatives for allied healthcare professionals and health subordinates began to be on solid footing. The feat of training Sudanese male medical orderlies as medical assistants was performed by Dr. Vincent Hodson, one of the early British doctors who joined the service. These men were given short courses in basic and simple medical knowledge to allow them to deal with simple medical and surgical problems, with clear instructions to refer intractable cases to a doctor's care. The project was coupled with the opening of dispensaries to be manned by those medical assistants. This enabled the health service to be extended to remote and rural areas. Furthermore, the establishment of the Omdurman Midwifery Training School in 1921 further strengthened the evolving network of what was described as 'the best of the best health service in the world'. However, most of these initiatives were taken in the northern half of the country; the southern frontiers had different colonial policies and received little, if any of the health services. The public services in the south stayed under the control of the military and remained rudimentary. On the other hand, the flocking of missionary societies from Europe (mainly Britain, Italy and Germany), and North America (both the United States and Canada), allowed the Condominium Government at Khartoum to pass on the task of education and health services to these societies. Since the days of David Livingstone, the coupling of mission and medicine among the pagan tribes of Africa was at the heart of the motion to spread the Gospel. This is covered in the second volume of this work.

The difficult first two decades of that service were followed by the founding of the Kitchener School of Medicine, the first medical school in the country (the third medical school in the whole of Africa, after Qasr al-Aini and Cape Town medical schools) in 1924. This medical school emerged from within the first modern school in the country, the Gordon Memorial College, and under the aegis of the SMS. From its inception, the Kitchener School of Medicine (KSM) enjoyed the full patronage of the SMS, and that continued till shortly before Sudan Independence in 1956. Such a unique relationship enabled medical education to be geared to the health needs of the Sudanese community and gave it the cachet of being the first academic institution of higher learning in the country, well in advance of the establishment of the first university in the country by over a quarter of a century. Another feature of the health service of the Anglo-Egyptian Sudan in its early phase was the birth of the Omdurman Midwifery Training School. This helped to transform a native system of midwifery by converting those traditional midwives, the *Dayas*, into a modern breed who were like 'Heavenly Messengers'. That feat greatly complemented the health services in the area of maternal and child health. Furthermore, it provided the much-needed venue for training young Sudanese medical students who were coming up through the ranks from the new Kitchener School of Medicine. The training of midwives superseded the training of nurses, which began in 1925 following the expansion of the health services and the availability of more medical staff. Prior to that, those two training schemes, coupled with the training initiative for medical male orderlies, vastly helped to extend the modern medical services to remote areas, hitherto uncovered, at a very low cost. Such an enterprise impressed many people who worked in the Sudan and it was a forerunner of modern primary health care. In addition to the pioneering training ventures, the SMD achieved other successes, especially in the public health domain. The epidemiology of two endemic diseases, the scourge of visceral leishmaniasis (*Kala-azar*) and the looming menace of sleeping sickness (trypanosomiasis), were at the heart of public health work since the early days of the Condominium. Both were well mapped, and prevention strategies were taken. Further, the novel idea of having a hospital ship was advocated, and by early 1922 the 'Lady Baker' was up and running. This later helped vastly in the provision of health care in areas hitherto unreachable in the Upper Nile and Bahr el-Ghazal regions of southern Sudan.

At its beginnings, the medical services benefited very much from Sir Henry Solomon Wellcome's benevolent donation of a tropical research laboratory. The laboratory helped the newly established service by providing the necessary bacteriology and other pathological tests for the newly established service. Dr. Andrew Balfour was the Medical Officer of Health for Khartoum. His public health work was key to the solid development of the medical service in general. Despite the work of Balfour and his team being completely independent of the medical department, it was executed with vigour and in harmony with others. Further, the excellent networking of Dr. Balfour and his successors, Dr. Albert Chalmers and Sir Robert Archibald, with the international tropical research community contributed immensely to the strong development and quality of the service. The feat of the WTRL in Khartoum set the scene for achievements that would have significant ramifications for the future development of medical research, as well as research in agriculture, soil, mineralogy, water, chemistry, veterinary medicine, entomology, and other domains. That research greatly helped the development in other government sectors. The laboratory's scientific reports published in 1904, 1906, 1908, and 1911, represented an academic face of the laboratory, not witnessed elsewhere across the domains of the British Empire. Further, its supplementary reports (published in 1908 and 1911), represented a pioneering continuous professional development for doctors in Sudan, well ahead of its time by many decades. The multifaceted activities of the WTRL made contributions to early works in fields like medical anthropology. Research in tropical medicine made an enormous contribution to the wealth of literature of that expanding discipline of clinical medicine, not only in Sudan but across the globe. It was a great historical shame that certain politics and possibly personality clashes curbed the survival and further evolution of the WTRL. Its premature demise—well before the political struggle for Sudan's Independence—had deprived the country of what was considered the only internationally renowned laboratory created by the Anglo-American tycoon, Henry Wellcome.

The first British, Syrian, and Egyptian doctors who worked in the Sudan were 'all-round' doctors. They were 'generalists', who were capable of dealing with any health problem. They were highly devoted and committed. An interesting irony was that one of the earliest military British doctors in the Sudan, Dr. Leonard Bousfiled, came to realize that there was no dentist in the whole of the Sudan. He went on to spend his three-month annual vacation in Britain to be the apprentice to a dentist in London, from whom he learned the tricks of the trade. This later helped him to deal with some general dental problems among his patients for the remaining part of his career in the Sudan. He could well be regarded as the 'first dentist' in the Sudan. The first leper colony in Sudan was established in Galabat, a remote outpost in eastern Sudan, by yet another highly devoted medical Corps Bimbashi, Dr. William Byam, who, interestingly enough, was the successor of Dr. Bousfield at Kassala. A third devoted British doctor, John Brian Christopherson, was among the first to have joined the service in the Anglo-Egyptian Sudan. Despite years of turmoil from personality clashes and rifts with military seniors and their circle, he devoted his efforts to research and discovered the first remedy for the devastating parasitic disease, bilharziasis (schistosomiasis). He also excelled in his clinical medical and surgical work and made a substantive contribution to the published clinical medical literature of the first quarter of the twentieth century. A few years ago, his great niece, Mrs Ann Crichton-Harris, published his biography and put him back on the map of medical history. Another magnate of the SMD, Dr. Oliver Francis Atkey, made unprecedented and devoted efforts to the cause of establishing and sustaining the first medical school in Sudan, the Kitchener School of Medicine, in 1924. He could be considered the first guarantor of that medical school. His efforts and the munificence of the Sudanese Persian merchant, Ahmed Bey Hashim Al-Baghdadi, were crucial to the securing of a smooth beginning of that medical school. Two Syrian doctors, Dr. Nesib Baz and Dr. Yusuf Derwish, who worked for the Sleeping Sickness Commission, were quite instrumental in keeping at bay the spread of this menace from Congo, Uganda, and

French Sudan into the southern frontiers of the Anglo-Egyptian Sudan. Dr. Derwish was awarded the MBE by the British monarch for his role in that Commission. Many Syrians and a few Egyptian doctors represented the backbone of the earlier health services in the Anglo-Egyptian Sudan. The great majority of them remained anonymous. Their names could not even be traced. The few who filtered through in various records were only mentioned in passing. Without their contribution, the health services in the first quarter of the last century could not have flourished and excelled. The contribution of those Syrians and Egyptians awaits full research. Other gallant characters in this amazing company, this time, were two women, Mabel and Gertrude Wolff. They were two English nurse/midwives who were born and educated in Egypt. They both made vital contributions to the evolving Sudan health service. The first sister, Mabel, was chosen to lead the Midwifery Training School in Omdurman and her sister was chosen as her assistant/deputy. Mabel helped accomplish the admirable feat of training traditional Sudanese midwives, called *Dayas*, and transform them into a new breed of modern midwives, who were regarded in their heyday in Sudan as 'heavenly messengers'. Gertrude led the establishment of the first female nurse school in Omdurman in 1926. Yet, the devotion and energies of the 'Wolves Sisters' (as they were known in the Sudan) set the foundation of modern nursing and midwifery services in the Sudan.

In writing this book, I have relied heavily on the available sources, kept in various places, especially in Durham, London, Cambridge, and Birmingham. The extracts of the Military Intelligence Reports of the Sudan Government were the major source for most of the earlier information on the health services. I also made use of some notes drafted by Dr. Robert Kirk, a very fine member of the SMS. These Military Intelligence Reports recorded the beginnings of the health services up to the time when Dr. Oliver Atkey took over as Director of the SMD in 1922, when the first independent annual report was published. I have also relied on the rich source of the annual reports of the SMS, which contain fine details of the scope and extent of the health service and its evolution. Copies of these reports are found both at the Sudan Archives in Durham and at the Royal Commonwealth Society Section of Cambridge University Library. The first volume of this work deals with the early evidence of medicine and the beginnings of modern medicine in the Sudan, focusing mainly on the SMD period. It also covers some aspects of the Wellcome Tropical laboratory. The history of the Laboratory was well covered in the documentary narrative by the late Professor Patrick D'Arcy. Part IV deals with some notable military doctors who were part of the Royal Army Medical Corps, the veterans who established the platform for early modern medicine in the Anglo-Egyptian Sudan. Those include the trio of Steven Lyle Cummins, Leonard Bousfield, and William Byam in the section titled the Medical Corps Bimbashis. A short summary of the life and times of Dr. John Brian Christopherson, the first director of the SMD, and a notable doctor who made an immense contribution to the advancement of medical sciences. An appendix on Sudanese native medical practices and superstitions is also included. This area is well researched and well documented by the Sudanese scholar, Professor Ahmed AlSafi; hence, we included in this treatise only what we felt was appropriate and relevant to the theme of the book. A sizeable part of this first volume is devoted to the origins and development of the geo-political relationship between Sudan and Great Britain, which in essence traces the origin of this relation back to the famous narratives of the Scottish Laird, James Bruce, who was the first Briton on record to have stirred the imagination of the Britons about Sudan and its people. Then came the subsequent writings of the Englishman, George William Browne, who attempted to verify the stories of Bruce and, fortunately for us, ended up going in the opposite direction, into Darfur. The major turn of events in the relationship took place following the writings of the prolific Anglo-Swiss scholar, John Lewis (Johann Ludwig) Burckhardt, who was the first to draw attention to the 'Clapham Sect' and alert the anti-slavery lobbying groups to the horrors of the slave trade in the Sudan and the rest of North East Africa. *Travels in Nubia* by Burckhardt and his personal friendship with Muhammad Ali Pasha may have unwittingly hastened the fate of the Sudan as the next target of the imperial ambitions of the Egyptian Viceroy. It was during the subsequent era of the Turco-Egyptian Sudan, when the relation between Sudan and Great Britain started to take a more cohesive shape, primarily through the complex relation between Muhammad Ali Pasha and his dynasty, and Imperial Britain. Into the mix came the quest for the abolition of the slave trade in Sudan, trade and commerce (a relatively trivial issue to Britain in the case of the Sudan), the discovery of the source of the Nile River. The climax was reached with the 'rise and rise' of British colonial ambitions and the onset of the race between the Great Powers known as the great scramble for Africa. The control of Egypt's finances and the subsequent invasion of Egypt by British troops, The Mahdist Revolution, Gordon of Khartoum, and the colonial genius Lord Cromer provided the required catalyst for the vivid political scene in the dying years of the nineteenth century. The outcome was the birth of a hybrid, a country governed by the 'co-domini', the Anglo-Egyptian Sudan, in its own right an unprecedented feat in modern history. This complex cascade is needed to give the reader the necessary background scene for the evolution of modern medicine in Sudan by the British at the turn of the twentieth century.

The forthcoming Volume 2 will include the era of the SMS; the history of the Kitchener School of Medicine and its antecedent, Gordon Memorial College; the evolution of academic medicine with the foundation of University College, Khartoum; and the birth of the University of Khartoum at the dawn of Sudan Independence. It also covers training schemes for doctors and allied healthcare professionals, the foundation of the Ministry of Health, and the beginnings of the Sudan Defence Force Medical Corps. It will also cover the evolution of medical research and includes a chapter on missionary medicine. It will finish by surfing through, highlighting some pioneering ventures and notable staff, concluding with an epilogue with some notes on contemporary medical links between Sudan, on the one hand, and Great Britain and Ireland, on the other.

Finally, I take full responsibility for the contents of this book. I have consulted all references. Any shortcomings are solely mine and they should lie at my doorsteps.

Dr. Tarik A A Elhadd
Doha, Qatar
March 2018

Endnotes

1 Herbert Chavasse Squires (1880-1964), (known as Paul Squires), was one of the pioneering British doctors to work in the Anglo-Egyptian Sudan. He entered the service of Sudan Medical Department in 1908 and retired from Sudan in 1930. He authored the first book on the foundation of the health services in the Sudan, 'Sudan Medical Service: an experiment in Social Medicine, Heinmann, London, 1958

2 C A Bozman, *Medical History,* 1959, April 3rd (3(2):171

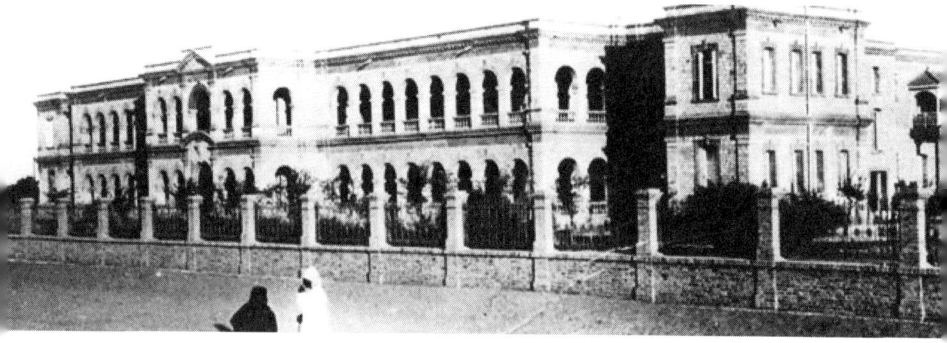

PART I

THE HISTORICAL BACKGROUND

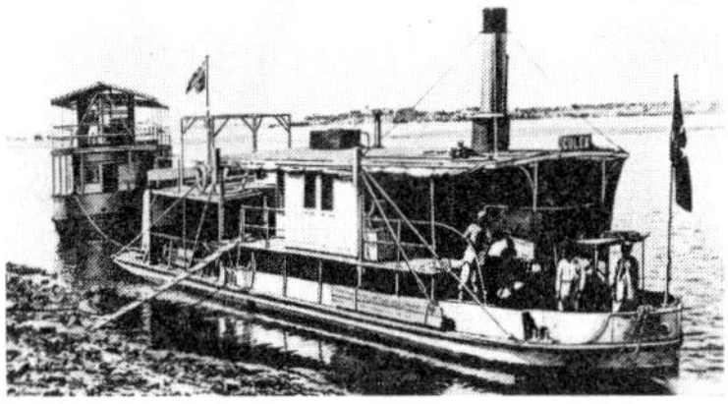

Chapter I

The Sudan, Up to the Nineteenth Century: A Brief Historical Account

Section I:

Sudan: The Land & Its People

The word'Sudan' has been used since ancient times to denote the belt of land that stretches from west to east, south of Sahara. In Arabic, the word has been defined as the 'land of the Blacks' (Arabic: *Bilad al-Sudan*). Up to the great colonial scramble for Africa, that land comprised the region which extends in the west from Mali down to Cameroon, and eastward to encompass all of the land up to the foothills of the Abyssinian plateau. By the twentieth century, this loose term had gradually disappeared and today the word 'Sudan' signifies what came to be known in the earlier part of the twentieth century as the 'Anglo-Egyptian Sudan'. 'The Sudan', by its current borders (up to 2011) (Map 1) occupied most of what used to be the 'Turco-Egyptian Sudan' (Map 2), which was created by Muhammad Ali Pasha, the great Egyptian Viceroy, in 1821. That land comprised what used to be the former Sudanese kingdom of Sennar or the Fung Sultanate. The Turco-Egyptian Sudan, which occupied most of what forms the current central and northern areas of Sudan in addition to Kordofan and the Red Sea littoral region (which included part of today's Eretria and Ethiopia). Southern Sudan and Darfur were annexed at later stages, during the 1850s and 1870s, respectively. The Mahdist State (1885-1898), which was established on the ruins of the Turco-Egyptian Sudan, consisted of a much-reduced area of land. The Anglo-Egyptian Sudan (Map 3), which came into existence in 1898, generally comprised the original regions of the Turco-Egyptian Sudan with the exception of Darfur, which was annexed in 1916.

This region exhibits a diverse topography. ranging from the 22nd parallel latitude to the north, down almost to the Equator. It embraces a heterogeneous population of culturally and ethnically diverse groups of inhabitants, heterogeneity that can be found even within the same region. The Western sector shows a barrier-nil extension into the central part of sub-Saharan Africa (present-day Chad and Central African Republic). Within this sector, containing the western part of Kordofan as well as Darfur and the northernmost part of the Bahr el-Ghazal region, the pattern of ethnic diversity reflects that of present-day Sudan. Nevertheless, the majority of the inhabitants here embrace Islam as a religion. The differences in ethnicity, culture, customs, and way of life are unprecedented, ranging from the cattle-owning Baggara nomads in the southern part, intermingling with the Nilotic tribes, to the Fur and the Massalit in the central and western part, to the Zhagwa, Meidoub, Berti, and the camel-owning Kebbabish Arab nomads to the far north. The eastern fringes of Sudan, on the other hand have a totally different ethnic admixture, comprising groups of the Beja, Beni Amer, and Hemran Arabs, to name but a few, who are more or less close to the rest of the Hamitic races of Eretria and Ethiopia. Probably the most homogenous group of people within the Sudan is exemplified by the inhabitants of the current central and northern part of the country, who have generally evolved from the admixture of the original Nubian and negroid races of these regions, through intermarriage with the migrant Arabs from Egypt, North Africa, and the Arabian peninsula, from the sixth century A.D. onwards. Heterogeneity returns on the southern frontiers with tens of tribes having different cultures and different ethnic admixture, from the Dinka of Bahr el-Ghazal and the Upper Nile, to the Shilluk and Nuer of the Lakes region, and along the northern and eastern Upper Nile regions, to the Anuak along the western borders of the Abyssinian foothills. These people belong to the Nilotic tribes of central equatorial Africa. Adjoining the borders of the former Belgian Congo, Uganda, Kenya, and former French Sudan can be found a multitude of tribes, like the Azande, the Bari, the Madi, the Mandari, the Latuka, and the Moru, all of whom ethnically belong more to the Nilo-Hamite (Bantu?) African groups of people. Adding to this fascinating mesh of diversity are the peoples of the Nuba Mountains in south central Sudan, and the heterogeneous group of tribes that inhabit the region along the Blue Nile at its entry from the Abyssinian mountain ridge. To throw more complexity into an already complex mix, a group of West African people, the Fulani and Hausa tribes, who migrated over the last few centuries, have settled in scattered cantons in various regions of the Sudan. These were mainly in the west, central, and southeast central parts of the Sudan, but also with a significant presence in the Gezira and along the main tributaries of the Blue Nile, the Rahad and Dinder seasonal rivers.

The geography of this subcontinent shows a gradual passage from a Saharan to sub-Saharan climate in the far north and centre, to a subtropical region and tropical rain forests in the far south. Rain falls accordingly, varies consistently and follows a pattern similar to the geography, with significant variation from year to year. The country thrives along the banks of the two great rivers, the Blue and the White Nile. These two rivers join at Khartoum and form the main Nile River. Both the Blue and the White Nile have many tributaries. The main branches of the White Nile are the Sobat, which arises from the southwestern hills of Ethiopia, the Zeraf, and the Bahr el-Gebel. The latter two flow from the eastern part of Central Africa. The principal tributaries of the Blue Nile are mainly the Rahad and Dinder Rivers, which also flow from the central and the west Ethiopian mountains. The main stream of the Nile is further supplied by the Atbara River, which also flows from the Abyssinian Mountains. The Atbara is fed by several other seasonal tributaries, including the Setit and the Basalam which also arise from the Abyssinian Mountains. Other small seasonal rivers that seasonally flow in the eastern part of the Sudan are the Ghash and Baraka Rivers. The Sudan has few mountain ridges, mainly to the far east, the far west, and the far south. The one on the far east includes a range of interrupted hills that are a natural extension of the Abyssinian mountains that run along the Red Sea region. A small elevation rises to the west of this ridge, around the region of Kassala, the largest of them, the highest of which are the Taka Hills, which overlook the town of Kassala. In western Sudan is the plateau of the Jebel Marra hills, and in the far south the ridge forming Amatong Hills. Agriculture depends on the rainy season, which extends to a variable degree from May-June to August-September in most central and south-central areas, with relatively longer periods in more southerly latitudes. Canal-based irrigation schemes are centred primarily along the Gezira peninsula in central Sudan and along the White and Blue Nile banks, mainly in the central and northern Sudan.

Time Immemorial

The beginning of the history of this part of Africa is not exactly known. The central and northern parts of the current Sudan, from circa 4,000 to 5,000 B.C., appear to have been inhabited by a Negroid race that, like their counterparts elsewhere, were mainly hunter-gatherers. They they possibly belonged to the 'brown race' that inhabited this area as well as Upper Egypt, the Beja area of eastern Sudan, the Abyssinian Mountains, and the Somali-lands, and were found to have acquired the knowledge of making pottery. These Sudanic people were conquered by the Pharaonic kings of the 3rd Dynasty around 3,000 B.C. According to MacMichael (1954)) and others have hypothesized that the aboriginal people of north and central Sudan shared a common culture. Along the great bend of the Nile in the northern fringes appeared the old town of Dongola, which signalled the beginning of the great Kingdom of Kush, around 2,000 B.C. The Egyptians then reappeared and their 18th Dynasty reconquered the Kushite Kingdom and extended Egyptian Dominion as far south as the area now adjoining Berber (circa 1530-1520 B.C). The great Temple of Gebel al-Berkel rose as the epicentre of the Egyptian theocracy in the region. This period of Egyptian rule began to decline circa 1,100 B.C. and this allowed the Kushites to break away and take their destiny back into their own hands. Later, the Kushite Viceroy, Heribor, became Pharaoh and made his son 'Viceroy of Nubia'.

The Kushite Kingdoms: Napata & Meroe

Following the aforementioned events, an uncertain dynasty rose to power in Kush, thought to have descended from the original royal line. Their first king, by the name of 'Kashta', took control and led the Kushites to conquer their former masters, sweeping through the Egyptian Kingdom up to Thebes circa 850 B.C. Then Piankhi (or Piankha), his successor, established the 25th Egyptian Dynasty. Piankha 'the Great' established his capital, Napata, near the Barkal Temple of Amon. He went on to build a string of pyramids and temples and, at a later stage during his reign, the centre of gravity of his Kingdom moved further south to the region of Meroe. This sprang up quickly around the current region of Atbara and Shendi on the eastern bank of the Nile. His successor, Shabaka (707-697 B.C.), moved his capital back to Thebes and he was later involved in wars against the Assyrians in what came to be known as Palestine. His successor, Taharaka (688-663 B.C.), was defeated by the Assyrians and were driven entirely out of Egypt in 671 B.C. The last of the 25th Egyptian Dynasty, Tanutamon, retreated to Napata following his final defeat by the Assyrians in 663 B.C. Thereafter, Meroe prospered, and Napata became the religious capital. The Kushite Kingdoms survived for over a thousand years following that final encounter with Pharaonic Egypt, but their way of life, religion, and civilization remained very much Egyptian. The Greek traveller, historian and geographer, Herodutus, travelled as far south as Aswan in Upper Egypt in 460 B.C. and mentioned of Meroe and the source of the Nile River in his *Histories*. This was the first evidence of interaction between Nubia and the Hellenic Civilization that later reigned over Egypt from the time of Alexander to Julius Caesar, and remained influential in Egypt through roman times and during the dawn of Christianity. Indeed, Theodora, wife of the Byzantine Emperor Justanian is credited with the spreading of Christianity among the Nubian kingdoms and the Sudan. Throughout the Greek and the Roman eras in Egypt, trade along the Red Sea and the Nile continued, largely without hostilities, except on a few occasions when the

Kushites dared to plunder the southern frontiers of first Greek and then Roman Egypt. They once raided as far as Aswan, which led the Roman governor of Egypt, Publinus Petronius to invade the Kushite Kingdom in 23 B.C., only returning after he had plundered and destroyed Napata in 22 B.C.

We owe a great deal of the information about Nubia during the Hellenic era to Eratosthenes, the Greek in charge of the Alexandria Library. Eratosthenes wrote a geographical manuscript about his travels in the area south of Egypt and suggested that the Blue and white Niles, flowed out of lakes located further south. Strabo, of Greek descent, preserved the work of Eratothenes and, like Herodotus, he himself travelled south and wrote of the geography of the Nile Basin in his Geography, written sometimes after 20 B. C. Pliny (23-79 A.D.) in his fascinating *Historia Naturalis,* left us ample descriptions of the 'Ethiopians', the people to the south of Egypt, and also recorded the habits of the Nilotic tribes. MacMichael, in the *The Sudan*, referenced the information gathered by Strabo about the architectural feature developed by the Niloteic tribes, known as the 'The King Beasts.' The same feature was used by the medieval architects as 'The King's Beasts' appears in various places in Britain, including two Cambridge Colleges, Hampton Court and the Royal Chapel of Windsor. However, it was the *Magnum Opus* of Claudius Ptelemeus (100-150 A.D.), a student at Alexandria University, that provided even greater details of the geography of Africa. Later this information was used by medieval explorers, discoverers, and sailors and by travellers of the eighteenth and nineteenth centuries, like David Livingstone, Richard Burton, John Speke, Samuel Baker, and Henry Morton Stanley, to 'discover' the 'Black Continent'.

Following the departure of Petronius, the Kushites rebuilt the Temple of Amon Ra'a at Napata followed later by building strings of pyramids and three temples at Naga'aa near Shendi. They also dug several artificial reservoirs of water along Meroe island, which lies between the triangle of Atbara and the Blue Nile Rivers, several artificial reservoirs of water were dug, as seemingly significant climate changes during that era resulted in less rainfall and water came to be in short supply. In the first three centuries after Christ, Napata and Meroe underwent gradual decline, and the weakness of the Kushites tempted their easternmost neighbour, Ezana, the first Christian King of Axum, to invade and plunder Meroe in 350 A.D. However, no lasting legacy of the Axumites was to be found at Meroe, as they apparently retraced their steps, returning to their Abyssinian stronghold. There is some compelling evidence to suggest that the Royal House of Meroe and Napata, or some of their descendants, went westward, where they established a kingdom in the area between present-day Darfur and Lake Chad, in Central Africa. Byzantine lamps of the 6th Century A.D. were found as far west as the current Ivory Coast.

The Christian Kingdoms of Nubia

Over the ruins of the Merotic Kingdoms, the Kinglets of Nobatia arose, becoming allied to the Roman emperor and rule of Egypt, Diocletian. As such, they helped their allies to offset the menace of the Blemmys nomads (the *Beja*) of the Red Sea Hills and eastern Sudan, who frequently raided the southern-most part of Roman Egypt. Not long after the Roman Emperor Justinian embraced Christianity, the priest Julianus managed to covert the 'Heathen Nuba' to the Gospel of the new religion. The conversion to Christianity of the Nubians and also adjacent inhabitants of central Sudan was almost total. Around this time, two main sub-kingdoms arose. The first was Mukkara, with its capital at Dongola (not far from Napata). Further south is twin kinglet of Aloa emerged, with its capital at Soba along the Blue Nile. Then, came the rise and rise of Islam. In the 7th Century A.D., Amr bin el-Aas conquered Egypt and swept through all of the Northern African territories in just a few years. He then sent an expedition, led by Abdalla Ibn Saad (Ibn Abi Al-Sarrah), to force the Nubians into submission, and his forces subsequently raided Dongola, destroying its church. A peace accord was reached, the famous 'Baqt Treaty', between the new masters of Egypt and the Nubians. According to that treaty, the Muslim forces were to return to Egypt, in return for which the Christian Nubians agreed to pay an annual tribute It would be several more centuries before any further major events occured in Nubia. This time, it would coincide with the ascendency of the Mamluks to supreme power in Egypt, circa 900 A.D. In the interim, slow but sustained migration of various

Arab tribes took place before, during, and after the establishment and expansion of the Islamic empires and the advent of its civilization. Such migration of Arab nomads came from different directions. Some of these Arab nomads came across the Red Sea from Arabia, or down the Nile from Egypt, or from other regions of North Africa, especially Morocco (*Bilad el-Maghrib*). These tribes settled in various regions of the north east, west, and central parts of the current Sudan and went to intermarry with the Negroid and Nubian people, including those of Mukkara and Aloa. With the definitive advent of Islam, those tribes settled gradually and are now represented by two large groups. The first group, known as the Juhaynyyia Arabs, comprised the Ja'aliyyien group of tribes, the Shukriyyia, the Kababaish, and others. The second group comprised the Fazzara Arab groups. They are mainly represented by the cattle-herding and camel-owning Arab nomads of Kordofan and Darfur. These include the Baggara Arabs, the Rizzigat, and others. Through intermarriage with Nubians and other indigenous negroid tribal groups, the current ethnic Sudanese people of central and northern Sudan emerged. This took place over several hundred years preceding the appearance of the Fung Kingdom of Sennar, the first large state that dominated the greater bulk of the current Sudanese territories, with the exception of Darfur and the far northern and southern Sudanese regions.

Gradual conversion of the Christian Nubians to Islam took place over several centuries and by the Year 1503 A. D. a major turn of events took place, the establishment of the Fung Kingdom of Sennar.

Section II:

The Fung Kingdom of Sennar

The origin of the Fung people and the dynasty of the Fung Kingdom of Sennar is clouded in historical mystery and records dealing with this issue are scarce. Those that have been traced largely derived from oral histories by two Sudanese writers: Mohamed Elnour Wad Daif Allah, a holy man; and Ahmed Alhaj bin Ali, an employee initially of the Fung and later of the new Turco-Egyptian rulers. However, further information have come from the writings of foreign travelers who entered the Kingdom. The writings of the Jewish traveler, David Ha-Ruebeni, who travelled to Sennar in 1523 before eventually being imprisoned by the Spanish Inquisition in the 1530's, is the earliest written records to she light on this Islamic Kingdom. The Fung Kingdom of Sennar, as it is known in English historical narratives, or the 'Black Sultanate', as it is known in contemporary Sudanese writings, attained hegemony in the early sixteenth century. The Kingdom dominated mainly the territories of the central parts of modern Sudan. The founding King was thought to be Ammara Dungus (or Dunkas), who reigned from 1504 to 1534. Amara, in alliance with the Abdallabi king, Abdalla Jamm'aa (or Gamma'a), waged an attack that resulted in the destruction of the last Nubian Christian Kingdom, Soba, in the year 1503.

The origin of the Fung remains mysterious, despite extensive research that was carried out during the last century. The first published work in English was the book *Tooth of Fire* by H. C. Jackson, which first appeared in 1912. The most comprehensive work to date on this Kingdom, *The Fung Kingdom of Sinnar*, is one written by Osbert Guy Stanhope Crawford in 1951. Crawford made use of earlier accounts in the extensive research done by other scholars, including Anthony J. Arkle, an amateur historian who contributed much to the historical and anthropological writings on ancient Sudan. Much of the research relied heavily on the writings of the foreign travellers mentioned earlier, including David Ha-Ruebeni and the Europeans, Charles Poncet, James Bruce, and Jesuit missionaries such as Theodoro Krump. The Fung Kingdom or Sultanate had its capital at Sennar, which was thought to have been founded during the reign of Amara Dungus in 1504. Abdalla Gamma'a, the Abdallabi king/chieftain, and the main ally of King Amara, entrenched himself in the subordinate Kingdom of the Abdallab with its base at Garri, an old trade post to the north of present-day Khartoum. The Fung managed to subdue most if not all of the tribes of central, eastern, and northern Sudan, up to the region of Dongola and the Red Sea littoral. These tribes were subdued either by force, by intermarriage (as in the case of the Shukriyya Arabs of the Butana plains) or through granting of lands (as in the case of the Shukriyya, the Ja'aliyyien and the Shaiggiyya). The Fung Sultans ruled supreme for over three centuries and their rule was characterized by flourishing trade and commerce with Egypt, Abyssinia, the Hidjaz, Wadai, and the Kanum Islamic Sultanate (Map 4). Their rule was also characterised by wars waged against their eastern Christian neighbour, the Abyssinian Kingdom of Axum. The last quarter of the eighteenth century witnessed an attempt by the Fung Kingdom to expand further west into Kordofan. An army led by the Hamj vizier, Abu Laikaylik, spent up to 14 years campaigning there to subdue the Musba'at, the suzerains of the Fur Sultans, who ruled Kordofan for several decades. They were thought to be a breakaway faction from the Royal Keira dynasty of the Fur.

During the dying quarter of the eighteenth century, from probably 1789, the hegemony of the Fung saw a significant decline coupled with the ascendancy of yet another mysterious central Sudanese clan, the Hamaj. Following the rise to dominance of the Hamaj clan, led by Mohamed Abu Likaylik, who was the Vizier of the Fung Sultan and his brother Adlan, the Fung monarch was deposed and then the Fung Sultans became puppets of the strong viziers of the Hamj. The dawn of the nineteenth century saw significant weakness of the Fung and loosening of their grip on their subordinates in the north and central frontiers. When the Turco-Egyptian troops of Muhammad Ali Pasha, led by his son Ismail Kamil Pasha, invaded the Sultanate, it was faced with little if any resistance and the fate of the Kingdom was finally sealed in 1821, when the last of the Fung Kings, Badi VI; submitted without significant resistance. The following periods of the Turco-Egyptian Sudan and its successor the Mahdist State shall be covered in Chapter 2.

The Western Sudanese Kingdoms: The Daju and Tunjur Kingdoms & The Fur Sultanate

The Daju people live in a wide belt of land that extends from eastern Chad to western Bahr el-Ghazal, Darfur, and Kordofan. The great Islamic geographer al-Idrisi in 1154 made the first reference to the people inhabiting this region as the *Tajuwiyyin* (= *Daju*). It is not clear whether the reference by MacMichael to a royal family (or maybe their descendants), who went west following the destruction of the Kingdom of Meroe by the Axumite King in the twelfth century, referred to the Daju. Their first king was thought to be King Gitar or Kosbur, and the last Ahmed al-Daj, whose life and times are still celebrated in western Sudanese folklore, although clouded in fiction. Several historical reports suggested a 'Daju-Tunjur transition' prior to the appearance of the Fur hegemony in the early sixteenth century. The transition to the Tunjur-Keira dynasties led to the appearance of the 'Keira' dynasty, the ruling house of the Fur. The Tunjur State appeared in Darfur and Wadai in the twelfth century and reigned until the mid-sixteenth century. There are several theories about the origin of the Tunjur. One is based on the claim that they were a faction of the Abbassid Arabs who crossed the Nile westward and established a kingdom in the central African sub-Saharan region adjoining the current northern Kordofan, Darfur, and Chad east of Lake Chad. Another is built on the possible migration of a group of 'Bani Hilal' Arabs from the North African hinterlands. Whichever theory is correct, it appears that the reign of the Tunjur dynasty preceded and led to the appearance of the Keira ruling house of the Fur.The beginnings of the Fur Sultanate are also hemmed with controversy. The oral and the historical records traced by O'Fahey and by Gustav Nachitgal, the German traveller, on the eve of the Mahdiyyia in the last few decades of the nineteenth century, suggested that the appearance of the Fur Sultanate in Darfur probably goes back to the mid-sixteenth century. Several theories claim Ahmed el-Maqour of Beni Hilal Arabs from North Africa, as the founding father of the Fur royal family. However, according to O'Fahey (2008), the credit of establishing the Sultanate itself is due to Suliman Solong (*Solongdungu*) and his two sons, Musa and Ahmed Bukr. Musa descendants went on to establish the Musaba'at, the kinglet that ruled Kordofan. From the House of Ahmed Bukr came the Keira dynasty of the Fur Sultanate. The two sons of Ahmed Bukr, Mohamed Tayrab and Abdul-Rahman 'el-Rasheid', were credited with the expansion of the Fur Sultanate, both eastwards and westwards. The grandson of Mohamed el-Fadul (son of Abdul-Rahman el-Rasheid), Ibrahim Garad, was the last of the first hegemony of the Fur Sultans. This hegemony was ended by Zubair Pasha Rahama Mansour in 1874. Zubair by then was the governor of the Bahr el-Ghazal Province of the Turco-Egyptian Sudan. Zubair, on October 25, 1874, at the battle of Manawashi killed Sultan Ibrahim Garad and annexed the Fur Kingdom to the Turco-Egyptian domain. This preceded the rise of the 'Mahdiyyia' by only a few years. A series of battles and bloodshed was to follow in 1874-1875. The rising power of Zubair was seen by Ismail Pasha Ayyub, Governor General of the Sudan, as threatening. Ayyub did his best to subdue Zubair by opposing several of his plans, especially his advocacy of re-instating Hasab Allah, uncle of Ibrahim Garad, as the Fur Sultan under the crown of the Egyptian Viceroy. Zubair, in protest, committed the deadliest mistake of his life by travelling to Cairo to complain about his adversary. He was forced to stay at Cairo and prevented from returning back to Sudan. His son, Suliyman, revolted in Bahr el-Ghazal and the new claimant of the Fur throne, Mohamed Haroun Rasheid b. Seif-eldien b. Mohamed Al-Fadul, came to his support. Both were defeated and killed. Then came the Mahdiyya, when the Fur suffered much bloodshed. It was not until the decisive defeat of the Khalifa by Lord Kitchener, when Ali Dinar (son of Zakariyyia b. Mohamed Al Fadul), had the golden opportunity to restore the throne of his forefathers and ascend as the last of the Fur Sultans. His reign lasted from 1898 till 1916, when he was killed by Hubert Huddleston at the battle of Bringiyyia, in the southern foothills of Jebel Marra. Huddlestone was later to become general Officer Commanding (GOC) Sudan in 1924, and between 1942-1947, one of the last (and possibly least popular) of the British Governor Generals of the Anglo-Egyptian Sudan.

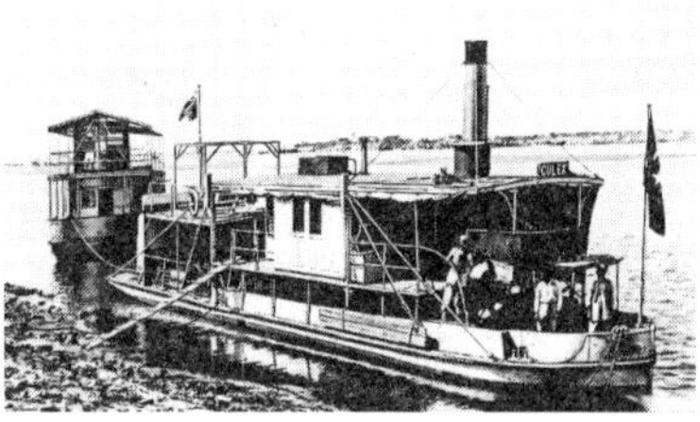

Chapter 2

Sudan & the United Kingdom (1700-1898): A Short History of the Relationship

Early Beginnings

Prior to the adventures of the Scottish 'Laird' James Bruce (1), there doesn't seem to be any specific mention or knowledge of the Sudanese territories in English literature. Indeed, there was more or less ignorance about the 'Sudanese Kingdoms' on the part of both the public and the state as late as the last quarter of the eighteenth century. By then, the British Empire was in a state of ascendancy; the British had already been to India and they had sound knowledge of northern African territories and the Levant. However, their knowledge of the inner African hinterlands was negligible. Further, there was not any specific interest on the part of either the government or the public to explore this mysterious continent. The adventures of James Bruce were not to be public knowledge or of general interest until 1792 when an account of them was first published. This then tempted the Englishman William George Browne to set off for the Sudanese frontiers to verify the stories of James Bruce and gain personal glory (2). However, due to tribal war and unrest in Nubia he was unable exactly to follow Bruce's route and was able to reach only the area of Dongola and, due to some local tribal wars and unrest in Nubia, Browne was compelled to continue down the old caravan route, 'Darb al-Arbaeen', and ended up in Darfur. At Darfur, Browne spent three years (from 1796 to 1798). Nevertheless, in 1789, the Committee of Trade and Plantation of Great Britain wrote to the British Consul at Alexandria asking for information about 'Sudan'. The Consul-General then wrote a memorandum based on 'frequent conversations with people, by some means acquainted with the "Sudanese Kingdoms".' The document went on to state: 'your Lordship's questions extended to matters not yet sufficiently in my possession to work upon, but I shall lose no time in obtaining them and of obeying your instructions to the best of my skill' (3).

Earlier on, and in the eighteenth century, the first Briton to have trudged the Sudanese hinterland was James Bruce, the Scottish traveller/explorer. Bruce had had a dream since childhood: to discover the source of the Nile. To accomplish his dream, he embarked on extraordinary adventures between Europe, North Africa, and the Levant until he came to Abyssinia. He passed through the Sudan in 1768, where he spent some time at Sennar, which, by then, was the waning capital of the Fung Kingdom (See Part II, Chapter1, Section1). It took some further time for awareness of Sudanese affairs to come under greater scrutiny in London, at least until an account of the travels of Anglo-Swiss scholar John Lewis Burckhardt were published in 1817. Burckhardt travelled into Nubia in 1814, reaching as far south as Berber and Shendi before crossing the desert to Suakin, and his writings about the slave markets in Berber and Shendi were the first to draw the attention of the lobbying groups of the Anti-slavery movement in Britain to this rife trade in the Sudan (4). Following the Turco-Egyptian invasion, more British travellers would traverse the Sudan. These included Lord Prudhoe and Major Felix in 1829, followed by George A. Hoskins in 1833 and Arthur Holroyd in 1836-1837.The first Briton to stay for an extended period was Mansfield Parkyns, who stayed from 1845 to 1848, principally in Kordofan (5). Parkyns came to the Sudan from Abyssinia and went first to Khartoum and then to Kordofan and el-Obeid, where he lived with the Kababish Arab nomads. His manuscript of the Fung chronicles has been useful to some of our contemporary historians in tracing the history of that illustrious Kingdom. Parkyns also made notes on the history of Kordofan and the Nuba. In the 1850s, a Liverpool man, George Melly, travelled to the Sudan with his family and stayed at Khartoum for a good spell. On his return journey, he passed Berber and came near to Abu Hamad. Melley's father passed away and was buried near the Nile. His grave was later visited by the first British Consul at Khartoum, John Petherick. The earliest description of Khartoum in English literature was given in Melly's travel book, *Khartoum and the Blue and White Nile*, published in London in 1851 (6).

The official relationship between Sudan and Britain started in a sketchy manner a few decades after Khartoum, the capital of the Turco-Egyptian Sudan, was founded in 1821. This relationship took a significant turn during the reign of Mohamed Ali and his dynasty in the Sudan. The rise of British colonial ambitions and the annexation of Egypt itself by Britain in 1882, which effectively politically controlled the affairs there (jointly with France), till Egypt became effectively a British Protectorate in 1914 with the advent of the First World War. The annexation of Egypt by Great Britain in 1882 moved the Anglo-Sudanese relationship into new territory. This coincided with the climax of the Mahdist revolt and the death of General Gordon at Khartoum. In the next section we shall highlight the era of the Turco-Egyptian Sudan, which had very much set the scene for the eventual annexation of Sudan by Great Britain and the creation of the Anglo-Egyptian Sudan.

Section I:

The Turco-Egyptian Sudan

> One can arrive at a fairly coherent understanding of a campaign that lacked all the coherence and was colonial warfare at its worst.
>
> –From *The Blue Nile* by Alan Moorehead

According to several contemporary historians, the modern history of the Sudan begins with the establishment of the Turco-Egyptian Sudan. Here, the ongoing geopolitical links between the Sudan and Egypt since time immemorial took a major turn during the reign of Muhammad Ali (Mehmet Ali) Pasha (b. 1769, d.1849). This era marked the beginning of the future relationship between Sudan and Britain and set the scene for the later territorial and political ambitions of Imperial Britain during the rise and rise of British colonial interests in Africa in the last quarter of the nineteenth century. Muhammad Ali, an officer in the Ottoman Army in Egypt around the time of Napoleon's defeat in 1801, was given a mandate by the Turkish Sultan to help finish off Napoleon's remaining troops in Egypt. Following the defeat of the French fleet by Admiral Nelson and the return of Napoleon to France, Egypt went into turmoil, with warring amongst the various Mamluk parties. In 1805, Mohamed Ali declared himself governor of Egypt, in complete defiance of the Mamluk Beys[1], and this was soon accepted by the Porte[2].. Muhammad Ali continued to gain ground and popularity among the Egyptian people, especially after he made several reforms in the laws governing taxation and ownership of lands. In 1811, Muhammad Ali invited the Mamluk chieftains to a banquet in the Citadel in Cairo which ended in the slaughter of all the guests. In the wake of the massacre, those Mamluks who survived fled to southern Egypt and the adjoining parts of the Sudan, especially the Dongola region. The Ottoman Sultan bestowed upon Muhammad Ali the title of 'Viceroy' of Egypt, which in a sense guaranteed that the heir of the throne in Egypt would continue in his own family line, despite the fact that he assumed the title of Khedive without official recognition from Turkey. Such a title was officially conferred by the Porte on his grandson, Ismail 'The Magnificent', in 1867 (Professor Ahmed Abou Shouk, personal communication). Muhammad Ali Pasha had the ambition of establishing an empire of his own, a far more glorious aim than merely ruling Egypt. His eyes were fixed upon the south, where stories of gold mines and strong men captured his imagination. He coveted the means to fuel the machinery to establish an empire that would cover sizeable proportions of the Arabian Peninsula, the Levant, sections of north Africa, Eritrea, the Sudan, the western coast of the Red Sea up to Somalia, and, later, even further, reaching deep south into central Africa.

The motives of the Pasha in invading Sudan were several-fold. First, he was in dire need of strong men, slave soldiers, who would form the military backbone of his '*el-Nizam al Jadeed*[3]'. Second, he dreamt of amassing the gold revenues and the wealth of those southern hinterlands were essential financial resources needed for his territorial expansion and imperial aspirations. Third, trade and commerce would enrich his treasury and provide the means for a much-needed economic boom. Fourthly, the discovery of the source of the Nile would guarantee the water supply needed for his new irrigation schemes that he planned for Egypt. And finally, he was keen to pursue and defeat his old foes, the Mamluks, who had fled to the area of Dongola and continued to pose a threat to the stability of his rule. The Egyptian viceroy was clever to send an envoy to the King of Sennar in 1815 around the time of Burckhardt's second trip into Nubia. The covert mission of the envoy was to gather first-hand information about the state of the country and its people before executing the actual conquest in 1820 (7).

To conquer the Sudan, the Pasha planned two expeditions. The first one was to be led by his third son, Ismail Kamil Pasha, and the second by his son-in-law, Mohamed Bek Khusru '*el-Dafterdar*[4]'. The one led by Ismail's force advanced to the south-east and within a short period managed to defeat the weak Sudanese kinglets along the Nile on his way to conquering the crumbling and ailing Fung Kingdom of Sennar. Mohamed Bek Khusru headed southwest to Kordofan and Darfur. Beginning his advance in autumn 1820, Ismail was accompanied by three Westerners, an American, a Frenchman, and a Briton, and it is through the writings of these three that we came to know the details of Muhammad Ali's military conquest of the Sudan. The American, George Bethune English, from Cambridge, Massasuchetts, was commissioned a second lieutenant in the US Marine Corps during the war of 1812, assigned to the Marine Corps headquarters. English sailed to the Mediterranean and was among the first US citizens to have visited Egypt. He landed in Alexandria in 1820, became a Muslim convert, resigned from his job at the US Navy, and joined the service of Mohamed Ali under the name of 'Mohammed Effendi'. He was then assigned to Ismail's expedition, in charge of the artillery. His book, *A Narrative of the Expedition to Dongola & Sennar*, provides a first-hand account of the details of the enterprise (8). The Frenchman, Frederic Caillaud, a geologist from Nantes, earlier joined Mohamed Ali's service as a geologist before the Dongola and Sennar Expedition. He was initially assigned by the Viceroy to obtain emeralds from the Red Sea. He was enlisted in the expedition as the geological expert, to guide the extraction of gold from the hills of Fazogli beyond Sennar. He subsequently published his surveys and some details of Ismail's expedition in books he wrote after returning to France in 1827 (9). The Briton, George Waddington, a Fellow of Trinity College, Dublin, was in Egypt at the time on an aquatarian mission with another Englishman, Reverend Barnard Hanbury. Waddington and Hanbury were granted permission by Mohamed Ali to accompany the expedition to hunt for antiquities in Nubia. By summer of 1820, what was described by Moorehead as a 'monstrous raid' had begun.

Ismail progressed amid little opposition down the Nile, and met his first resistance in 'Dar Shaigiyia' at the Battle of Korti on November 4, 1820, when a Shaigiyia girl, Meheira Bint Abboud, played a major role in raising the morale and zeal of her people to stand up to the invading troop. A second round was to follow when another girl, Safia, herself a daughter of a Shaigyie Chieftain, King Subair, played a similar role to that of Mehiera but was captured, and her fellow soldiers annihilated. Here we quote Alan Moorhead from his scholarly book, *The Blue Nile*: 'Ismail ordered her to be washed, perfumed and dressed elegantly and then sent back to her father. Her father was relieved to see her alive, but he muttered after he saw her, 'all this is well, but are you still a virgin?'. Safia assured her father that she was indeed still a virgin. The father, satisfied with this fact, he swore that he would never fight the man who spared the honour of his daughter, and later went and submitted to Ismail (10). Following this, Ismail attained the submission of the two Shaigiyya chieftains, Mek Shawish and Mek Subayer. In actual fact, the Shaigiya became useful allies and helped Ismail in his campaign down the Nile. The Shaigyia '*Bashi-Bazuq*' soldiers later provided the backbone of the military rank and file of the 'new Turkish order' in the Sudan. Next, the town of Berber, whose chieftain, 'Mek Nasr-eldien' of the Mirafab section of the Ja'aliyyien tribe, readily surrendered. An earlier conflict between Nasr-eldien and other Ja'alie chieftains, Mek Nimr of Shendi, and Mek Musa'ad of al-Matamma, greatly helped the cause of Ismail. There were some suggestions that Mek Nasr-eldien, following the invasion of his 'Dar' by Nimr and Mus'ad in 1818, in favour of his Mirafabi rival Mek 'Ali wad Tumsah', led him to flee to Egypt and to urge Mohamed Ali to invade the Sudan (11, 12). The advance of Ismail Pasha towards Sennar was met with little resistance. Again, the divided Sudanese made the task of Ismail an easy one. He met no significant resistance when he took Qarri and Halfayat el-Muluk, the seat of the Abdallabi king. Finally, Ismail had little trouble conquering the Hamaj and the Fung of Sennar. In the last few decades of the eighteenth century, the Fung Sultans became puppets of the Hamaj Viziers after the Sultan was deposed by Mohamed Abu Likaylik and his brother Adlan in 1764 (shortly before James Bruce's visit to Sennar in 1772). At the western front, the other army led by Mohamed Bey Khusru al-Istambouli, known as '*el-Daftardar*', conquered the Musaba'at of Kordofan after several skirmishes and with hardly any major resistance against a far superior force. The rest of the nomadic tribes of the central, eastern, and northern Sudan, e.g., the Shukriyya and Beja, put up some resistance, and some, like the Ababda camel-nomads even collaborated with the new order. The Ababada men became guides for the invading troops through the maze of the Sudanese desert and, after the conquest, formed the backbone of the camel postal service and were given the right to guide and tax caravans along Berber-Dongola-Kursuku trade route to Egypt (13).

Having finished his task at Sennar and campaigning later at Fazugli to investigate the presence of the gold mines, Ismail went to Shendi on his way back to Egypt. Here he made a demand of Mek Nimr, chieftain of the Ja'aliyyien, to pay a tribute of 100,000 dollars in cash plus slaves and other commodities. When the Ja'aliyyien Mek tried to explain his inability to meet such a hefty demand, Ismail became furious and threw his long pipe into the Mek's face. It also transpired that he had insulted the daughter of Mek Nimr. The Ja'ali notable was restrained from taking revenge at once by the Mamluk bodyguard around the Pasha (14). On that same night, November 3, 1822, Ismail and his entourage were invited to a dinner party when they were all burnt alive. The assassination of Ismail and his men set off a limited revolt among the Ja'aliyyien and others, in which the invaders were hunted and killed. This sparked a reprisal by the twin Turkish army led by *el-Daftardar*. Hearing the news of the assassination of his brother-in-law, Mohamed Bek Khusru rushed through the Kordofan lowlands, committing horrific atrocities, killing whomever he met. On his rampage of revenge en route to Shendi, villages were burnt, and lands were plundered. At Shendi and its twin town al-Matamma, on the western bank of the Nile, the atrocities committed by Daftardar and his army left deep wounds and bitter memories among the Sudanese for many decades to come. Furthermore, the revenge campaign of Daftardar left long-lasting effects on the 'Ja'aliyyien Dar', which became desolate and depopulated, following the dispersion of the tribe into various parts of the Sudan, especially the central and eastern towns.

The new order took some time to be established. Muhammad Ali's adventure in Egypt's southern frontiers proved a success, but at a hefty price, namely, the loss of his youngest son. A new system of administration was to be foiled. However, this turned out to be a painstaking experiment that lasted decades, even beyond the lifetime of Muhammad Ali himself. The era of the Turco-Egyptian Sudan was clouded by a system of taxation which was both unrealistic and tagged to a string of corrupt 'Turkish' officials. This eventually led to an easy downfall for Muhammad Ali's Sudanese empire in 1885. Muhammad Ali's principal intention of stocking the treasury of Egypt with the 'Sudan surplus' was to be executed only for the first few months following the invasion.

The Turkish way of administration and development were seen by the Sudanese as an instrument of injustice and oppression, alien to their moral, cultural, and religious values (15). Over the ensuing years, the system of administration was open to experimentation and subject to a series of forward and backward organization and re-organization. Initially the administrative hierarchy was built around the Turkish model of 'The Kashifs' and their assistants (the Qaim-maqams) at the district level, followed by the 'Mamurs', who were then the provincial governors. They were later replaced by the 'Mudirs' (Arabic, plural, meaning 'managers') and the provinces were called the 'Mudiriyyas'. The rest of the administrative hierarchy clustered around the Kashif, with the cascade of the 'Mubashir' (chief clerk), then the Mu'allim (clerk), the Sarraf' (Arabic = cashier), and finally the 'Katib' (Arabic = inscriber). Tied to this was the system of taxation, which began operating in the first few months, during the advance of the conquering army. The first architect of this system was an Egyptian Copt by the name of Hanna el-Taweil, who was assisted by several others, including Mohamed Saeed Effendi (the personal secretary of Ismail Pasha) and a Sudanese *'Arbab'* and a court official, named Dafallah wad Ahmed (16). The taxation system began as flawed and continued as such, being run by a terrifying squad of tax collectors, the Shaigiyya *'Bashi-bazuq'* (Buzuq; Turkish = cracked brain). To satisfy their tax obligations, the Sudanese had to sell their properties to meet the hefty tax demands. Others, especially those living along the strip of the Nile from Dongola to Khartoum, had to abandon their '*saqiyya*' fields and migrate to towns like Khartoum, Kassala, Gedaref, Sennar, and Wad Medani to make a living and evade the tax collectors. The Ja'aliyyien tribe, in particular, was hard hit following the earlier destruction and massacre of their people by Daftardar in the wake of the assassination of Ismail Pasha. This second wave of redistribution scattered their tribal natives in various regions of the Sudan. The Frenchman, Ferdinand Lafarque (c. 1800-1871), who lived in the Sudan for nearly a quarter of a century, wrote vivid description of the state of affairs, translated by Bejerkelo: 'The Turk has miscalculated the resources of the country, and preferred to exploit the people rather than to encourage them. There was a year of shortage in every three, and in every five there was one of famine'. (17). On the other hand, the slave trade flourished to meet the demands of the Egyptian army for 'slave soldiers'. When Mohamed Sai'd, the Egyptian Viceroy (r. 1854-1863), abolished the slave trade, a private one opened along the White Nile in the 1850s and beyond (see next section).

Mohamed Sai'd, the Egyptian Khedive, during his visit to the Sudan in 1857, realized the poor state of the country and its desolate inhabitants. The reign of his predecessor, Abbas I (r. 1848-1854), was characterised by an uneven policy towards the southern dependency of Egypt, with five governors at Khartoum being appointed and removed during the last six years of his rule. Mohamed Sa'id Pasha tried to make reforms, including the ouster of corrupt and unpopular 'Turkish' officials and the appointment of some Sudanese to share in the governing of their home country; as a result, few Sudanese went on to hold executive positions. Despite that the Turks managed to reinforce the authority of most of the tribal elites (such as the Shoukriyya and the Kababish), they aimed to curtail the tribal chiefs who opposed them and to promote others from the periphery or from the trader class, as in the case of Shaikh Bashir Ahmed Aqid, who was appointed Sheikh of the Ja'aliyyien. The first Sudanese to hold a distinguished government position was Mohamed Bey Rasikh, who belonged to a village near Berber. Rasikh became Governor General in 1861 and remained in office for a short spell (18). He was followed by Shaikh Ahmed 'Bey' Awad al-Kariem Abu Sinn, the 'Nazir' of the Shukriyya tribe, who became Governor of Khartoum from 1863 to 1870. Others included Hussein Bey Khalifa, the Sheikh of the Ababda, who was appointed Governor of Berber (1869-1873), and Alyas Bey Um-Berier (a Ja'alie notable), who was Governor of Kordofan on the eve of the Mahdiyya. However, Sudanese employment in the senior ranks was not confined to the above.

It is worth noting that the Turco-Egyptian rule was not without credit. The regime unified the scattered and dispersed Sudanese regions into one unit. The northern and central parts (Dongola/Berber/Khartoum and the Fung districts), the eastern regions (Takka 'Kassala', Red Sea, and Suakin) were joined to Kordofan in the west.

In the 1850s and 1860s, the south was annexed and, in 1874, Darfur (the last to be annexed). This provincial system of the administration was to be adopted initially in the first few years of Anglo-Egyptian rule in 1898. Further, there were significant developments in irrigation and industry. Several factories were built, and new towns came into existence or flourished. It was during the Turco-Egyptian era that Khartoum and Kassala were established (*vide infra*). The river transportation system was another positive accomplishment of the era; likewise, the postal system and telegraphic communication, which was not much different than that of Egypt itself. During the reign of Ismail Pasha (1864-1879), an ambitious plan was conceived to link Cairo and Khartoum by a railway line, with a view towards having part of the line go from Dongola to Darfur. The building of the line began energetically. It was planned to run from Aswan to Kurusko, and then to follow the Nile down to Khartoum. The project was abandoned shortly after it began, however, as Khediev Ismail became effectively bankrupt.

In conclusion, the Turco-Egyptian era in Sudan in general was marred by heavy taxations and the tyranny and corruption of the ruling officers. Here, we quote Bjorkelo, whose scholarly thesis 'Prelude to the Mahdiyya' summed up that era:

> A striking feature of the {Turkish} administration in the Sudan was the combination of an Ottoman formal structure with unstable tenures of office, unclear demarcation of authority and uncertain guidelines on how to deal with the Sudanese. There were clear racist undertone in the attitude of the Turks in order to categorise and differentiate the Sudanese and dispense their unequal justice, they used the degree of Islamization as a yardstick which meant that only a thin layer of Orthodox, 'proper' Muslims, reinforced from Egypt, were to be treated as fully civilized human beings, while the majority unless they are regarded as allies, deserved no particular pity, as they were either superstitious Suffis, pagans or just Black slaves. (19)

Thus, the Turco-Egyptian period was viewed by many as 'little better than a chapter in the history of crime' (20). The corrupt conduct of government and heavy taxation in the last two decades of the Turco-Egyptian Sudan set the scene for the uprising of the Mahdiyya (1881-1885) and, at the same time, made the times ripe for the climax of the Sudanese-British relationship. This eventually paved the way for the creation of the Anglo-Egyptian Sudan on the ruins of the Mahdiyya and the eventual annexation of the Sudan into the British Empire in 1898.

Section II:

The Consul Agents & Slave Trade: European Merchants & Missionaries

Khartoum of the Turco-Egyptian Sudan:

The story of how Khartoum came to be established is controversial. It was thought that the town have been founded by Ismail Pasha in 1821, when he ordered the building of the town to serve as the capital of the Turco-Egyptian Sudan before he was murdered. There is little support for such claim, but it is true that Ismail ordered a small garrison to be stationed at the confluence of the two Niles on his way south in 1821. It is well established that after Ismail took over full control of the Fung Kingdom, and following the submission of its last Sultan, Badi VI, he established his headquarters at Sennar and the city became the first capital of the new order (21). However, due to its bad climate and a series of epidemics of malaria and dysentery, which greatly reduced the number of invading troops, with over two thousand invalided and over six hundred dead, and after consultation with his father, Ismail decided to move the capital once more to Wad Medani (22). According to a Sudanese civil official, Ahmed bin Ali, who served both the Fung and the Turkish Administration, following the ordeal of Ismail Kamil Pasha's troops and their great sufferings, his father sent a group of expert physicians from Egypt who, following deliberations, decided that the capital would better off if moved either to Shendi or to Wad Medani, for geo-political and climatic reasons (23). Ismail then moved the capital initially to Wad Medani and built a palace, and beside it he established barracks, officers' quarter, and a hospital (24). However, Ismail was forced by circumstances to move the capital again, to Shendi, as a few month after he settled at Wad Medani epidemics broke out among his troops and that city's climate too was deemed to be unhealthy (25). However, subsequent tragic events prompted the capital to be moved to Khartoum, after the treacherous murder of Ismail Pasha and his entourage at Shendi on November 4, 1822.

In any case there has always been some tribal settlement at the site of present-day Khartoum, especially on Tuti Island and the adjoining northern fringes (current suburbs of Khartoum North [Bahri]). Migration of the Mahas from their abode in the north took place around the sixteenth century. In ancient chronicles, it was mentioned that they had been sending their children to the 'religious school', *'The Khalwa'*. of Sheikh 'Arbab Al-Agayid', a famous religious scholar and teacher in medieval Sudan. According to some recent sources, the site of the Khalwa of Sheik Arbab Al-Agaid' was located at the site of the present-day 'Farouk Mosque' in the heart of modern Khartoum (26). Following Ismail's massacre by Mek Nimr and the return of his brother Ibrahim al-Wali to Cairo in 1822, Mohamed Bey Khusru Daftardar became the commander-in-chief until 1824, when he eventually left for Cairo. His successor, Uthman Jarkas al-Biringi (a Circassian), established his headquarters at Khartoum; during his rule, Khartoum expanded and when he died in 1825 Mahu Bey Urfali (a Kurd) took over but he was also soon to die (in 1826) during a smallpox epidemic. He in turn was succeeded by Ali Khurshid Agha, during whose governorship Khartoum flourished and became the capital of the new regime. It was Khurshid Agha who organized the provincial system of administration in Sudan and he was the first Governor General (*Hikimda'r*) of the Turco-Egyptian Sudan (1833-1838).

Khartoum was regarded as the last outpost of civilization in 1847 when visited by the Welshman John Petherick. In 1850, a Liverpool man, George Melly, visited the town with his family, including wife, son, daughter, and both parents. Melly wrote one of the earliest descriptions of the town in English literature (27). Petherick first came to Khartoum on his way to Kordofan when he was commissioned by Mohamed Ali to explore the iron ores of Kordofan. Since 1845, Petherick was appointed as a mining engineer by Mohamed Ali and he spent his first two years between Cairo and Sinai before being sent to the Sudan. Petherick formed a good relationship with Mustafa Pasha Kiridilli, then Governor of Kordofan, and also befriended Georges Thibaut, a French gum-trader. Before Petherick could finalize his mining mission, his employer, the Egyptian Viceroy, entered his final illness. While he was intending to return back to Britain, Thibaut was persuaded by the British Consul General at Cairo, Charles Murray, to stay at Kordofan as a gum trader. Those years were full of tensions between the Egyptian government and the consuls of the European Powers. Since 1827, Egypt had held a trade monopoly in the Sudan. By 1838, the Porte signed a treaty with the European Powers to end the trade monopoly in Egypt, but Mohamed Ali argued that Sennar and Kordofan (his southern dependencies) were not part of the Ottoman Empire. The European Powers were arguing that Mohamed Ali himself was a subject of the Porte. All attempts to enforce the treaty on the trade in the Sudan failed. This disagreement continued until the final illness of Muhammad Ali (b.1769-d.1849), when his successor, Abbas I, became his regent in 1848. Following the death of his uncle Ibrahim Pasha, he ended the trade monopoly in the Sudan. Murray intended to use the new role of Petherick as a lever to enforce the monopoly's abolition. Petherick accepted, and an arrangement was made between him and Murray that Petherick was to hold the post of British Honorary Consul Agent or Vice Consul to protect British subjects and British interests in the Sudan. The British Government agreed to the arrangement, as it cost them nothing (28). Despite these arrangements, Petherick remained at Kordofan until 1854, running his own business alongside Georges Thibaut. This period saw significant developments in the Sudan following the opening up of the country for trade with many European, Syrian, Greek, Egyptian, and Turkish traders operating from Khartoum by obtaining credits from various companies and individuals in Egypt and Europe. Famous foreign traders at the time in Khartoum including the Frenchmen Antoine Brun Rollet, Alexander Vaudey (A Savoyard like Brune-Rollet), de Malazac, Vayssiere, the Maltese de Bono, the Syrian Ibrahim Baz, and the Egyptians Ali Ammouri and Al-Aqqad (29). To protect trade with their European subjects, several European consuls in Cairo emulated Charles Murray by appointing consul agents from among their native traders in Khartoum. Georges Thibault became the consular agent for France, Joseph Natterer for Austria, and even Alexandré Vaudey (who started his career in Egypt as a secretary to the famous Clot Bey) managed to obtain the post of the consular agent for Sardinia and moved to Khartoum as a trader. He subsequently brought two nephews, Ambroise and Jules Poncet, who later became very successful slave traders in the south (30).

By the mid-1840s, the Vatican decided to send Catholic missionaries to proselytize in the Sudan, especially among the pagans of the south. The Vatican was alerted to a concerted move among their Protestant rivals of plans to send missionaries to central Africa. David Livingstone (a Protestant missionary) had already been to South Africa since 1843. Further, the Vatican was anxious about the spread of Islam into the heart of Africa. The '*de Propaganda Fide*', whose official title is "*sacra congregatio christiano nomini propagando*" or the 'Red Pope', initiated the creation of the Apostolic Vicariate of Central Africa by Pope Gregory XVI in 1846. Prior to this, events in Abyssinia helped the Catholic Church to gain a foothold in the heart of the Sudan. Father Luigi Montuori, who was expelled from Ethiopia following a feud with the leaders of the Orthodox Church in Gondar, crossed over to Khartoum in fall of 1842. In less than two years, Montuori had established good relations with the ruling and merchant classes in Khartoum. Here, Montuori established a school and a church (31). Following the success of Luigi Montuori, the Vatican decided to send Catholic missionaries to gain a foothold among the pagan virgin lands of southern Sudan. The forces of Christian missionaries and European traders acted in concert with each other. A party led by Ryllo, a Polish Jesuit and three other priests—Knoblecher, a young Slovene, Angelo Vinco from Verona, and Pedemonte, an old Jesuit priest—was dispatched to the Sudan. The group reached Khartoum in February 1848 and four months later Ryllo died and Knoblecher became his successor (32). The Catholic missionaries at Khartoum would be assisted in their mission by several European traders. Antoine Brun Rollet, a Savoyard ivory trader, who first came to the Sudan in 1831, provided an invaluable support to Knoblecher and his colleagues when they moved up the Nile to establish their first mission station at Gondokoro, to start proselytizing among the Bari tribe (33). This coincided with the flourishing trade in ivory and further opening of the White Nile by European (and other) traders. Those traders were financed by creditors who were usually based in Egypt. Some were financed by big trading companies; e.g., Brun Rollet was financed by the British mercantile firm Joyce Thurburn & Company, based at Alexandria. Others were financed through individuals based either in Egypt or in Europe. The Frenchman Alphonso de Malzac was financed by Franz Binder, a Transylvanian who later went on to be the richest European in Khartoum, with a wealth estimated at £8,000 (34). The interest paid on these finances was quite hefty and stemmed from the ongoing restrictions imposed by one or the other of the Governor Generals in Khartoum. Several of those traders faced financial ruin. This may have been the motive behind many of these traders resorting to the slave trade to boost their income (35). Hence, the slave trade in the White Nile was practiced not only by the northern Sudanese '*jellaba*', but also many European traders. The Frenchman de Malzac, for instance, became so wealthy from the trade in slaves and ivory that he was nicknamed 'The King of the White Nile' (36).

The opening up of the southern frontier waterways took place in the 1850s. These navigation channels were not known to the Europeans or the Turks until the venture undertaken by the Copt Habashi, an ivory trade agent of John Petherick. Habashi unravelled the waterways of Bahr el-Ghazal in November 1855 and early 1856. He was later joined by John Petherick, who subsequently claimed fame and distinction as the first European to navigate the waterway channels of Bahr el Ghazal. Habashi sailed past Lake No and down Bahr el-Zaraf, the entrance to which was obscured from the sight of Captain Selim Quputan by the dense Sudd at Lake No (see next section). Pethrick and Habashi reached the point which later came to be known as *Meshra el Rek*[5]. From there, in January of 1856, they crossed Bahr el Ghazal by land to reach Wau and later to explore the southern frontiers of Bahr el-Ghazal until they reached the lands of the Luo and Bongo (37). Perhaps only a few days later, Pethrick and Habashi's footsteps were followed by Brun Rollet and his wife There was even a suggestion that the Aswani trader Ali Amouri was the first one to sail down these waterways well ahead of Pethrick, Habashi, and Brun Rollet (38). The opening up of Bahr el-Ghazal further widened the sphere of trade in ivory and slaves and witnessed the beginning of the appearance of the 'Bahr el- Ghazal Zaribas[6],' which became the hub of ivory trade and slave hunting. These '*zaribas*' became known by the individual traders. Among the famous *zaribas* were 'Zariba de Malzac', 'Zariba Ghattas' (a wealthy Copt), 'Zariba Kuchuk Ali' (a Turk), and 'Zariba Aqqad' (an Egyptian) (39). In late 1850s appeared Zubair Rahma Mansour. Zubair, who belonged to the Ja'aliyyien tribe, was born in 1831 in a small village north of Khartoum and was educated there before joining the service of Ali Ummori, an Egyptian ivory and slave trader in Bahr el-Ghazal. Soon his star was on the rise, and later he became a powerful merchant and a dominant figure in Bahr el-Ghazal. Zubair went on to play a decisive role in the history of his country. However, Zubair was a controversial figure and often cited as a gruesome slave trader. Here we quote A. B. Theobald who wrote a rather unbiased statement about his qualities as a leader, a ruler, and a trader:

> Zubair was no ordinary slave trader. Although he rose to power and wealth by the usual means of trade in ivory and slaves, yet when he reached a position of authority, he did not himself raid for slaves..........He was himself so humane and generous that the slaves of others sought eagerly to join him. He was a warrior and administrator of remarkable talent, an adventurer of bold ambition, and above all a mighty leader of men. He was in fact a kind of brilliant, unscrupulous figure of whom the moralist must disapprove, but who nevertheless throughout the ages has drawn to himself the passionate hero-worshipping, and devoted obedience of ordinary men. (40)

With more news filtering out about the slave trade and reaching Europe through the regular reports from the Consular Agents in Khartoum and the correspondence from Knoblecher, the Catholic Chief missionary, the Anti-Slavery Movements, and pressure groups, specially in Exeter Hall, stepped up the pressure on the Egyptian Viceroy to abolish the slave trade. The government of Sudan itself, however, had been involved heavily in these cruelties since the conquest. One of the major objectives of Mohamed Ali himself was to obtain slave soldiers for his '*Nizam el Jadeed*'. Despite the fact that Mohamed Sa'id Pasha issued a decree abolishing the slave trade in Sudan in 1857, the practice continued. By the late 1850s and the early 1860s, slaves were a major commodity for traders in the southern frontiers. Nevertheless, the 1860s saw the climax of the efforts to discover the source of the Nile. This climax accompanied the quest to abolish the slave trade in the Sudan and East Africa. This further pushed the Sudan into the backyard of the European colonialists. This will be the theme of the next section.

Section III:

The Quest for the Discovery of the Nile & the Dawn of the Great Scramble for Africa

> In the eighteenth century The British Empire had been at best amoral. The Hanoverian had grabbed power in Asia, land in America and slaves in Africa. Native people were either taxed, robbed or wiped out. The Victorians had more elevated aspirations. They dreamt not just of ruling the world, but of redeeming it.
>
> –Niall Ferguson, *Empire: How Britain Made the Modern World*

David Livingstone & Earlier Beginnings

By the late eighteenth century, a renaissance was at its zenith; many explorers had already explored several continents. The British Empire was on the rise and rise, and the scramble for Africa had not yet begun. Britain had already been to India, China, and parts of the Middle East. However, to most Europeans, the 'black continent' was still a mystery. Although several explorers had been adventurous in traversing several frontiers of the New World and Asia in the preceding centuries, the 'dark continent' remained clouded in mystery. The travels of the Frenchman Poncet in the early days of the eighteenth century and those of Scottish explorer James Bruce in the last decade of that century continued to stir emotions but several more decades would lapse before these writings triggered a more energetic move to open the continent for commerce, introducing the 'light of the Gospel' and civilization to the 'heathens'. As elegantly described by Niall Ferguson, it is a historical irony that the movement to embrace the 'Dark Continent' under 'the wings of Christendom' coincided with other movements to subject it to colonialism. In Britain, the movement to send missionaries to Africa was started by men like Zachary MaCulay and the 'Clapham Sect', which included others like Thornton and the parliamentary orator William Willberforce. Here the religious fervour to 'do unto others as you would have others do unto you' (Matthew 7:12) was on the same wavelength as the teaching of the Enlightenment. This all set in motion a movement against slavery. A few more activists joined in. Men like William Pitt Jr, Edmund Burke, the poet Samuel Taylor Coleridge, and the king of the potteries, Josiah Wedgewood, were to play a crucial role in these activities (41).

Nevertheless, the source of the Nile was a great mystery until the second half of the nineteenth century, when serious efforts to unravel this mystery began to be made in an orchestrated manner, primarily instigated by the Royal Geographical Society of Great Britain. The appeal to discover the source of the Nile had captured the imagination of many explorers since time immemorial. The writings of Ptolemy reveal an interest in the subject, and the subsequent military expedition sent by the Roman Emperor Nero in 66 A.D. to discover the source of the Nile resulted in reports that the Roman Army reached the area of the Nile but were unable to proceed further. This became common knowledge. Further, there were some legendary stories about the Greek merchant Digenes, stating that he had stumbled on some great lakes off the coast of Zanzibar following his return from a trip to India in the first century A.D. which added further to the excitement. The magnificent writings and the map drawn by Ptolemy remained a major reference. Ptolemy hypothesized that the Nile draws its source from two great lakes in the centre of Africa, and that these lakes are fed by some mountains which he called the 'Mountains of the Moon' (*'Montes Lunes'*). Ptolemy map (42) remained a reference till the time of James Bruce. Bruce, who drew other maps that were of great help to European explorers in years to follow. Some early missionaries, especially German and Austrian, in East Africa wrote about several great mountains that resembled those of the '*Montes Lunes*' mentioned by Ptolemy. Then the stories of Arab slave traders who mentioned several great lakes inland from the coast of Zanzibar further fueled the imagination of British explorers in the 1850s and beyond (43).

Several explorers were destined to play a vital role, and their adventures and rivalry culminated in a saga of personal feuds, conflicts, long-lasting hostilities, and even personal tragedies. Those events overlapped with the first waves of missionary activities in Africa. An interesting corollary is that the first missionary/explorer to have a prime role in setting the scene for the quest for discovery of the source of the Nile was also a medical doctor, the Scot David Livingstone. Son of a tailor turned salesman, Livingstone was born in 1813 in Balantyre, a small village in Lanarkshire, in the south-western fringes of Glasgow, six years after the abolition of slavery in Britain. He was educated at Anderson College in Glasgow (later to be University of Strathclyde), qualified in medicine in 1840 from the Royal College of Physicians and Surgeons of Glasgow, and went on in the same year to be ordained as a minister for the Church of Scotland. Having been inspired by the 'Clapham Sect', Livingstone was in regular attendance at their meetings in 'Exeter Hall', of the London Missionary Society. Livingstone, for the rest of his life, was destined to spearhead the motion of 'Embracing the Black Continent into the light of the Gospel', and introducing 'Christianity, Commerce and Civilization' into the heartland of the 'heathens and pagans' of Africa (44). Livingstone's missionary activities were considered a failure by his first sponsors, the London Missionary Society. Following his return from his first trip, he could not manage to secure more funding from the Society. However, he eventually succeeded in getting sponsorship from the Royal Geographical Society for his third expedition, with a primary aim of discovering the source of River Nile. He was also appointed by Queen Victoria as 'Her Majesty Consul for the east coast of Africa'. Livingstone made notes about several diseases he encountered during his hard years in southern and central Africa, including his hypothesis of the tsetse fly as the possible vector of the lethal disease, sleeping sickness, which the Zulu natives of south Africa call *'the nagana'*. Livingstone, was posthumously proved to be correct, by another Scot, Dr. David Bruce, during the last years of the Victorian Era. The discovery of the source of the Nile occupied much of the energies of Livingstone in the last years of his life. However, when he set forth to find the great lakes to the west, off the shores of Zanzibar, he was only to stumble on other lakes, and later to be lost in the swamps of the Congo River basin. The last years of Livingstone's life were full of tragedies. He lost the chief of his missionary group, Father Mackenzie, and then his wife, who succumbed to malaria; he failed to abolish the slave trade; and eventually he became lost in the middle of nowhere. Livingstone was rescued in 1863 by Henry Morton Stanley, another character who was destined to play a pivotal role in the discovery of the Nile's tributaries. The rescue mission of Livingstone by Stanley was widely publicized in Europe and America in Stanley's book, *How I Found Livingstone* (45). The famous phrase uttered by Stanley when he found Livingstone at Ujijii in 1864, 'Dr. Livingstone, I presume', went into history. Livingstone's eventual demise in 1873 followed disease and despair as he failed to achieve any of his dreams. Despite Livingstone's never having reached the proper heartlands of the Nile, his observations and the relentless attempts of the British Government to find him set the scene for the discovery of the origins of the Nile by John Hanning Speke, Richard Francis Burton, and James Grant. Stanley was to make the final fingerprints of those discoveries, and Samuel Baker was later to join in from the north.

Muhammad Ali Pasha & the Nile Discovery: Captain Selim Qupitan Expeditions (1839-1842)

> The ambition of Muhammad Ali is to possess all the banks and islands of the Nile, and to be master of all who drinks its water from Abyssinia to the Mediterranean; an ambition worthy of a great Prince if its origins not to be traced to avarice.
>
> –George Waddington, *Journal of a Visit to Some Parts of Ethiopia*, 1824

As already mentioned in earlier sections, one of the several objectives of Mohamed Ali in invading the Sudan in 1820 was to discover the source of the Nile. For Egypt, the Nile is its lifeline. Mohamed Ali, with help and planning from mainly French engineers, forged an evolution in agriculture with plans to construct several projects in the Delta to regulate the flow of Nile water, maximize its utilization, and minimize its loss. The expedition up the White Nile to discover its source in Central Africa was part of these plans. That expedition was led by one of Mohamed Ali's able engineers, a Turkish Bimbashi by the name of Selim Qupitan. Selim made three trips. The first left Khartoum in 1839 and included two Frenchmen, the merchant Georges Thibaut and J. P. d'Arnaud Bey, an engineer employed by Mohamed Ali. The accompanying troops were led by Suliman Agha Abu Daud, Kashef of Kerri (46). According to Hill, the Royal Geographical Society in London contributed £50 towards the cost of that expedition (47). Reaching the Shilluk town of Kaka and later down to Lake No, the expedition's advance further south was hampered by the thick Sudd Swamp. They could only reach as far south as the vicinity of Bor and returned back after the Sudd made any further advance impossible. The second expedition set off in November of 1840 and this time Qupitan was accompanied by other Frenchmen in addition to his earlier comrade Thibaut d'Arnaud. These included L. Sabatier and F. Lafargue, and a German named Ferdinand Werne. This expedition, like the previous one, had limited success. In a third voyage, the group managed to reach the southern frontier of Gondokoro in January of 1841. This town was the southern limit of the geographical discoveries of Selim Qupitan. In his annual address to the Royal Geographical Society of Great Britain for the year 1939, its president, Mr W. R. Hamilton, mentioned that 'The Council of the Society have, in the course of last year, appropriate the sum of 50 L. from the funds of the Society towards a project, formed by a society of gentlemen interested in Egyptian and AEthiopian (sic) discovery, for sending out a native of Dongolah (sic) to explore the sources of the Bahr al Abyad, or the western and principal affluent of the Nile.' (48) According to the version of Richard Hill, of a committee in England that was keen on the issue of discovering the source of the White Nile, thought of sending a Sudanese 'Dongolawi' by the name of Mohamed Effendi Abdelkariem, who was in London at the time, in disguise, to make the discovery for them. However, Abdelkariem turned out to be not up to the job, as he decided not to accompany Selim, and instead asserted that he would reach the source of the Nile via Kordofan and Darfur! (49).

Bimbashi Qupitan wrote several reports, which were compiled into journals and later translated into French by Jomard, a member of the Société de Paris (50, 51). Thibaut and Werne both wrote separate accounts of the journeys and their books were later translated into English. The Royal Geographical Society, which was founded a few years earlier, in 1830, found great appeal in the writings of d'Arnaude, Werne, and Jomard, which sparked efforts to discover the source of the Nile. The maps drawn by members of Selim Qupitan's expedition were used by Burton, Speke, and Grant, and later by Stanley and Baker.

The Forgotten Speke & the Charismatic 'Ruffian', Dick Burton

In the footsteps of Livingstone appeared Richard Francis Burton, who was a special man of that era. Charismatic and controversial, but certainly a multitalented Victorian, Burton was famous for being a prolific writer, linguist, explorer, poet, fencer, and diplomat (52). He was born in England in 1821 (the year Muhammad Ali's troops completed the conquest of the Sudan). His family, of Anglo-Irish descent, travelled extensively in Europe when he was a young boy, and it appears that those travels and exposure to several cultures and languages may have nurtured the multi-lingual talents that distinguished Burton later in his life. Burton mastered several European languages, including even Romanian, after it filtered out that he had a passing affair with a Romani 'gypsy' girl and he then mastered the rudiments of her language too! Burton started his education at Trinity College in Oxford, but he was dismissed after he antagonized his teachers. He then joined the East India Company as a Captain and served under Sir Charles Napier. There, he mastered several Indian dialects, including Guajarati, Urdu, Hindustani, Persian, and even Arabic. In toto, he was believed to have spoken 29 languages. He travelled in disguise to make Hajj (pilgrimage) to Mecca and Medina and he wrote two volumes about these adventures. He fought as a soldier in several places, including the Crimean war.

In 1855, Burton was commissioned by the Royal Geographical Society to explore the interior of East Africa and selected John Hanning Speke as his partner in this venture. Speke, an Englishman from Somerset (b. 1827), first met Burton in 1855 in Eden before their first adventure in Somaliland in that year (53). By then, Burton had been commissioned by the RGS to start his quest to discover the source of the Nile. The first part of that journey, through Somaliland, had to be called off as they were lucky to survive following an attack by a group of Somalis that nearly cost them their lives. In a second journey, Burton and Speke set off from Zanzibar in the direction in which they thought the presumed lakes to be. However, both fell ill by the time they reached the shore of Lake Tanganyika. Burton was so ill that Speke went northbound alone. Speke became the first European to see the great lake, which he named after Queen Victoria. Judging by its size, Speke thought that it must be the source of the Nile, but he failed to properly survey it, enabling Burton and others to contest his claim and leading to a rift in the relationship between the two companions. Speke later returned in a second journey commissioned by the Royal Geographical Society with the aim of proving his initial findings. He was accompanied by a Scotsman, Captain James Grant. Speke and Grant were able this time to traverse Lake Victoria on its western side, and they continued northbound, where they saw the great Falls that Speke named 'Rippon Falls', after the President of the Royal Geographical Society. They then sailed down the Nile till Gondokoro, inside the southern frontiers of Sudan, where they were met by Samuel Baker and the British Consul John Petherick in 1863. They travelled to Khartoum before proceeding to Alexandria. Speke's discovery was contested by Burton and others, and he published his 'journals' shortly before his tragic death a day before his famous contest with his famous debate with Burton was to take place at the Society for the Advancement of Science in London in 1864. Speke shot himself on a hunting trip, probably by accident, although suicide cannot be ruled out.

Section IV:

The Evolution of Political Relation: The Anti-Slavery Movement, Samuel Baker, and Charles Gordon

By the time the anti-slavery movement in Europe and Britain became a powerful lobby, the rulers of the Turco-Egyptian Sudan, beginning with Muhammad Ali himself, were deeply involved in the slave trade. As mentioned in previous sections, one of the major motives of Muhammad Ali in invading the Sudan was to secure slave soldiers to supply the required military might for his imperial ambitions. Following the subjugation of most of central and northern Sudan in the first few years of the conquest, regular expeditions to the south were waged by the rulers at Khartoum under direct pressure from the Egyptian Viceroy himself. Since the conquest, Muhammad Ali imposed a monopoly on trade and commerce in his new dependency, banning foreign traders from business in the Sudan without government permission, arguing that Sudan was now part of Egypt and therefore not subject to the agreement between the Grand Signior and the European Powers. The third governor of the Turco-Egyptian Sudan, Ali Khurshid Pasha (r. 1826-1838), was instructed to carry out raids for slaves. As early as 1827, he waged an expedition from the town of Rossiers, on the southern fringes of the Blue Nile close to the Abyssinian border, deep into the territories of the Dinka and Nuer, to capture slaves.

A second expedition in 1830 was to follow, this time into the adjoining area of the Shulluk around the Sobat River. In the last years of his successor, Ahmed Pasha Shamli (Abu Widan) (r. 1838-1843), the government monopoly on trade in the Sudan was to come to an end under sustained pressure from the European Powers. This period saw the growth of foreign traders, European and others, in Khartoum, especially Levantines, Greeks, and Italians. As mentioned earlier, by the early 1850s the expansion of the government territories into the south had already taken place and with it the opening of trade deep into the equatorial region and into Bahr el-Ghazal, both regions known as sources for slaves. On the other hand, and despite continuous pressure from the European Powers on the Egyptian Khedive to abolish the slave trade, it continued unabated and expanded further and further. Mohamed Said Pasha (r. 1854-1863), who succeeded Abbas Helmi I (r. 1849-1854), ordered a stop to the slave trade in 1854; however, his orders were not heeded, and the trade continued and expanded into deeper areas. It is worth mentioning that Mohamed Ali himself had earlier issued an edict, in the last days of his rule, to end the slave trade in the Sudan, but it also was not enacted. The first practical steps to abolish slavery in Sudan were taken in 1862 by Ismail Pasha, the successor of Mohamed Sae'id Pasha, when he was his regent in Egypt. Musa Hamdi Pasha, the 'Hikimdar' of the Sudan, accordingly issued orders in 1862 to allow boats to leave Khartoum only for ivory trade. Later, in 1864, more measures were taken by establishing a river police to confiscate all boats with slaves. However, that proved to be a failure, as traders learned to bribe the police and escape with their booty. Further, the authorities in Khartoum would levy capitation tax on trade into the South, which eventually drove the European merchants out of trade, and led to creation of merchant princes with subsequent flourishing of the slave trade. Several figures sprang up, including the 'merchant-prince' Sheikh Ahmed al-Aqqad, and others, who started initially as ivory traders and then changed direction into the slave trade (54). A major turn of events took place in 1869. From direct pressure of the European Powers to curb the slave trade and during a visit of the Prince of Wales to Cairo, Khedive Ismail appointed Samuel White Baker to lead an expedition to expand his control into Central Africa with another mandate to suppress the slave trade (*vide infra*):

> We Ismail, Khedive of Egypt, considering the savage conditions of the tribes which inhabit the Nile Basin; Considering that humanity enforces the suppression of the slave-hunters who occupy those countries in great numbers.... We have decreed and now decree as follows: To suppress the slave trade, to introduce a system of regular commerce.... The supreme command of this expedition is confined to Sir Samuel White Baker.... (*The Firman of Khedive Ismail to Sir Samuel White Baker*) (55)

Samuel White Baker is considered the doyen of all British explorers, and was also a prolific writer. He came twice to the Sudan. The first time was in 1861, as an explorer, adventurer, big game hunter, and ivory trader. However, he was one of the first of his generation of explorers to have mapped the various tributaries of the Blue Nile in a journey that had taken him nearly eleven months. When Speke and Grant were heading back to Egypt, Baker met them at Gondokoro in February of 1863. Baker later managed to discover an important tributary of the White Nile, Lake Albert '*Albert N'yanza*', which he named after Prince Albert, husband of Queen Victoria (56). Baker was born in London on June 8, 1821 into a wealthy family from Worcestershire. He was educated at a private school in Gloucestershire, Tottenham, before studying at Frankfurt University to graduate with a B.A. in civil engineering in 1845. Earlier in his life, he had taken several posts as Royal Superintendent in the Balkans and Central Europe, designing and planning railways and bridges. He had several children from his first wife, who died in 1855, of typhoid fever. Following his wife's death, he went to Mauritius and Ceylon (present-day Sri Lanka), before going on a hunting trip in Central Europe and the Balkans with a friend, Maharaja Duleep. At the end of that adventure in 1859, in Budapest, Baker met his second wife, Barbara Maria Finnian von Saaz, a Hungarian whose family were killed during the Hungarian Revolution, and had been acquired by an Armenian slave trader who intended her for the 'harem' of the Ottoman Pasha of Vidin (now in Romania). Baker fell in love with her but had been out-bid by the Pasha, so he escaped with the girl to Bucharest, Romania. She later accompanied him in his travels to the Nile valley, and they later married in 1865.

Khedive Ismail, during a visit of the British Crown Prince, the Prince of Wales, and under pressure from the European Powers to abolish the slave trade, appointed Baker as governor of Equatoria. Baker was given the titles of Major General, Pasha of the Ottoman Empire, and Governor of the Equatorial Province, with a mandate to stamp out the slave trade from central and east Africa. This mission lasted from 1869 to 1874. In his writings, Baker made many useful observations about the state of health of Sudan (*vide infra*). Both Baker and Gordon played a major role in furthering British interests in the Nile Basin in the prelude to the Mahdiyyia and in the build-up to the 'Great Scramble for Africa'. Baker's mission to suppress the slave trade wasn't very successful, despite earlier successes. According to Holt, Baker was not a good administrator despite his excellent qualities as an army officer (57). While he was campaigning vigorously in the Upper Nile, the slave trade flourished in Bahr el-Ghazal. Khedive Ismail attempted to extend his rule into Bahr el-Ghazal by appointing Mohamed al-Billali (or al-Hilali), a former suzerain of the Darfur Sultan, as chief of the district of Bahr el-Ghazal. Despite early friendship with the chief of the slave traders in Bahr-el-Ghazal, Zubair Rahma Mansour, they later fell out with each other and, during a battle with some slave traders in 1871, al-Hilali was killed. In 1873, Khedive Ismail realised the true power of Zubair and appointed him as governor of the Bahr el-Ghazal after he gave the district the status of a full province. Zubair thereafter would play a decisive role in annexing Darfur and extending the rule of the Khedive into this Sultanate, which remained outside the Turco-Egyptian Sudan for more than fifty years. In that same year, 1874, Baker's mandate and mission in Central Africa came to an end, and he was succeeded by another Briton, Charles Gordon Pasha, who took as his lot the task of completing the work of Baker in equatorial Africa. Following the rise of the Mahdiyya, Baker stood firmly against the advocacy of Sir Evelyn Barring (later Lord Cromer) of abandoning the Sudan following the major victories of the 'Mahdi of Sudan', and in later years became a strong advocate for the Reconquest of the Sudan (*vide infra*).

The Terrible Stanley: The Journalist Turned Explorer

Another character who was destined to play a decisive role in furthering British interests and extending the dominion of the British Empire into the Sudanese heartlands was the Anglo-American Henry Morton Stanley. Stanley appeared on the imperial scene initially through his background as a journalist and a reporter. He was born John Rowland, illegitimate son of a Welsh mother, was raised in poverty, and worked as a youth in Liverpool before trying his luck as a cabin boy aboard ship on a voyage to New Orleans in 1859. Here, a wealthy American merchant, Henry Stanley, adopted the boy and gave him his name and a job. Stanley had several postings to Ethiopia and Ghana as a reporter to a New York–based American newspaper. His 'turn of luck and fame' came after his successful mission to find and report on the missing David Livingstone, all trace of whom had been lost for several months. Stanley, after a 'mission finding trip' funded by David Bennet, owner of *New York Evening Star*, succeeded in finding the debilitated Livingstone, and the words he uttered upon meeting the frail and infirm missionary—'Dr.. Livingston, I presume'—went down in history. Stanley's book, *How I Found Livingstone,* which was published in 1871, shortly before the death of Livingston in 1873, brought him fame and fortune (58). Stanley became 'reporter turned explorer' and he went on to be one of the most successful explorers of his generation. Following his 'Livingstone finding mission', he was sponsored by the *New York Herald* and the *London Daily Telegraph* to explore the areas of central Africa. He circumnavigated Lake Victoria and he met the Kabaka (King) Metusa of Buganda (Uganda), and here he managed to summon missionaries to introduce Christianity in the region. That journey, which took three years (1874-1877), set the scene for the great 'Scramble for Africa'. Stanley was then commissioned by the Belgian monarch, King Leopold II, to explore the Congo River basin. But those same adventurers, which were publicized at the time as shear philanthropy came out to taint and smear his image when the true stories of the barbaric creation of the Congo Free State filtered out. Stanley then became more interested in advancing the interests of the British Empire in Central and East Africa. He was commissioned to execute the rescue operation of Emin Pasha (the German doctor Edward Schneitzer), who was under siege in 1888 by the Mahdist troops following the death of his predecessor, Charles Gordon, in Khartoum in 1885. Emin Pasha was the Governor of Equatoria on behalf of the Egyptian Khedive. Emin Pasha, during that rescue operation, which took most of 1888-1889, also involved Stanley in claiming vast territories of land under British control. It was during these travels that he found the link between Lake Edward and Lake Albert, the important tributaries/auxiliaries of the Nile. Stanley was famous for taking a ruthless approach against the native Africans whom he encountered in most of his explorations.

Later, it filtered out from several of his companions that he had committed many atrocities during his explorations.

Intriguingly, Stanley had strong personal connections with Henry Solomon Wellcome, the philanthropist Anglo-American who later played a decisive role in the medical history of the Sudan (see Chapter IV). The famous 'Tabloid Medicine' chest owe its publicity to the relation between the two. Stanley was one of the invitees during the famous dinner Wellcome organised in honour of Andrew Balfour before his first trip to Sudan. It was during that dinner that a row erupted between Sir Patrick Manson and Stanley, as the former accused him (not without reasons) of introducing trypanosomiasis to Uganda and the Sudan during his rescue of Emin Pasha in 1888-1889.

Section V:

Prelude to the Final Climax, the Eve of the Mahdiyya: Charles Gordon & The Mahdi

Following Samuel Baker's relative success in suppressing the slave trade in the Upper Nile and is expanding the dominion of the Egyptian Viceroy to include new territories in Equatoria, he recommended the British officer, Charles Gordon, who had amassed great fame in China and became known as 'Chinese Gordon'. Gordon, an imperial hero, was born in London in 1833, the son of a senior army officer. In 1852 he was commissioned with the Royal Engineers, and he fought in the Crimean war (1853-1856). He then became involved in Chinese affairs in the 1860s, where he succeeded in suppressing the Taiping Rebellion. Hence, on his return to Britain, he was cheered as an imperial hero. Gordon succeeded Baker as governor of the 'Equatorial Province of the Nile Basin'. He continued his predecessor's work and achieved much success, managing to further extend the rule of the Egyptian Viceroy into the heart of central Africa, whilst continuing his predecessor's policy of curbing the slave trade. The details of these events are beyond the scope of this treatise. However, the successes of Gordon and the repeated failures of the Turkish elite at Khartoum prompted Ismail, the Egyptian Khedive, to appoint Gordon as Governor General of the Sudan in 1877. Gordon, as usual, put much vigour and energy into his job. His days and nights were continuous work. His tenure at Khartoum was characterized by frequent journeysto the periphery, to pacify, suppress revolts, and even extinguish all-out war. However, Gordon resorted eventually to being aided by several Europeans and some Sudanese. One of those he employed was the Italian, Romolo Gessi. Gessi was instrumental in curbing the revolt in Bahr el-Ghazal and Darfur led by Sulayman, son of Zubair Pasha Rahma Mansour, the famous Sudanese notable and alleged slave-trader. Gordon's tenure as governor saw some improvement in the overall administration of the country and further curbing of the slave trade. However, it only delayed the inevitable and set the scene for the Mahdist revolt, which began in late 1880 and early 1881.

Following a series of conflicts between Khedive Ismail and the European Powers that culminated in his bankruptcy, then succeeded in persuading the Turkish Sultan to depose him. Ismail was sent into exile in Italy and the new Khedive, his teenage son, Twefig, succeeded him in June of 1879. Gordon left Sudan in 1880 and resigned six month later, deciding to return to England and never return. The efforts of Gordon to make reforms, curb corruption, and improve the ailing Sudanese economy all came to tatters and the situation would again pass into oblivion. By 1880, when Gordon left, he was succeeded as Governor General by Rauf Pasha, the same man Gordon had dismissed twice for incompetence and corruption. Here, following decades of a ruthless and unjust rule by the 'Turks' the Mahdist uprising took its toll and stormed the tyrants of the Turco-Egyptian rulers. Here, religious and patriotic motives were entwined. The oppressive regime was supposed to be replaced by a just one; but the false dawn of utopia was soon eclipsed by another regime and era which, in the memories of many Sudanese, did not carry happy memories. There were wars, famines, and evolving autocratic rule, which, if it had survived the rapidly changing regional and international scene of the late nineteenth century, would have materialised in a tyrannical family dynasty. However, all the ensuing circumstances suggested that the regime would not last long; the cascade of events would sweep it like a storm.

Then came the annexation of Egypt by British troops in 1882. Following this, events proceeded very quickly, with the rise and rise of the 'Mahdi' in the Sudan. The Mahdi, whose original name was Mohamed Ahmed ibn Abdallahi, was the son of a boat builder. He was born in 1844 at 'Labab Island' near Dongola. His father moved to work and live at Karrari, north of Khartoum, when Mohamed Ahmed was a young boy. He grew up eager to pursue a religious path among one of the Suffi '*Tarriga*' and he became a disciple of several Sheikhs. From 1860 he spent a spell of several years as a disciple of Sheikh Mohamed Sherif Nur-el Dayim, grandson of Sheikh Ahmed Eltayeb wad. el-Bashir, a revered sheikh of the 'Sammaniyya Order'. Mohamed Ahmed fell out with his Sheikh and later joined a rival Sheikh of the same order, Sheikh el-Gourashi Wad el-Zain, whose base was at Masallamiyya, a small town in the Gezira.

No doubt, Mohamed Ahmed, since his beginnings as a disciple, had a high reputation for extreme piety and asceticism (59). After the death of Sheikh el-Gourashi Wad el-Zain, followers began to gather around Mohamed Ahmed. He had earlier moved to reside at 'Abba Island' on the White Nile, as early as 1870. Gaetano Casati in his book, *Ten Years in Equatoria*, stated that:

> Michael Saad (a Copt), Chief Accountant of the Equatorial Province, told me that he was sailing upstream in company with the Egyptian Expedition under Sir Samuel Baker, he with others landed at the island Abba to pay their respects to the santon (sic). Mohamed Ahmed received them very courteously and as is usual complimented them with sucre and sweet milk. (60)

Casati himself, on his way to the Upper Nile in 1880, would pass by Abba Island and witness the members of the boat as 'they are rendering homage to a holy man who dwells here. He is immortal report says…the crew were saluting with reverence Mohamed Ahmed, the future Mahdi, who was destined to cause so much strife in the Soudan' (61).

The story of how Mohamed Ahmed claimed to be the long-awaited Mahdi is told in several versions which have been detailed by several historians on the Sudan. Worth mentioning is that the concept of the Mahdi in Sunni Islam is completely different from the concept of the Mahdi in Shiite Islam. It is important to point out the Mahdi declared his movement in several stages, which began in March of 1881. The details of these events are beyond the scope of this book. However, the time was ripe for a revolution against the foreign unjust rulers of the country. The 'Mahdi' was young, charismatic, and full of religious fervour. The people of Sudan were ready for a call to arms. What were the reasons for the revolt? The reader is referred to the books by Holt and Theobald on the Mahdiyya. The desolate regime of the Turco Egyptian rule had reached a stage of utter tyranny and corruption. The cry of 'Mahdi' to drive out the 'Turks' spread like a flame among the peasants and nomads of the country. The religious appeal provided the required catalyst to the masses. The administration initially took very little notice of this 'Dervish'. When the masses started to gather around him, however, military and political miscalculation eventually proved drastic. From his first appearance on the political scene in 1881, the Mahdi enjoyed successive victories. Several military expeditions sent by the rulers in Khartoum were either defeated or indeed completely annihilated. By January 19, 1883, the Mahdi and his troops managed to capture el-Obeid, a major town in western Sudan, after a long siege. The long rivalry and rift between two Sudanese notables, Elias Pasha Um Brier and Ahmed Bey Dafallah, helped to tip the balance of power in favour of al-Mahdi. Earlier, most merchants and traders, either Sudanese or foreigners, fled the city. Those foreign traders who stayed became captives, were placed under a Christian Syrian trader, long a resident of el-Obeid, by the name of Jurji (Georgi) Istambuli. Istambuli was forced to convert to Islam and was called Mohamed Sa'id al-Muslimani (61). The captured troops were used to enrich the army of the Mahdi for his subsequent rounds with the new Governor General of the Sudan, Abdel-Gadir Hilmi Pasha, who succeeded Rauf Pasha early in 1882. Earlier on, Bara, an important strategic town near el-Obied, was taken over by some troops allied with the Mahdi. Following the fall of el-Obeid, the revolt spread quickly to other parts of the country. Various tribes of Kordofan and Darfur swore allegiance to the Mahdi and began attacking and looting the garrisons. While the Mahdist troops were besieging el-Obeid, a group of Austrian nuns and priests led by Father Joseph Ohrwalder was captured by some allied troops in the Nuba Mountains. This group had arrived in the country in late 1881 and made their way to the Nuba Mountains and began proselytizing there. Ohrwalder and the nuns remained as captives in Sudan till 1892, when they eventually succeeded in escaping (63). Soon the revolt spread to the Gezira, and to the Blue and White Nile. Despite energetic efforts by the Governor General, Abdel-Qadir Hilmi Pasha, (of Syrian origin), who succeeded in achieving some victories, especially in Sennar and the White Nile, he was recalled to Egypt and was replaced by Alaa eldin Pasha Siddig, an officer of Circassian origin.

After the fall of el-Obeid the Egyptian Government began to realise the seriousness of the situation in the Sudan. Further, the Urabist crisis was extinguished by the interference of Britain at the Battle of Al Tell Alkabir. Britain now had an agent and consul general in Cairo, who was presumably directing affairs in Egypt, but Great

Britain was still reluctant to take any active involvement in the Sudan. More reinforcements were sent to help Abdel-Qadir Pasha Hilmi in his efforts to curb the revolt in Central Sudan, but the British Government repeatedly rejected any attempt to involve British or Indian troops in the Sudan, albeit eventually agreed to send a British Officer, Colonel Stewart, as an envoy to report on the situation in the Sudan. That was followed by choosing a British army officer, Colonel William Hicks, a retired officer of the Indian Army. Britain made no objection to that appointment. Hicks eventually managed to secure a large army; however, from the beginning he and his various Egyptian officers were not in tandem. Further, he was also in continuous disputes and disagreement with the Governor General, Alaa Aldien Pasha Siddiq. The entire army was annihilated by the Mahdists at Shaykan, near el-Obeid, in November of 1883. Both Hicks and the Governor General Alaa aldin Pasha Siddiq were among the slain (64). This decisive victory paved the way for the Mahdi to advance towards Khartoum. The consequences of Shaykan forced Rudolph Slatin, the Governor of Darfur, to submit to the Mahdi. His earlier efforts to hold ground were not successful. He even professed the Islamic faith and called himself '*Abdel-Qadir Salatin*', a name by which he was known throughout the Mahdiyya till his escape in 1894. The British governor of Bahr-el-Ghazal, Frank Miller Lupton Bey, who succeeded Gessi, had to follow suit, and he also had to profess the Islamic Faith and called himself Abdallahi. Both submitted and were taken as prisoners by the Mahdi. Lupton later died in Omdurman in May of 1888 (65).

Events in the west and southwest of the Sudan after the siege and fall of el-Obied were followed by the outbreak of revolt in the east. Osman (or Uthman) Digna, a half-Kurdish, half-Hadendawa trader, led the revolt and threatened Suakin and other towns in the Red Sea littoral. He acquired support from the religious family of the Majadieb of al-Dammer. Sheikh Eltahir Eltayib Al-Majzoub, of that revered family, who had long resided in eastern Sudan, gave Digna the invaluable support that helped to rally the masses behind him. His warriors had several skirmishes with the British and Indian troops stationed at the Red Sea. They defeated a small army led by Colonel Valentine Baker (brother of Samuel Baker). Rudyard Kipling's famous poem, 'Fuzzy Wuzzy', praising their courage and their breaking of the British square, has gone down in history. Digna harassed the Egyptian garrisons and managed eventually to cut off the important Berber-Suakin route to Khartoum, an essential lifeline of the regime. Late in 1883, after Shaykan, the new British Consul and agent at Cairo, Sir Evelyn Barring (later Lord Cromer) approached his government, enquiring what would be its response if the Egyptian Government asked for help from the British and the Indian troops to avail the crises in the Sudan. Lord Granville, the Foreign Secretary, responded by recommending the 'evacuation policy' which became a central component of the British policy in handling the rising threat of the Mahdi (66). It was Lord Granville who repeatedly offered the appointment of Charles Gordon to carry out the mission of evacuation of the troops and foreigners, with such tasks being laid down in a specific mandate. The British Government, under some public pressure and some effects tendered by the media, favoured Gordon to be appointed by the Egyptian Government to carry out such a task. Sir Evelyn Barring (later Lord Cromer) put great pressure on the Egyptian Government to accept such a proposal, despite Barring not being in favour of assigning Charles Gordon to such a task (67). The British Government made this decision after enough intelligence information was gathered to indicate that the government at Khartoum was collapsing and would not stand against the sweeping force of the Sudanese led by the Mahdi. Sir Evelyn Barring eventually agreed to Charles Gordon being the man for the mission, after he failed to convince Abdel Qadir Pasha Hilmi to accept that mission. Gordon was regarded by the British Government as the right person to enforce the policy in the Sudan and to restore law and order. Despite the fact that the mission had some clear endpoints and specific mandates, what actually happened was in complete variance with that understanding. Since Charles Gordon had left Sudan in July 1880, much water has passed under the bridge. However, Sir Evelyn Baring gave his famous advice for 'The Abandonment Policy' to the Egyptian Government. When the Egyptian Government with Sherrif Pasha as Head refused to comply, he was told by Sir Evelyn Barring to obey or forfeit office! Nubar Pasha Bohgos took office and began the process of evacuation of the troops by agreeing for Charles Gordon to be the right person to enforce this in Sudan (68). Gordon appeared on the scene early in January of 1884, coming via Cairo, where he met Zubayir Pasha. It became known that Gordon was inclined to assign Zubayr to take over a government that he would form after the evacuation was complete. However, the British Government repeatedly rejected the idea of involving Zubayr Pasha, who was regarded as *persona non grata* on account of his alleged involvement in slave-trade trafficking. Gordon, by accepting such a mission, thought he would be able to win the hearts and minds of the Sudanese and reverse the inevitable. He was wrong. A new chapter in history had already begun to be inscribed. Beyond doubt, Gordon had an admirable character, and was well respected when he had been in Sudan twice before. However; Gordon did not realize how much water had passed under the bridge.

Gordon at Khartoum: The Dramatic Finale

Gordon, after arriving at Khartoum, began to realize that the capital was becoming more and more isolated. He was beginning to grasp the actual situation. However, he had had a change of opinion, which now focused on the ultimate solution by involving the British Army, which would be able to destroy the Mahdi. He was advocating this both to the public and to the 'virtual ruler of Egypt', Sir Evelyn Barring (69). He exchanged correspondence with the Mahdi, offering him the post of Sultan of Kordofan. He felt this would pave the way for smooth evacuation of the troops and foreign nationals from Sudan. He also felt that this would help to pass the rule of the country back to the Sudanese notables. . The revolt began to spread quickly to the central part of the country and at Khartoum Gordon became more and more isolated as he became surrounded by the Mahdists hardliners and their sympathisers. Even those whom he felt would cooperate with him—like Shiekh el-Obeid Wad Badr of 'Um Dawan Bann' and Sheikh Abdel-Rahman eltayib Wad el-Basir, of the Halaween tribe, in the Gezira—responded by asking him to surrender. Further north, the Mahdi's former mentor, Sheikh Mohamed Al-Khayir, took over control of Berber and, with Osman Digna, consolidating his control of the Berber-Suakin route, and things began to look more ominous (70). Gordon, realising his futile and increasingly untenable position, began to change his mind about getting British troops to crush the Mahdi. He conveyed his thoughts to Cromer (71). He then issued a proclamation to the inhabitants of the Sudan, asserting that British troops were on their way thither. The clear goal was to reassure them as to the ultimate defeat of the Mahdists by the superpower that was Great Britain. In Holt's words, 'this assertion may have been a misunderstanding or a piece of bluff' (72). To begin with, the British Cabinet rejected this notion and repeatedly declined the nomination of Al-Zubayer Pasha Rahma Mansour as head of government of the Sudan. On the other hand, Gordon repeatedly declined the requests by the Mahdi for his surrender and his acceptance of Islam as a Faith. That led to a period of stalemate. Soon the Mahdi broke the deadlock by taking active steps to begin the siege of Khartoum as early as April of 1884. The Mahdist amir Mohamed Osman Abu Garja, Commander of the River Districts, was sent first, followed by another commander, amir Abdul-Rahman al-Nujumi. From then on, events began to progress very rapidly, with troops under Gordon losing ground and becoming demoralized. By August of 1884, the siege of Khartoum began to show its effects. By September, the Gordon rescue mission began its advance after the British Parliament finally agreed to fund a relief expedition. Gordon's communications suffered a lot, and in the same month as the urgent measures were taken to rescue him, he sent his *aide-de-camp*, Colonel Stewart, in a steamer to Egypt. The latter mission proved to be mortal as he was ambushed, surrounded, and slaughtered with all his men past Abu Hamad. Earlier, in August, the Mahdi had left his mammoth camp outside el-Rahad, a town to the south east of el-Obeid, and the major siege of Khartoum reached its climax after he camped with his main army at the fishing village of Abu-Saa'ed on the western bank of the White Nile, opposite Khartoum. By then the relief expedition, 'the Desert Column', was advancing slowly down the western side of the Nile, past Wadi Halfa, led by General Sir Welsley, only to go beyond Kurti on January 5, 1885. The Desert Column faced intermittent resistance, but it managed to take over the strategic town of el-Matamma shortly before the fall of Khartoum. It took several days for Sir Charles Wilson to organize his troops before sending a steamer up the Nile to rescue

Gordon, only to arrive on January 28, 1885, too late for Gordon, as the town had been stormed by the Ansar[7], the Mahdi's followers, two days earlier. Gordon stood his ground and fought to the last minute. He was slain on the staircase of his Palace at Khartoum in contravention of the clear instructions of the Mahdi. By midday of January 26, the take-over of the city was complete. Gordon's death sent shock waves into the core of the pride of imperial Britain. The deep wound of his death would not heal until thirteen years later, when the campaigns of the Reconquest set forth. A new chapter in the history of Sudan would begin.

Section VI:

The Reconquest: Cromer, Kitchener & Wingate and the creation of the Anglo-Egyptian Sudan

> He was never in a hurry, never anxious to make an effect or sensation. He sat still and men came to him. He watched events until their combination enabled him to intervene smoothly and decisively.... He rejected all high-sounding titles; he remained simply the British Agent. His status was indefinite; he might be nothing, he was in fact everything. His word was law.
>
> –Winston Churchill on Lord Cromer

The Mahdist State: The Prelude to the Condominium

Following the fall of Khartoum and the death of Gordon, the Mahdi ruled supreme. A new capital was established at the site of Fort Omdurman on the western bank of the Nile. It didn't take much for the rest of the country to submit to the new order. Within a few months, the remaining parts of the Turco-Egyptian Sudan became incorporated into the new state, with the exception of Suakin and Wadi Halfa, which remained under Anglo-Egyptian control. After a very short rule, the Mahdi died following a short illness and the reins of power passed to Khalifa Abdullahi el-Ta'aishi, a very able character, a longtime supporter of the Mahdi. Abdullahi had been second in command of the Mahdist movement since the beginnings of the revolution. Abdullahi, who rose from humble origins, was destined to play a decisive role in the history of the Sudan. His father, Mohamed Adam, nicknamed *'Tor Shayn'*, came from the land which lay beyond Darfur, between Wadai and the Bornu kingdom. On his way to pilgrimage to Mecca, he settled in the land of the Gubarat clan of the Tai'isha tribe and married the mother of Abdullahi. He was famous for his piety, and as a skilled diviner. The tribe relied upon his foresight in planning their raids on neighbouring tribes. Abdullahi inherited his father skills as soothsayer. During the conflict between Zubair Pasha Rahma Mansour and the Rezaigat tribe, Abdullahi fought on the side of the latter, and was captured by Zubair. He was lucky to escape death and later approached Zubair to try to convince him that he (Zubair) had many of the characteristics of the expected Mahdi, only to be rebuked by Zubair. He then heard of Mohamed Ahmed, the eventual Mahdi, and decided to join him at al-Massallamyia, when Mohamed Ahmed was building a tomb for his mentor. There was some controversy over whether Abdullahi may have suggested the idea of the Mahdi to Mohamed Ahmed after he joined him at the Gezira. What was important in that encounter was that Abdullahi soon rose to be *primus inter pares* among the closed circle of the adherents of the Mahdi. He would later command the largest part of the major military forces of the Ansar.

The task of the Khalifa to reign supreme proved to be rather tough. From the outset, he was faced with jealousy and intense rivalry, which was mainly waged by the Mahdi's kin, known as the Ashraf, and their allies. Within the first year of his rule, through skilful manoeuvres of opportunism but also due to certain events that took place in the new state, Abdullahi managed to neutralize their power and attack them piecemeal. By late 1886, Abdullahi had diluted their military power via one of his intelligent military commanders, Hamdan Abu Anja (who was one of the military commanders of Zubayr Pasha). However, the Ashraf were not completely neutralised and sidelined until 1892. Abdullahi, feeling vulnerable, resorted to putting relatives and members of his own Tai'isha tribe in key positions of high command. But in those posts that they were not capable of handling, he had to place members of the riverain tribes. This created a degree of division among his ruling structure and made the state weak and vulnerable for external powers to exploit. The militant nature of the Mahdist state itself led to a continuous cascade of campaigns involving several frontiers. Part of the 'Mahdist Ideology' itself involved the spreading of its doctrine into other countries. The origin of this preceded the Khalifa's reign. The decisive and swift victories of the 'Mahdi' deepened his personal conviction that his mission should go beyond local frontiers. Letters were sent to the

Egyptian Khedive, to Queen Victoria, to the Sheriff of Mecca, and to the Ethiopian emperor to accept the 'Mahdist Faith' or risk destruction. Abdullahi, after he secured his own personal hegemony, began to prepare for a campaign that would both invade Egypt and wage war on the Abyssinians. As early as 1885, during the life of the Mahdi himself, Abdul-Rahman al-Nujumi, who was leading troops chasing the Relief Expedition force, was ordered to stay at al-Matamma in order to begin the mission of invading Egypt. However, events at Omdurman and elsewhere delayed the beginning of this task for some time. Some historians believe that the eventual creation of this mission, which began sometime after the Khalifa Abdullahi began to feel the threat of the Ashraf and *'awalad al-balad'*, was played carefully by the Khalifa to weaken his opponents. However, due to many factors, that army was annihilated at Tushki in southern Egypt by 1889, and its leader was killed.

Since the earlier days of the Khalifa's reign, the western parts of the country, Darfur and Kordofan, were inclined to mutiny. The tribal structure of the region was not diluted once the Mahdiyyia reigned supreme. The eagerness of the tribal shieks and chiefs for independence would set the scene for the tribal revolts, especially in the west. Further, the subjugation of the Darfur Sultanate as early as 1874 by Zubair Pasha Rahma Mansour on behalf of the Turco-Egyptian hegemony and the continuation of the status quo after the Mahdists' victory did not deter the claimants of the Darfurian throne to abandon the pursuit of their lost dynasty. Despite initial good relations with the Khalifa, one Yusuf Ibrahim, son of Ibrahim Garad (who was killed by Zubair at Menwashi in 1874), openly revolted. He was eventually routed and killed in early 1888. As early as 1886, unrest amongst the Rezaigat tribe, led by their chief Madibbu, became apparent to the Khalifa. Their longing for independence and freedom led them into open revolt. This did not last long; their leader Madibbu was captured and was killed by Abu Anja, an old adversary. Around the same time, the Kabbabish, who were one of the largest tribes in the western frontiers of Kordofan and Darfur, persisted in their disobedience of the new order at Omdurman. It is an historical irony that this tribe remained a foe of the Mahdiyyia movement since its early days. Following a temporary submission of the tribal leader to the Khalifa, its chief, Salih Fadallah Salim (brother of al-Tum Fadlalla Salim, who was killed by the Mahdi at el-Obeid in 1883), also openly revolted. Like his fellow Rezaigat chief, he was eventually surrounded and killed in May of 1887. Its complex tribal structure made it tough for the Ansar to impose its full authority. Out of the blue in the fall of 1888, a charismatic figure appeared among the Massalit tribesmen, claiming that he was the deputy of the fourth Khalifa of the Mahdiyyia, *al-Mahdi al-Sanaussi*. The man became known as 'Abu Jummaiza'. He soon acquired massive support from the many tribes of the far west and he inflicted heavy defeats on the Mahdist armies that were sent to defuse his movement. His threat remained rife till his untimely death from what seems to have been a haemorrhagic fever. The remnants of his troops were then defeated by a large army sent from Omdurman in winter of 1889.

On the Abyssinian front lay most of the glorious victories of the Mahdist State. Despite the fact that the area (which comprised mainly the Buttana valley, the hub and heartlands of the Shukriyya tribe) was difficult for the Ansar to get a strong foothold, the help of Sheikh Abdallah Awad el-Kariem Abu Sinn made the subjugation of the area around Kassala and el-Gedarif possible. His father, Sheikh Awad elKariem Ahmed Abu Sinn, in contrast to his son, remained hostile to the Mahdiyyia and was imprisoned in Omdurman, where he died in 1887. The Abyssinians and the Ansar went into several rounds of war and battles, and in most of them the Ansar emerged victorious. In one encounter in 1889, King John of Abyssinia was killed. This opened the way for the Italians to extend their dominion beyond Musawa'a, which later cost the Ansar the control of Kassala, which was occupied by the Italians in 1894. On the north-eastern front, repeated attempts to drive the only remaining Anglo-Egyptian post at Suakin never succeed in accomplishing that mission. It was there that Kitchener, who was appointed as Governor of the Red Sea littoral as early as 1886, became well known to the Ansar. As a junior officer, Kitchener was among the troops of the Gordon Relief Expedition whose task failed to rescue the British imperial hero in 1884-1885. Throughout the Mahdist era, this front remained rife with interrupted skirmishes that waxed and waned according to the circumstances. It is worth mentioning that the Anglo-Egyptian dominion was even extended into the Mahdist heartlands by capturing Tokar (Tukar), the eastern headquarters of the Mahdist state, as early as 1891 (73). That front remained very vibrant, probably reflecting the military desire of the British to restore the imperial pride that had been wounded after the failure of the Gordon rescue mission, and the continuous failures to capture Osman Digna, who remained a threat to the military outposts in the region.

Then events proceeded very quickly. The French started to forge their plan to expand their imperial dominion beyond the central African belt of what came to be known later as the French Sudan (extending from the Atlantic Coast of West Africa into present-day Chad). The concealed aim of the French was to extend their dominion and to annex the heart of Africa, including the Nile Basin. In Britain, there was a change of government and with it a change of hearts. Gladstone and his Liberal Party would lose power and a Conservative Government led by Lord Salisbury took over. In the meantime, the military enterprises of the Khalifa went to tatters. His armies that were invading Egypt were defeated at Toshki, in Upper Egypt, in 1889, and here one of his best military leaders, the Mahdist amir 'Abdulrahman el-Nujumi', was killed. Britain by then had foiled a treaty with Italy. The Italians had gone into Abyssinia and their troops were rounded up at Adawa. In the meantime, significant propaganda was unleashed by Colonel Reginald Wingate, the director of military intelligence of the Egyptian Army. Wingate exploited fully the stories of 'horror and desolation' associated with the 'barbaric regime of the Khalifa' in Omdurman. This was fuelled by two books. The first, *Ten Years of Captivity in the Mahdi's Camp*, written by an Austrian priest, Fr. Joseph Ohrwalder, who had been a captive and prisoner of first the Mahdi and then the Khalifa (74). Ohrwalder managed to flee Omdurman in 1892, in an escape that was masterminded by Wingate himself, who utilized some men from the Ababda tribe to provide the escape tools and guide him through the desert to Egypt. The Khalifa's alienation and mistreatment of several Sudanese notables and tribes helped to seal his eventual demise and the collapse of the Mahdist State when the moment of reckoning came. The second book, *The Fire and Sword in Sudan*, was written by the Austrian Rudolph von Slatin, another famous European captive and prisoner of the Khalifa. Slatin also managed to escape with the aid of Wingate in 1895 (75). The two books were both translated into English by Wingate and, in addition, Wingate himself wrote a book of sheer war propaganda, *Mahdiism and the Egyptian Sudan* (76). These books and the publicity that surrounded them collectively fueled public and political support for the re-capture of the Sudan from the Mahdists. By 1896, Lord Herbert Horatio Kitchener, the new Sirdar of the Egyptian army, was leading his troops along the Nile. His initial aim was to distract the attention of the Mahdists from the eastern front, where the Dervishes were gathering at Kassala to lend support to their 'new allies', the Abyssinians, against the Italians. Kitchener, who had earlier been the governor of the Red Sea littoral, based at Suakin, was trying tirelessly to weaken or capture the Mahdist emir, Uthman Digna, but to no avail. Thus, Kitchener was no stranger to the Sudanese territories and the political landscape in the Sudan since the death of Charles Gordon.

The Reconquest & the Nile Campaigns, 1896-1898

> That a new and better Soudan will be raised up over the ashes of Gordon, and all those brave officers and men who have perished in the loyal performance of their duty.
>
> –Wingate, *Mahdiism & the Egyptian Soudan*, 491

By then, the international political scene was ripening. The European superpowers were in an all-out race characterised as 'The Great Scramble for Africa'. The British imperial ambitions for extending their territories into the heart of the Nile Valley and further into Africa began to take its final shape. Uganda and the rest of east Africa had already been annexed by 1894. Further, an agreement was reached with the Belgian monarch to limit his territorial claims. On the other hand, the treaty with Italy—which had begun its imperial adventures decades before by annexing Eritrea at the expense of Ethiopian hegemony—had a significant impact on future events.

Further, the British desire to secure a major foothold against the efforts of the French to extend their African dominions from the shores of the Atlantic Ocean in West Africa to the Red Sea littoral would be proven to be more decisive by subsequent developments in the dying years of the nineteenth century. In 1894, the French took active steps to gain a foothold at Fashoda (which by then was under the Mahdists' control). On March 13, 1896, the political game at Whitehall reached a climax when the Sirdar of the Egyptian army, Herbert Horatio Kitchener, received instructions to advance towards Dongola Province and occupy it. The move was made in response to the news that the 'Dervish Forces' were gathering momentum at Kassala to support the Abyssinians, who had inflicted a heavy defeat on the Italians at Adowa early in March of 1896. On the other hand, another motive stemmed from the emerging rivalry between the French and the British over territorial claims to the Nile Valley and the heart of Africa beyond. The race to gain control over these regions was in full stride from 1894 onwards. Britain had claimed Uganda as a protectorate in April of 1894, and the French had already established a strong presence in French Somaliland, whence they began to lend support to the Abyssinians in their conflict with the Italians. Further, the French were sympathetic to the Abyssinians' territorial claim of sovereignty over the right bank of the White Nile from 5° to 14° N. The French supply of weapons to the Abyssinians proved crucial in their victory over the Italians at Adowa. Earlier in 1891, the Anglo-Italian Agreement over the British interest in the Nile Valley made them allies.

The first phase of the Reconquest was the advance of the troops that Kitchener and Wingate had been organising for some time. The bulk of the first troops was made up of Sudanese soldiers, who were mainly southerners, and some remnants of the old *Jihadiyyias* who later changed allegiance. These Sudanese battalions were under the command of British officers. Egyptian troops formed the rest. The advance of the troops was paralleled by laying a railway line down the east bank of the Nile. The first major encounter took place at the Battle of Fiket (Farka) on June 7, 1896. The Ansar were defeated. The next major town, Sawarda, was taken shortly thereafter. The advance of the invading army was halted after a cholera epidemic broke out among the troops in mid-July. By September 23rd, the whole of Dongola Province was taken over by the invading troops. The Nile Expedition took a major turn of fortunes when Kitchener decided to change tactics and began to construct a different railway line, one that ran from Wadi Half across the Nubian Desert towards Abu Hamad. This move caught the Khalifa by surprise. That helped the quick deployment of the troops into the heart of the Mahdists' territories. Before the beginning of the second phase of the Nile campaign, major developments at Omdurman took place. The decision of the Khalifa to move the bulk of his army to camp at the town of al-Matamma, the capital of the Ja'aliyyien tribe, drove the tribe to revolt. On July 1, 1897, the rebellion was fiercely crushed, the Ja'aliyyien men were massacred, and their heartland was plundered by their fellow countrymen, the Ansar. That led to a major crack in the unity of the Sudanese against the invading army (77). In the wake of these events, the advance of the invading army towards the strategic town of Berber was met with little resistance. Berber was taken over by a faction from the Ababde tribe, led by Adelazim Bey Hussein Khalifa and Captain Hunter on September 6, 1897. By then, the major Mahdist army was advancing slowly after re-enforcements arrived, mainly from the west of the country, the heartland of the Mahdist movement. However, the large army that eventually encamped near the present-day city of Atbara was decimated both by famine and by repeated desertion of its soldiers. Kitchener's task was all but done on April 8, 1898, with nearly three thousand dead and over four thousand wounded. The way to Omdurman had been well paved for the conqueror to mount his final assault on the Khalifa at Omdurman.

It is worth mentioning that an alliance between the Abyssinian Emperor, Menelik, and the Khalifa of the Mahdi had been long sought by the former but was met with few positive gestures from the latter. Envoys and message exchanges had begun as early as 1895, when Menelik first sent an envoy, a certain Abyssinian Muslim, Mohamed al-Tayyib (78). The Abyssinian monarch felt that he was more threatened by the Italians than by the Sudanese. Such an invitation was renewed following the battle of Adowa in June 1896, by which time the mighty threat of Kitchener was looming against the

Khalifa. A major encounter of historical significance took place late in 1897, when the same envoy came to Omdurman and, in a secret audience, presented a French flag that had been given to al-Tayyib by Lagarde, the French Governor of Somaliland, in the presence of Menelik. The Khalifa clerk, advisor, and confidante, Yusuf Mikha'il, asserted that: 'The ambassador told the Khalifa to raise this flag on the frontiers of his kingdom in order to be an independent king in his kingdom and France would be a protection to him' (79).

The final stage of the Reconquest reached its climax at Karrari on September 2, 1898. Following the defeat of Mahmoud Wad Ahmed at the Atbara, the Khalifa decided to defend his capital by letting the invaders come as near as possible. The epic battle was documented by the historic narrative of Winston Churchill, *The River War*, that candidly witnessed to the bravery of the Sudanese (80). The day was destined to be won by the Maxim gun. By midday, the Ansar were either dead or maimed, wounded or captured. The day before, Omdurman had been subjected to intense bombardment from the gunboats on the Nile. A faction of Ja'aliyyien irregulars, encamped with some of the invading troops on the opposite bank of the Nile, participated on the final assault on the town. The Mahdi's tomb was a major target. When the Maxim's lips were silent, the Khalifa slipped hastily towards the south for another round against his future assailants. On September 8th, Kitchener took a Nile steamer in haste, to settle the score with Jean-Baptiste Marchand, the French General who had set foot at Fashoda earlier in the summer. On the other hand, the Khalifa remained a nuisance to the new order after he succeeded in reaching the eastern parts of the Nuba Mountains and remained at large till he was finally routed and massacred at Um Diewiakrat, near the present-day town of Kosti, in November of 1899. Earlier, in January of 1899, the Condominium Agreement had been signed, a hybrid Anglo-Egyptian state would be placed on the map of the world, and a new era would unfold.

Endnotes

1 *Bey*: Turkish, a title of honour (pl., *Beys*).

2 *Porte*: central government of the Ottoman Empire.

3 *Nizam el-Jedid* (Arabic, new order) refers to the regular army of the early nineteenth century established by Muhammad Ali Pasha.

4 Turkish, chief of finance.

5 *Meshra el Rek:* Arabic, Harbour of Slavery.

6 *Zariba*: a Sudanese Arabic word meaning a guarded courtyard usually surrounded by thorny bush trees.

7 'Ansars was the name given to the followers of the Mahdi, and the name is retained to this very day for the followers of the 'Umma' Party.

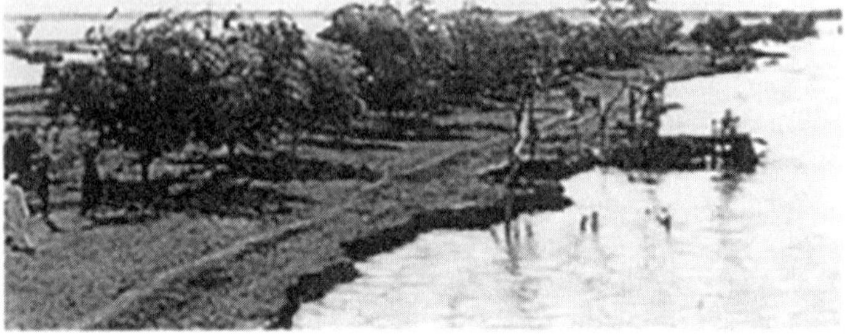

1. Al Khartoum. The mud bank where it all started

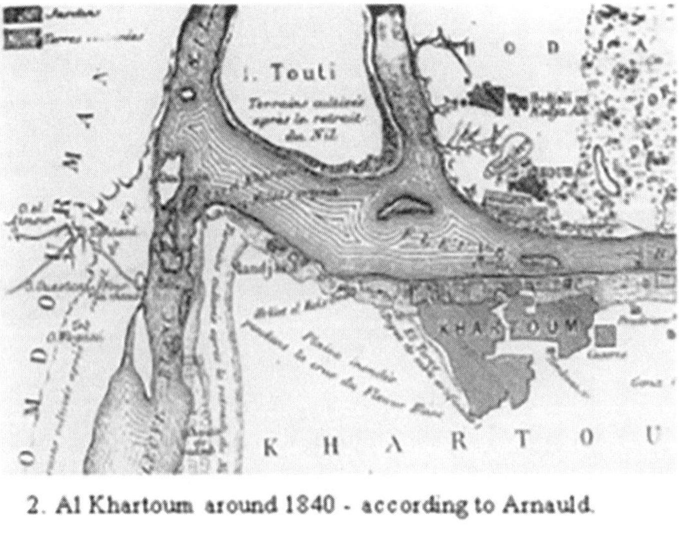

2. Al Khartoum around 1840 - according to Arnauld.

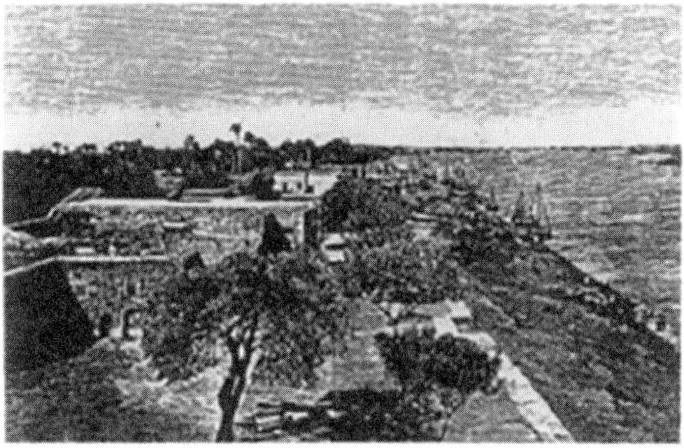

3. Khartoum of the mid-1800s.

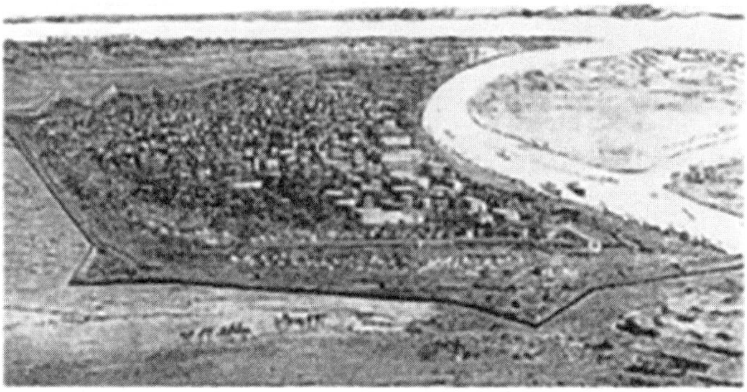

4. Al Khartoum at the end of the Turkiya.

(Above Photos are courtesy of B. E. Babiker, *Khartoum: Past, Present and the Prospects for the Future*, Durham Middle East Papers, Sir William Luce Publications Series, p.9.

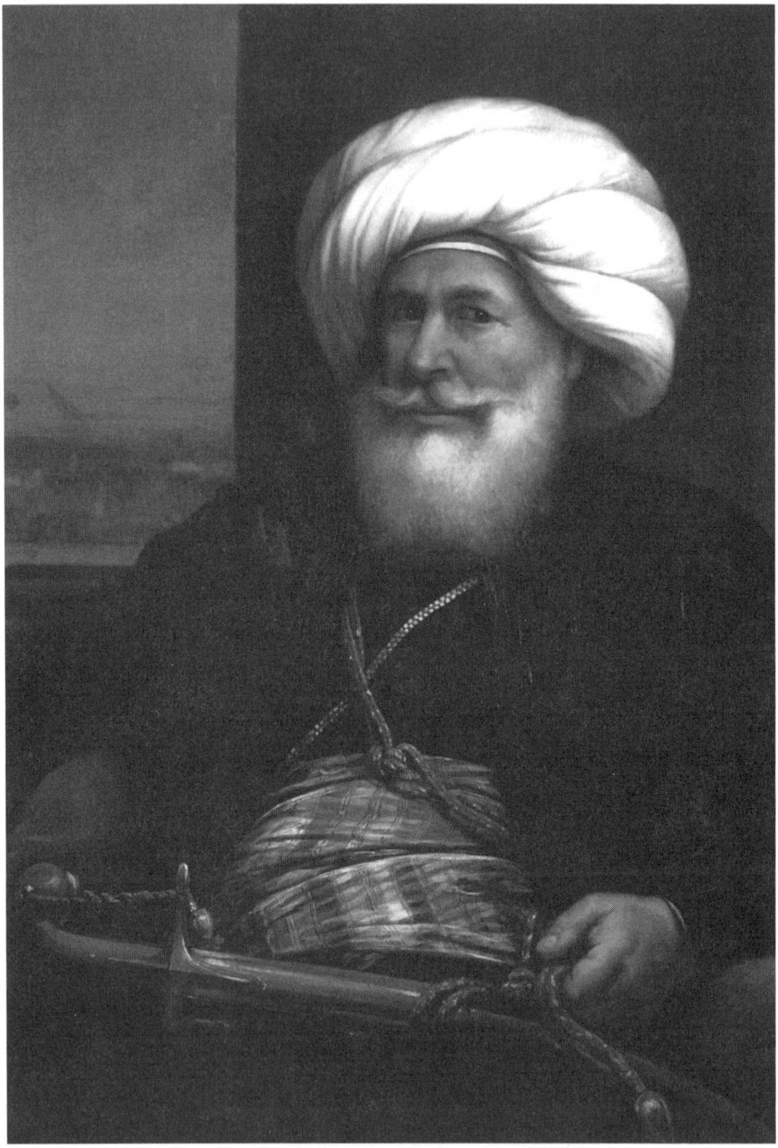

Muhammad Ali Pasha of Egypt
(Courtesy of Wikipedia)

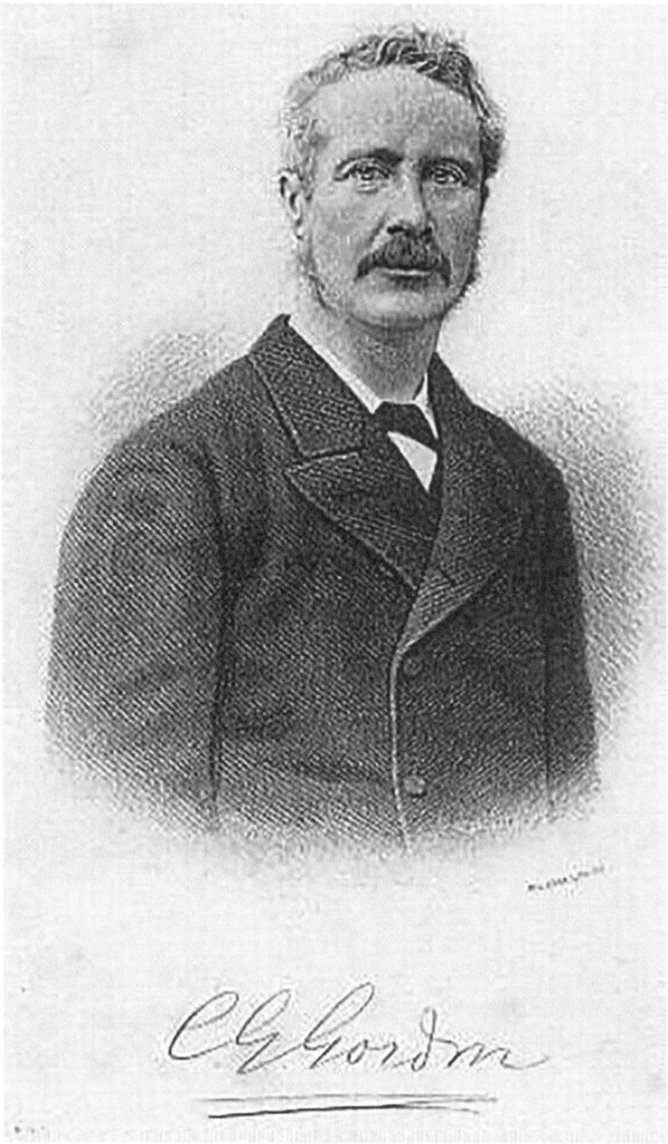

Charles George Gordon 'Gordon of Khartoum'
(Courtesy of Wikipedia)

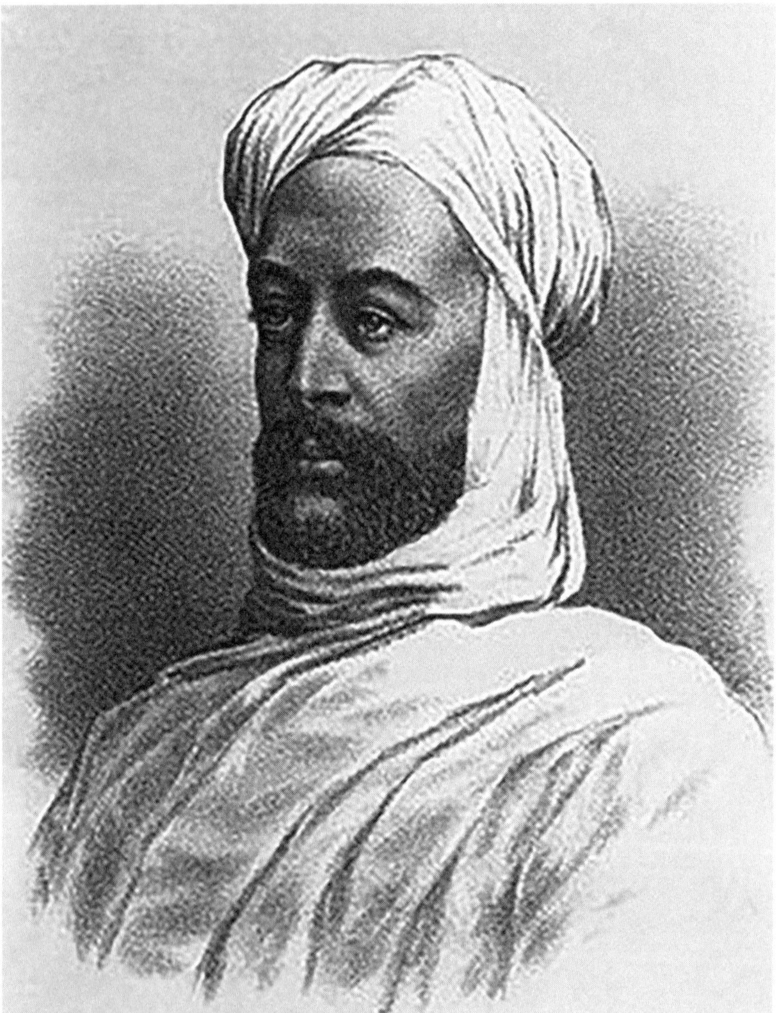

Muhammed Ahmed el-Mahdi
(Courtesy of Wikipedia)

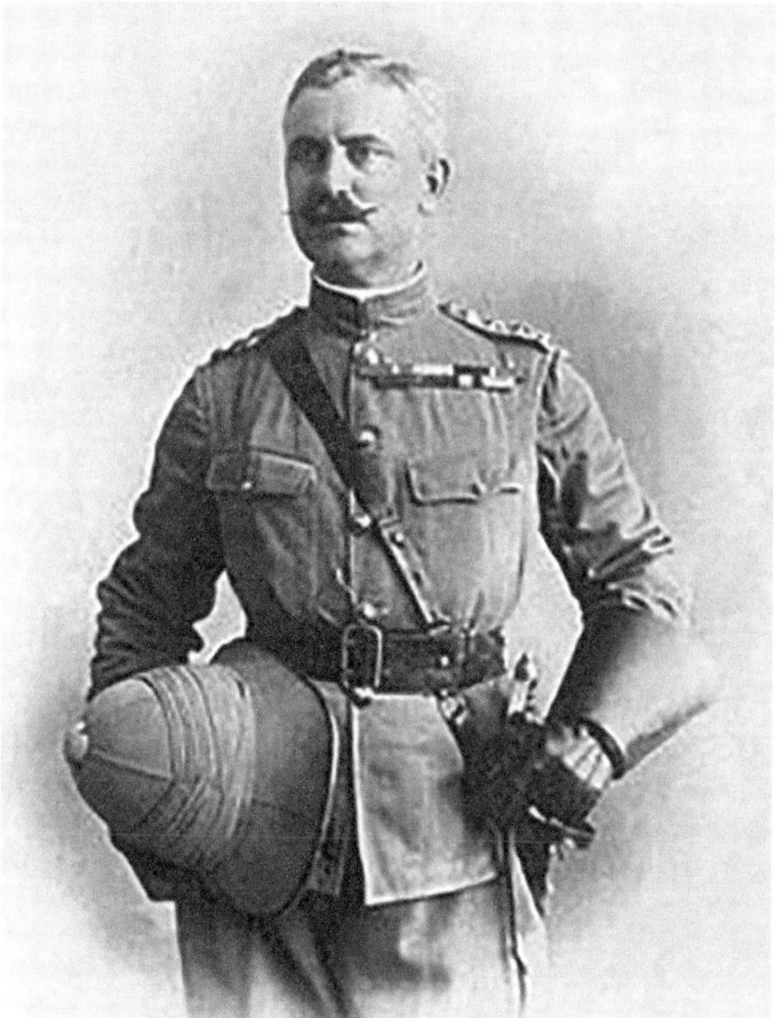

Sir Francis Reginald Wingate
(Courtesy of Wikipedia)

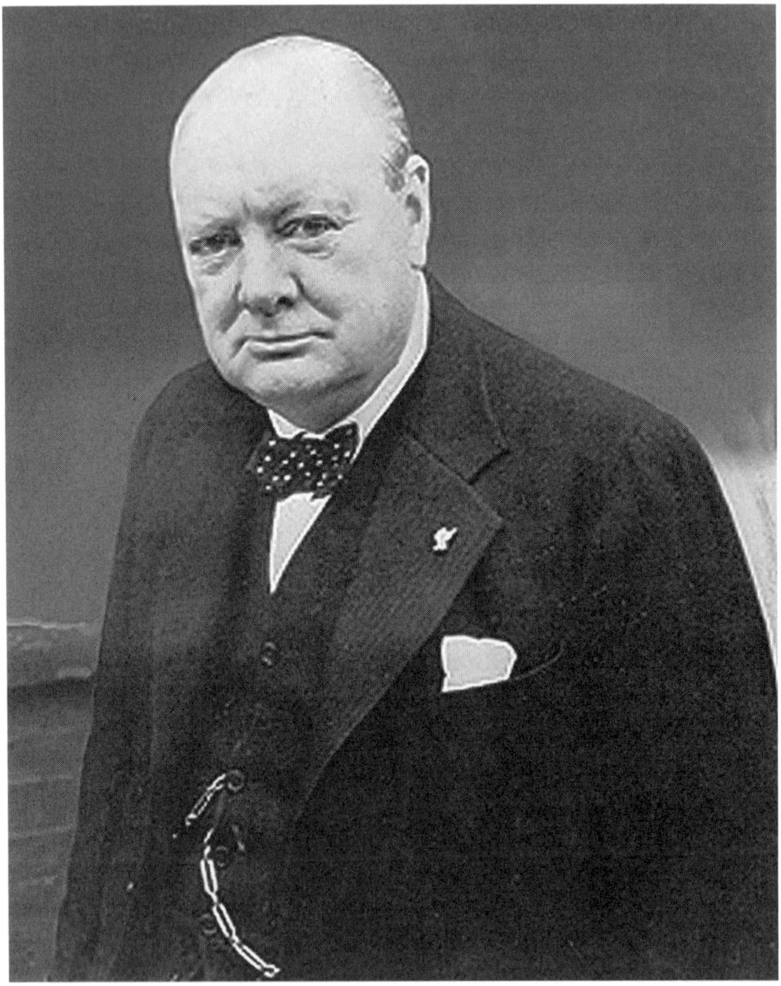

Winston Churchill
(Courtesy of Wikipedia)

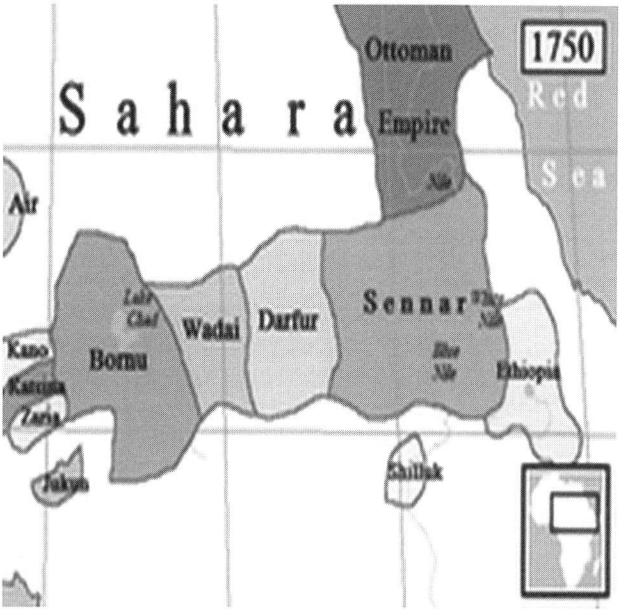

Map of the central African Kingdoms
(Courtesy of Wikipedia)

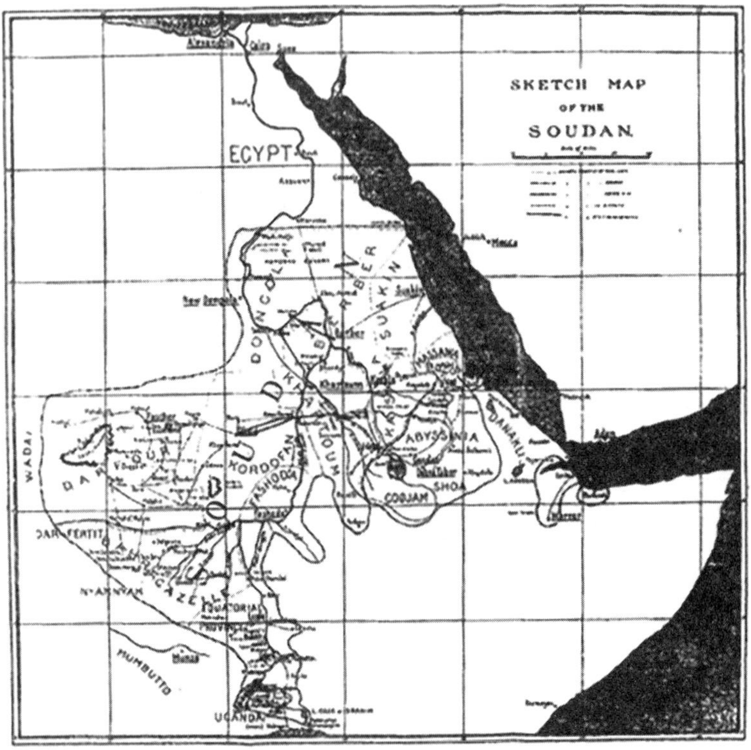

Map of Turco-Egyptian Sudan
(Courtesy of Wikipedia)

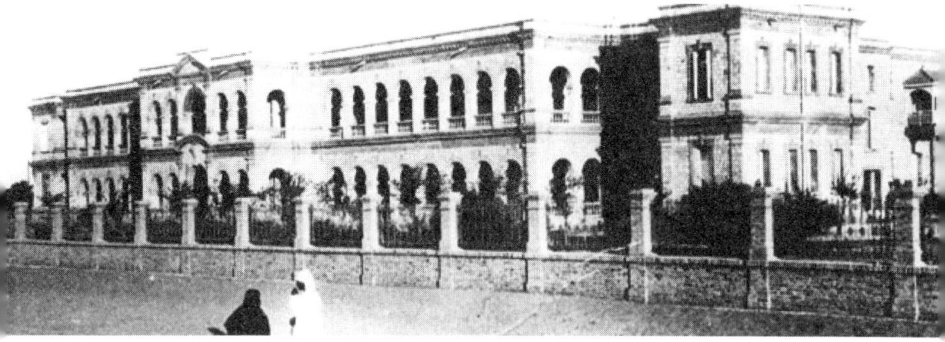

PART 2

MEDICINE IN THE SUDAN, 1504-1898

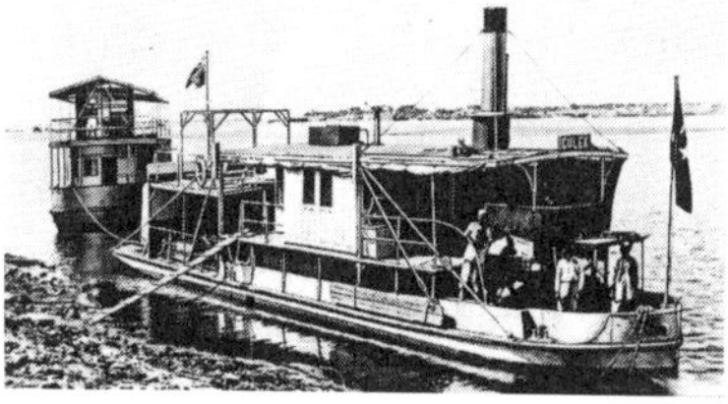

Chapter I

Early British & European Medical Encounters during the Fung Kingdom of Sennar & the Pre-Turco-Egyptian Sudan

Section I:

The Earliest European Medical Encounters in the Sudan during the Fung Sultanate: Dr. Charles Jacques Poncet & Fr. Theodoro Krump

Since medieval times, several European explorers or travellers had assumed the role of physician while travelling through the North and East African hinterlands. The major reasons were to gain an easy pass, to secure help, and to impress. During the era of the Fung Kingdom of Sennar (1503-1821), and following the travels and writings of David Ha-Rubeini, a controversial figure and possibly a Jew of Yemenite descent (1), the first documented encounter of the Sudanese people with Europeans was with the French physician Charles Jacques Poncet. Poncet passed through the Sudan in 1698-1699 on his way to Gondar as an envoy of the French monarch, Louis XIV, to the Abyssinia monarch, Iyasu I, 'The Great' (2). Poncet, who was a physician by training and an apothecary by practice, had gained a reputation in Egypt amongst the Turkish elite and the European residents since his arrival in Cairo in 1691. In his journey to Gondar, he was accompanied by Father Charles Francis Xavier de Brevedent, a Jesuit priest, and by Haji Ali, an Abyssinian Muslim merchant sent by Iyasu to guide his European guests on their journey. The group left Cairo in November of 1698 and travelled towards Nubia down the bank of the Nile. Their journey coincided with a plague that hit Egypt and reached the upper fringes of Nubia in the late seventeenth century. Poncet wrote about its devastating effect, as it wiped out the entire population of many villages. This was probably the only recorded time that a plague reached and affected the Sudan. Poncet and his companions then passed through 'Hafir Maschu', an important caravan outpost on the eastern bank of the Nile. Here they were hosted by the 'Nubian Prince of Argo', whom Poncet 'treated from an ailment'. This was probably the first European medical encounter in the Sudan. The group then passed through Dongola where they were hosted by its King, eventually reaching Sennar in February 1699. At Sennar, they spent three months as guests of the Fung monarch before leaving for Gondar. Poncet's subsequent writings about the city, its inhabitants (which he estimated were a hundred thousand souls), the royal family, their entourage, and the trade in Sennar, is probably the first European first-hand account of the Fung Kingdom of Sennar. Intriguingly, Poncet did not mention in his book anything about the art of medicine and medical practice in the Sudan or Sennar, despite the relatively long spell he spent there. The only remark in this respect was his earlier treatment of the vassal of King of Dongola, the Prince of Argo (which was only mentioned in passing). One interesting incident was when a six-month-old girl (whom Poncet referred to as a 'Turkish' girl; probably the child was very light in colour) was presented for treatment. The child was dying, and Poncet could do little to help her.

Following this successful venture, the French monarch Louis XIV sent a diplomatic mission to the Abyssinian Emperor with several Jesuit missionaries in 1700. This mission included Theodoro Krump, a Bavarian Catholic missionary, whose subsequent writings, titled *Palm-Baum,* represented a rich treatise on life in Sudan on the eve of the seventeenth century and contains the earliest evidence of medical practice in what Krump referred to as the 'Kingdoms of Dongola and Sennar' during the zenith of the Fung Sultanate (3). According to Jay Spaulding (2008), the writings of Theodoro Krump:

> ...in many ways represents the most important single written source concerning the pre-colonial history of the Sudan as it has provided an invaluable testimony about the structure functioning of the Funj government before the fall of the Unsab dynasty.... and contributes data of unparallel quality on the organization and conduct of the trans-Saharan caravan trade, the commerce in slaves, Sudanese medical practices, Sudanese relations with Ethiopia and a wide array of often unexpected vignettes of daily life.' (4)

We also know from Krump's accounts that, prior to his arrival in Sennar in May 1701, there was already a group of Jesuit missionaries who possibly arrived shortly after the trip of Charles Poncet. Amongst them was Father Pasquale da Montella, whom Krump referred to as the 'Private Physician' of the Fung Sultan (5). It is not clear whether Krump had had any formal medical training or whether his 'expertise' in medical practice in the Sudan was that of an amateur. However, several of the names he used for various remedies and medicine he administered to various people whom he treated were medical names in Latin (6). So, it is highly likely that he had some sort of medical knowledge and, in his own statement, he was selected to replace Father Pasquale da Montella, when the Abyssinian Emperor requested the Fung Sultan to send him to be his private physician (7). Krump, explained why he was chosen to be the new King's physician, as the Fung Sultan agreed to let Pasquale go, on the condition that the Jesuit would find him a replacement. Krump stated that:

> Father Prefect was therefore compelled to assign one of us to Father Pasquale place in Sinnar.... The Father Prefect came to me, explained his motives, and asked me to stay here, since I had practiced medicine for two years at the Sanctus Spiritus [Hospital] in Rome as well as supplied with medication. (8)

Whether his skills were acquired through apprenticeship (in preparation for his missionary journeys), or whether he had them through specific training, one cannot be certain. It appears that it was a common practice in those days to prepare travellers or those involved in specific discovery missions to gain some medical knowledge of common diseases, especially those encountered in the tropics (*vide infra*). The writings of Krump about the medicines he used, the cases he treated, and the illnesses he described implies that he had a good grasp of some form of medical knowledge, at least by the standards of his day.

Both Krump and Pasquale were given the 'revered heyday title' of *'Mu'allim'*, which apparently was the common title used at that time for professionals (in both Egypt and Sudan). Furthermore, both were given Arabic names. Pasquale was called '*Mua'llim Yusuf*', and Krump was named '*Mua'llim Yunus*'. From Krump's work, *Palm-Baum*, translated and summarised by Jay Spaulding, Krump used the practice of 'cupping' and leeching and he mentioned that the same practice was done by Sudanese native doctors. Krump went on to treat the Fung monarch himself from an accidental wound he sustained in his right foot. In his journals, Krump writes: 'The year 1702. On the twelfth of January the king sent me a 'mursal' (messenger) ordering me to come to him to treat a wound which he had carelessly given himself in the right foot with his sabre. Fortunately, I healed him within a few days with the balsam of Innocent XI' (9). Krump would be summoned to treat notables as well as common people. He mentioned that during his stay in Sennar, he was called almost daily to attend the sick. He once cured 'Sheikh Idris', son of the viceroy, from jaundice, and managed a major wound of 'an Arab' injured by a horse 'by applying a mixture of butter, and finely ground snuff tobacco and honey' (10). He was summoned one day to treat syphilis in the son of the Qadi of Sinnar and an Arab sheikh. He went on to state that syphilis was very common in Sinnar, where the natives called it 'the French disease' (11). He would even use their technique of cauterization, as he used it to treat a fellow priest when they were travelling back to Egypt in 1702.

A few months after he resumed his new role in Sinnar, Krump was requested by the King to go to Qarri to treat its Sheikh, the

Abdallabi king and vassal of the Fung Sultan, from an illness. One could guess, from Krump's description, that the illness was a possible urosepis and prostatic disease, which he said he treated with the 'panacea pill' (12). He had to treat the Abdallabi king once again from what he described as possible seizure or toxic confusional state. In this later episode, he used the method of bleeding his vassal host (13). Krump spent the time from July 1701 till December the same year at Qarri. He described how, when he first arrived at Qarri, he was received with excitement by the natives, and during the period he spent there he treated many with various illnesses and gained credit and respect. However, it appears that he was kept at Qarri for a long time against his will and certainly he was not pleased about it (14).

Krump, following his return to Rome, retired back to his native land of Bavaria in Germany. His journals were published in 1710. In 1705, the French monarch decided to send a second mission to the Abyssinian Emperor. That included another group of Jesuit missionaries. The mission, led by Le Noir du Roule, had the Paris graduate, the Zantiote Greek physician Agostino Lippi, among its members, which consisted of several Jesuit priests. Dr. Lippi (1678-1705) was sent as a private physician to the Abyssinian Emperor, Iyasu I. The mission was to travel through Sennar, but, for reasons that are unclear, the group was plundered, and its leader was murdered (15). According to Wallis Budge, there appeared to be a form of dispute and rivalry between various Christian sects in Egypt, which may have played a role in this tragedy that befell the diplomatic and religious mission of de Roule (16). It was also likely that the incident occurred during the clash between Badi, Al-Ahmar 'The Red', and his adversaries at a time when there was significant turmoil in Sennar. One can only speculate.

Several decades later, in 1772, the first Briton who is known to have travelled into the Sudan was the Scottish Laird, James Bruce, of Kinnaird. Bruce assumed the title of '*Hakim Yagoub*' (Ar. *Hukim* = physician; *Yagoub* = Jacob) during his travels in Africa. This will be the theme of the next section.

Section II: 'El Hakim Yagoube': James Bruce, the Explorer Turned Physician

> In disgust he left London for his Scottish estate, to marry, to litigate, and finally, in his widower-hood, to pour out the long, confused, brilliant book of his travels which was read throughout Europe and revived the stream of criticism and satire again which was to flow till long after he was dead.
>
> –J. M. Reid, *Traveller Extraordinary: The Life of James Bruce of Kinnaird*

To our knowledge, James Bruce was the first British explorer to travel into the Sudanese hinterlands. This man had an interesting story. Of a noble background, belonging to a notable line of Scottish Lairds (Lords), James Bruce was born in 1733 and was brought up on the family estate of Kinnaird which belonged to his family. His father was a senior judge in the court of Scotland, and although he was eager for his young son to follow in his footsteps and be a judge in Scotland, James had other ideas. Since his teenage years he was keen on adventure and travel and become fascinated by the thought of discovering the source of the Nile. He lost his mother at an early age, so was sent to London where he was looked after by a relative. Bruce was educated at Harrow (as was a much later British visitor to Sudan, Winston Churchill), and showed talents in languages, becoming the school Latin orator at age 12 (17). Bruce's fascination with travel became more pressing after he lost his first wife, and he decided to set off to satisfy his dream of discovering the source of the Nile. He taught himself Portuguese, Spanish, and the principles of astronomy. He also befriended the French monarch, Louis XVI, and learnt some aspects of draftsmanship in Italy. Being kin to the English and Scottish monarch, King George III (r. 1760-1820), he succeeded in being appointed as the British Consul in Algeria early in 1763. There he learned the Arabic language as well as some principles of medicine from Dr. Bell, a British military doctor who was attached to the naval ships that patrolled the Mediterranean from Algiers. In summer of 1765, Bruce resigned his post as consul and headed east along the North African coast, travelling through Tunisia and Libya, where he boarded a ship heading towards Crete. The ship was wrecked, and after rescue he travelled in Asia Minor, learning Greek at Constantinople, and then left for Syria. At Aleppo, he was treated by a British physician, Dr. Patrick Russell, a specialist in tropical illnesses. From Dr. Russell, Bruce learned more principles of medicine and medical treatment (18). Here, the British Ambassador to the Ottomans obtained a *firman* (safe passage document) from the Sultan of Turkey that would be helpful to Bruce in his future endeavours.

In summer of 1768, Bruce landed at Alexandria under the title *'El Hakim Yagoub'*, accompanied by his Italian assistant, the painter Luigi Ballugiani. The French monarch had earlier supplied him with astrology and astronomy tools to aid him in his future travels. In Egypt, Bruce approached the Mamluk Governor, Ali Bey Abu Al-Dahab, and befriended him, offering his services as a physician. Following a short spell at Cairo, and with Ali Bey's help, he crossed the Red Sea after he travelled up the Nile to Assiut. He then travelled down the eastern coast of Arabia, boarded a British battleship from Jeddah, and went to Yemen. From there he crossed the narrow strait of the Red Sea to Mussawaa, the main port of Abyssinia, arriving there in late 1769. Following various risky journeys through the Tegrai land, Bruce eventually reached Gondar, where he was taken in as the emperor's private physician. In those days, Abyssinia was witnessing a turmoil of inter-tribal wars and several conspiracies to depose the emperor. Bruce, during the time he spent in the Abyssinian Royal Court, had the opportunity to describe this important chapter in the history of Abyssinia in his journals (19). At Gondar, the capital, Bruce thrived for several years, escaping many dangers and conspiracies and making many friends and foes. He gained trust and love after his success in treating several members of the Royal family using his "magic" purgative, *'brucea anti-dysentrica'*. Amid all this, Bruce managed to satisfy, as he believed, the main purpose of his adventure and his life's dream and ambition of locating the source of Nile. Coming in sight of Lake Tana, from which the Blue Nile flows, Bruce writes:

> I remembered that magnificent scene in my own native country, where the Tweed, Clyde and Annan rise in one hill; three rivers, as I now thought, not inferior to the Nile in beauty, preferable to it in cultivation of those countries through which they flow; superior, vastly superior to it in the virtues and qualities of the inhabitants, and in the beauty of flocks crowding the pastures in peace, without fear of violence from man or beast.... (20)

Early in 1772, Bruce travelled into the Sudanese hinterland of the Fung Province of Atbara, passing through the frontier district of 'Ras Al Fil' and its main village, 'Hor Cacamoot' (translated by Bruce as the valley of shadow of death, today it is the town of Gallabat). He received some help from its chieftain, Erbab Gimbro, and proceeded to the main town of the province, Teawa[1] and had to deal with the Fung governor of the Fung Atbara Province, Shiekh Fidele. Bruce treated the governor's several wives with his purgative (21). The administration of emetic produced such a good effect, that a further attendance was ordered. Of this occasion, Bruce wrote:

> ...the ladies all disrobed, and standing before me naked, each demanded to be examined. Not content, with this they then demanded that I, likewise should disrobe!! I have been to more than one battle, but surely would have taken my chances again in any of them to have been freed from that examination. (22)

Bruce escaped death in 'Teawa', when 'Sheikh Fedail' exercised all avenues of extracting 'whatever treasures Bruce may have had'. However, he eventually succeeded in reaching Sennar after travelling via Beyla (present-day Jebel Beyla), where he treated its Sheikh 'with his purgatives'. The Sheikh, so grateful, helped Bruce to reach Sennar safely.

At Sennar, Bruce wrote what is most likely the first writing of a British man about the Fung Kingdom of Sennar. He narrated his various encounters with the Fung's King and his entourage, he befriended the 'Vice-Vizier' Adlan, brother of the powerful Vizier, Abu Le Kaylak, who was away at the time, involved in a long war at Kordofan to conquer it for the Fung Sultanate. Following several months at Sennar, Bruce travelled north along the banks of the Nile, where he met 'Wed Agib' whom he described as the Arab chief responsible to Sennar for the northern sheikhs and kinglets. He then reached Shendi, where he spent a few days as a guest of Wed Agib's*[2] sister, 'Lady Sittana', who help the Scotsman prepare for the long journey via Berber to Aswan, crossing the desert at Abu Hamad, which he described as a journey full of 'sand and simoum*[3]'.Bruce's writings about 'King Ismain' and the people of the Fung and their origins was used as reference in the subsequent attempts to document the history of the last Sudanese Kingdom before the Turco-Egyptian conquest (23).

Despite the fact that James Bruce was not a doctor, it is an irony that he 'rode' over the glory of 'their status', claiming to be one, and making use of the simple knowledge he gained from the two British doctors he befriended. Medicine and its practice in Bruce's day were still in their infancy. However, Bruce, with an impressive wit and with an observant eye, made very useful descriptions of various diseases and ailments he observed during his stay in the Sudan. Bruce described the symptoms and incidence of guinea worm infection, the 'Medina worm' (*Dracunculus mediensis*), with which he himself became infected (24). He noted that the disease is called 'Farenteit' by the locals and was prevalent where people drank from stagnant water. He asserted that 'this extraordinary animal only afflicts those who are in constant habit of drinking stagnant water, whether that water is drawn out of the wells, as in the Kingdoms of Sennar, or found by digging in the sand where it is making its way to its proper level the seam, after falling down the side of the mountains' (25). A similar observation was given by his fellow Briton, William George Browne (*vide infra*), who gave a detailed description of this ailment and the contemporary native methods of extracting it by winding it around a piece of cloth or bird feather, commenting that once he saw a 'length of five feet or more of this extraordinary animal, winded out with invincible patience in the course of three weeks' (26).

Stemming from his rudimentary knowledge of medicine gained in his apprenticeship with two British physicians in Algiers and Aleppo, Bruce made detailed descriptions of common diseases he observed in the few places he had been to, including lower Arabia,

Abyssinia, and Sennar. He described a form of fever known by the natives as '*nedad*', which, he stated, prevails in the Red Sea coastal areas and also in Sennar (27). It is possible that this could well be either benign tertian malaria or Dengue fever. Interestingly, Bruce stated that elephantiasis was common in the hinterlands he been to in Africa, and he wrote an excellent description of its morbid anatomy and commented that it is not a contagious condition as 'the wives of those who were in a very inveterate stage of this illness… had borne them several children who were yet perfectly free and sound from any contagion' (28). Bruce also made records of dysentery, the bloody flux, and fevers at Sennar, which were probably malaria and other viral illnesses. He also mentioned hepatomegaly, venereal diseases, and smallpox epidemics. He described the native method of vaccination against smallpox, which the natives called 'buying the pox'. Here a rag would be wrapped around the arm of an infected person, and the person wanting to be 'vaccinated' would be standing by. Usually the old women of the tribe were the ones who carried out the procedure. A price had to be placed on the 'rag' and, after haggling and bargaining on the price, when it was agreed to, the rag would be taken away by the person wanting to be vaccinated. The rag would be tied on the arm and when the recipient contracted the disease he would only have the number of pocks he paid for! (29). Bruce went on to give advice about health issues to potential European travellers and, interestingly enough, he gave strong advice against consuming local liquors, which he commented should be regarded as poisonous (30). Bruce was one of the first to have gathered a collection of tropical plants, an entity which at the time was not known in the West. Ironically, he used some of these plants as medicines and purgatives during his travels into the Fung Kingdom of Sennar. These plants later came to be known as *'brucea dysenterica'*. Many of the plants he collected during his trips in Abyssinia featured in his journals (31).

Following his successful return to Egypt, Bruce eventually went back to London, where life did not treat him well. His stories were disputed, he was cast as a liar, and he went into dispute with powerful figures in London at the time. Men like Samuel Johnson and James Boswell were his adversaries. It was not until 1790 that, urged by his friend Daines Barrington, he published his treatise of what are considered to be extraordinary. His travels would very much stimulate later explorers to follow in his footsteps and verify his stories. After the substantial accuracy of his travels were thereafter demonstrated, his quest to discover the source of the Nile captured the imagination of other British explorers in the second half of the nineteenth century, inspiring them to eventually succeed in fulfilling the same dream. The substantial accuracy of his Ethiopian and Sudanese travelogue has since been demonstrated, and it is now considered a real addition to the geographical knowledge of his day.

Section III:

The Prelude to the Turco-Egyptian Period: Browne & Burckhardt—William George Browne's Medical Encounters in Darfur

> If any medical professor should chance to advert to them, the writer is too conscious of the superficiality of his own knowledge not to perceive that little satisfaction will be derived. But persuaded that the art of healing, even at this day, abounds little less in experimental than in the age of one of its brightest ornaments, who makes the confession, he is induced to believe, scarcely any fact relative to it, or any experiment, faithfully narrated, can be wholly destitute of its use.
>
> –W. G. Browne, *Travels in Africa, Egypt & Syria from the Year 1792-1798*

The English explorer, William George Browne, who was born in London, became fascinated by travels into the interior of Africa after he read Bruce's journals. Following his studies at Oxford, Browne used the fortune left to him by his father to finance his trip to the Middle East and Africa. In his travels in Syria, Egypt, and Africa, Browne described vividly some diseases he had seen or opted to 'treat' (32). Like many other European travellers in his day, he billed himself as a 'Frankish physician'. Browne travelled from Egypt into the Sudan, aiming primarily to follow the route of James Bruce into Nubia, then into Abyssinia via Sennar. However, due to some local troubles in the region of Dongola, he changed his plans and went to Darfur as '*Daif-es-Sultan*'[4] ('Guest of the Sultan') (33). Browne arrived at Kobbe, the caravan market town in Darfur, and reached el-Fasher in summer of 1793. He remained in Darfur till 1796 and then he returned to Egypt. In his book, *Travels in Syria, Africa and Egypt* (1799), Browne devoted a full chapter to his medical observations. He began this chapter by asserting: 'from the following detailed remarks, the result chiefly of personal observations, if the physiologist can derive any amusement, or the traveller the smallest investigation of the his personal suffering, the purpose of committing them to paper is answered' (34). Browne described a broad range of diseases and medical conditions, from spring catarrh (known at the time as the Egyptian ophthalmia), to smallpox, plague, leprosy, Guinea worm, syphilis, and scurvy, to name but a few. In this section we shall confine ourselves to those he had described from his time in Darfur.

Browne wrote extensively about spring catarrh from his own observations as well as those of the contemporary concepts about its causes and treatment. He stated that he had not witnessed this common cause of 'defective vision' in Darfur. It is noteworthy that his observations were very accurate and typical of those made by British doctors who worked over a hundred years later in Sudan, who reported that the 'Egyptian Ophthalmia', tends to be less seen the more southward from Egypt deeper into the Sudanese territories' (See Part III, Chapter 2). Browne also stated confidently that plague, a dreadful scourge especially in the Mediterranean and the Levant, has not been witnessed in the Sudan. With the exception of a few cases amongst the returning pilgrims from Mecca early in the twentieth century, the Sudan remained free through the centuries from the menace of plague which has devastated other countries in the Middle East. In contrast, Browne described smallpox as 'a disease much dreaded by the people of the Soudan, whether Moors or Negros' (35). Interestingly, he noted that the fatality rate among the 'Negros' tended to be much higher. Browne attempted to inoculate five slaves, all under twelve years of age, from the Fertit tribe in the southwestern part of the Sudan, as desired by their master. He gave them a strong dose of senna prior to the procedure. He stated" 'Three of them had not in the whole forty pustules, and soon recovered. The other two suffered much, and the eruption, though not confluent, prove fatal to one of them' (36). Browne also mentioned that Guinea worm (Medina worm) was called by 'the Mohammedans of Fur and the Arabs' '*Fertit*', probably because it was common in those days amongst the slaves who belonged to that African tribe. Interestingly, the disease is still called by the same name amongst the Sudanese to the present day. Browne gave an elaborate description of this ailment and of how it was treated by the natives. Interestingly, he made the excellent observation that 'the disease seems to originate in the water, which is replete by animalcules, and which no care is used to purify!!' (37). Later in the ninetieth century the disease life cycle was described by the Bulgarian Physician Hristo Stambloski, in Yemen (1877-1878), which proved that Browne's observation was correct as Cyclops: a water parasite is the vector in disease transmission (38).

Browne went on in his interesting medical accounts to describe several other medical conditions as he saw them amongst the people of Darfur, including scurvy. He referred to syphilis, which he commented was less formidable in Darfur than in Egypt. By contrast, he observed that leprosy was not uncommon in Darfur and was once intrigued to witness a case of early leprosy cured under his observation by a 'salve, native of a Kingdom called Baghermi, but the means he had used he could not be prevailed on to disclose' (39). Interestingly, he stated that 'complaints proceeding from too copious secretion of bile are extremely common both in Egypt and Darfur'. He was referring to jaundice, which he quoted using the word used by the Darfur dwellers as '*Saffafir*', which is a corrupted version of the same name used by the natives of Sudan to the present day, refereeing to jaundice collectively as '*Suffair*'[5], meaning 'yellow discolouration of the eyes and body' (40). He went on to elaborate on the ways people treat such a syndrome in Darfur by using senna leaves as a purgative, and also prescribing his own use of 'James' powder'[6] (41). Browne also described cases of 'splenic tumours', by which he probably meant cases of splenomegaly (42). He also described cases of haemorrhoids and fistula-in-ano, mentioning that in Darfur it is treated by cautery in the case of the former and topical application, but without incision, in the latter. He also remarked that abdominal hernia, which he referred to as umbilical hernia cases, were very common in Darfur and that they were treated with cauterization (43). He mentioned the way women delivered their babies, remarking on excess cases of foetal and maternal morbidity in Darfur (44). Those remarks were probably the first ever historical records in English literature about the Sudanese native methods of parturition. Browne also described means of medical treatment, including what he referred to as phlebotomy, as the means of treating several diseases. He stated that ' ""Scarification" (sic), or superficial incision of the skin, is commonly recurred to (sic) for various diseases, and at all ages, from two years till sixty' (45). He also referred to other mode of bleeding by using horns, not dissimilar to leaching by cupping. A similar technique was described during the early years of the Anglo-Egyptian rule amongst the primitive races of south-eastern Sudan by Alexander McTier Pirrie (see Part IV). Contemporary medicines used by the natives to treat various disease conditions were also documented by McTier Pirrie, ranging from *'natrun'* to 'tamarind', to phlebotomy, to the ancient practice of leeching and the use of some substances as aphrodisiacs. This last he remarked were on high demand, unsurprisingly. Finally, Browne made some crude 'anthropological 'remarks on the characteristics of the 'negroes' (sic). He also commented on the practice of male circumcision, commenting that 'among the Furians circumcision appears to be no other than a religious ceremony, performed in compliance with an express command of the author of their faith; and it is very doubtful whether it was ever practiced among them before their conversion to Mohammedism (sic)' (46). He also made extensive accounts on the practice of female circumcision, which he stated is less practiced in Darfur. Finally, he also wrote a short account on the practice of castration of male slaves, in which he stated that those slaves destined for Cairo or Constantinople were castrated in Upper Egypt, where the practice was normally conducted by members of families who seem to have it as a hereditary profession (47).

Browne was forced to stay in Darfur and his requests to travel to Sennar were declined repeatedly by Sultan Abd el-Rahman el-Rasheid, but eventually he was allowed to go back to Egypt, in 1796. Following his return to Britain in 1798, in 1800 Browne made another spree of travels into Asia Minor and Persia, where he travelled to Tibriz, where he was murdered in 1813.

John Lewis (Johann Ludwig) Burckhardt & Travels in Nubia

In the footsteps of his two predecessors, but with a rather different intention—to discover the source of River Niger—the Anglo-Swiss traveller, Johann Ludwig Burckhardt, who is widely known in English literature as John Lewis Burckhardt, was born in Lausanne in 1784. Burckhardt made landmark contributions to our understanding of the Middle East and the Sudan in the build-up to the reign of Muhammad Ali Pasha. Burckhardt was descended from a noble Swiss family from Basel. He was the eighth child of John Rudolph Burckhardt, who suffered greatly during the French Revolution and, fearing ruin and destruction of himself and his family, took his young son to study at Leipzig and later Gottingen in Germany. Young Johann's qualities were attested to by his acquaintances and his learning talent and genius were recognized by his mentors. Life and destiny led both father and son to seek refuge in Britain. In 1806, young Johann arrived in London carrying letters of recommendation from his mentor, Professor Blumenbach of Gottingen University, to Sir Joseph Banks, President of the Royal Society and an active member of the Association for Promoting the Discovery of the Interior Parts of Africa (48). At the time, the association was looking to recruit a talented traveller into the interior parts of West Africa, with the intention of exploring the Bournu Kingdom. Burckhardt learnt Arabic at Cambridge and London also received lectures in chemistry, astronomy, mineralogy, medicine, and surgery in preparation for his travels. Early in 1809 he was sent to Aleppo, where he received further education in the Arabic language, studied and learned the Koran and Islamic theology, and learned the ways and customs of the 'Mohamedans'. Here, Burckhardt became disguised as *Hajji Ibrahim Abdalla Al-Shami*, a Turkish merchant, having extensively practiced the style of such dress and customs whist back in Cambridge and London. During the two years he spent in the Levant, he made some explorations into Palestine, Lebanon, and present-day Jordan. Burckhardt was considered the first European to have witnessed and documented the historical city of Petra (in present-day Jordan). After just over two years in Syria, Burckhardt was instructed by the Society to go to Egypt to join some caravans that normally travelled into the Bournu country through Fezzan in Libya. He reached Cairo in September of 1811, the year when Muhammad Ali Pasha completed his successful campaigns against the Mamluks. During winter of 1812, and having missed the Fezzan caravan, he wrote to the association as follows:

> The delay thus occasioned in my Fezzan expedition, I shall endeavour to make profitable to African geography, in another quarter. I mean to set out next month, by land for Upper Egypt, as soon as the state of the Nile renders the voyage practicable. I shall push on beyond the first cataract and follow the course of the river by the second and third cataract, towards Dongola. That country farther up than Derr, has never been visited by any travellers…; yet I am informed by many of the natives, that the borders of the river are full of ancient temples and other antiquities, resembling those of Luxor, and the Isle of Philae…. were it not for the Mamluks who have settled at Dongola, and taken possession of that country, I might hope to reach that point. (49)

During that time, Muhammad Ali Pasha was strengthening his grip on Egypt and the Mamluks had fled south to Upper Egypt and deep into Nubia. Having befriended Muhammad Ali Pasha, who gave him a *firman* to aid him in his travels to Nubia, Burckhardt set off on his first trip in January of 1813. He took a route down the bank of the Nile with the help of a guide from the Aga of Aswan through Upper Egypt into Wadi Halfa. He then passed the Island of Say, the Sukkot[7], and then into the Mahass[8] homeland, reaching the upper frontiers of Dongola. He returned back to Aswan by March 1813. After a year of waiting for a suitable caravan to join, Burckhardt then executed a second journey that began on March 2, 1814, this time taking a different route, crossing the Nubian Desert from Aswan to Berber. A future conqueror of the Sudan, Lord Kitchener, would use the same route to surprise his Mahdist opponents. At Berber, Burckhardt stayed for two weeks and then travelled further south, where he stayed for a few days at 'Damer', an important town on the eastern bank of the Nile. He finally reached Shendy on April 17, 1814. After spending one month at Shendy, Burckhardt set off again for Suakin, the old medieval port on the Red Sea, taking the route along the Atbara River via 'Goz Radjab[9]' (sic) He passed through the 'Taka' region and finally reached Suakin on June 26, 1814. After crossing the Red Sea to the 'Hijdaz' in Arabia in July of 1814 and staying at 'Dijidda*' (sic) (*Jeddah), Burckhardt performed 'Hajj' in November of 1814. He finally returned to Cairo in June of 1815, after spending some time in 'Medina', the second holiest city in Arabia after Mecca. While in Arabia, Burckhardt suffered a diarrhoeal illness which became chronic and lingered for the next two years and eventually leading to his untimely death in Cairo on October 17, 1817. He was barely 31 years of age.

Burckhardt's journals of his travels in Nubia and other places were published posthumously in 1819 by his employer, 'The Association of Promoting the Discovery of the Interior of Africa'. Burckhardt's ingenious writings became a major source for the geography and history of the Nubian Sudan in the prelude to the Turco-Egyptian invasion of 1821. In his treatise, he wrote extensively on the people's habits, the climate, and trade and commerce as he saw them in Berber and Shendy. He gave some accounts of the oral history of various inhabitants of the Sudan. Burckhardt witnessed an important era in Egypt and Sudan, rich in historical events. It was soon after that Mohammed Ali Pasha ascended to power and the time of his great imperial conquests in Arabia and his bloody conflicts with his rivals, the Mamluks. Burckhardt very much followed in some of the travel footsteps of James Bruce in the Nubian Desert. He also befriended and was guided by another Briton, George William Browne, whom he met in England prior to setting off on his travels. What is relevant here is that Burckhardt had made ingenious observations on various medical conditions during his travels in the Sudan. This, when taken together with the writings of Bruce and Browne, form the backbone of what we know about medicine and diseases in Sudan in the eighteenth and nineteenth centuries.

Burckhardt, like his predecessors Bruce and Browne, portrayed himself as having some medical knowledge, claiming the status of a physician. He took that in addition to his 'persona' of Hajji Abdalla Ibrahim Al-Shami. He was disguised as Hajji Al-Shami from the time that he was in Aleppo, Syria, in 1809-1812. 'I got myself introduced to one of their chiefs as a physician in search of medicinal herbs…' (50). Burckhardt kept full records about various medical problems he saw or heard of during his travels. Whilst he was in Egypt, and in the wake of the massacre of Shahin Pasha and 120 of the Mamluks in Cairo Castle in 1812 and their flight south, a famine broke out in Upper Egypt and Nubia followed by a smallpox epidemic. According to Burckhardt, half of the population of Nubia perished in its aftermath. While in Berber, Burckhardt made interesting remarks on the health of Berber inhabitants:

> The people of Berber appear to be a healthy race. There seemed to be few invalids, and the place being situated on the skirts of the desert, the air is certainly wholesome. I was told of fever called wardé, from woid (rose) which seems to be epidemic, and often proves mortal; the people of Dóngola are very subject to it; it exists during the time of high water, but it does not make its appearance every year. (51)

Likely Burckhardt here was referring to 'malaria' as per the typical description. He went on to remark that 'plague was unknown, and from what I heard during my former journey in Nubia, I have reason to believe that it never passes the cataract of Assouan. (52) On the smallpox epidemics of 1813 and 1815, when he was back in Cairo he wrote:

Smallpox is very destructive whenever it gains ground. Last year it was added to famine, and death was very numerous. It had been brought to Berber by the people of Taka, who had received it from the Souakin traders; it spread over all the country up the Nile….Grown people were attacked as well as children; it was observed, even that the latter suffered less and that most of them escaped. About one thirds of those who were attacked recovered, but they bore the mark on their skin, especially on the arms and face, which were covered with innumerable spots and scars; very few instances happen where the disease is of mild kind, or where it leaves but few marks. (53)

Such intelligent observations by Burckhardt provide invaluable epidemiological accounts of smallpox in the Sudanese people on the eve of the Turco-Egyptian period. It gives: insight to how the population was affected to various degrees according to their age. He described the periodic outbreaks of epidemics every eight to ten years, he also described the method of inoculation that was practiced in the Nile Valley was called *'dak-el-Jedri'*[10] (54), and the medicine used by the natives to attempt to cure those infected, by stating 'the only cure for the smallpox was to rub the whole body with butter three or four times a day and to keep themselves closely shut up…' (55). Burckhardt also mentioned the smallpox outbreak that occurred in 1815 and he stated that the epidemic took the lives of fifty-two persons of the 'Temsah' family of the Meyrafabs[11], amongst whom was Mekk Idries, his host while in Berber. He also recorded that the nearby town of 'Damer' suffered less during the smallpox epidemic than Berber, and that 'in "Shendy Slave Market", the slave who bears the smallpox marks would bring more money than the one who doesn't' (56).

Burckhardt's observant eye helped him to record other diseases as he saw them. He mentioned that he saw few cases of ophthalmia, and that he did not observed the disfiguring facies of 'tertiary syphilis', as he had encountered them commonly in Egypt, prompting him to state that venereal diseases were not common at Berber (57). He also remarked that, as the methods of irrigation in Nubia were not as efficient as in Egypt, the variability of the Nile flood may result in periods of famine now and then. He stated that there was a famine in the year prior to his second visit to Nubia, early in 1814 (58). He stated that, amongst the slaves, the practice of castration was carried out on some of them, especially those destined for 'export' to Turkey and Arabia as 'guardians of female virtue'!! 'Two years ago, Mohamed Aly Pasha caused two hundred young Darfur slaves to be mutilated, whom he sent as a present to the Grand Signior' (59). Burckhardt witnessed these operations during his stay in Upper Egypt, whiltst waiting for his second expedition in Nubia, which he stated that 'it is carried by two Coptic monks (who excelled their predecessors in dexterity) in Siout[12], and that only the slaves brought from the Borgho, to the west of Darfur were mutilated prior to them been sold and sent elsewhere'. He went on to describe those mutilated slaves in what can be regarded as a typical medical textbook description of hypogonadal males (60). Interestingly enough, Burckhardt also wrote extensively in his journals about the practice of Pharonic circumcision[13] (Synonym: Female Genital Mutilation), in what could be also regarded as important testimony to the history of this dreadful practice in the early nineteenth century. He remarked on the arrival of some…

…Slave girls to Shendy who were called mukhayet (consutae) from an operation which has been described by Mr Browne. I am unable to state whether it is performed by their parents in their native country, or by the merchants, but I have reason to believe by the later. Girls in this state are worth more than others; they are usually given to the favourite mistress or slave of the purchaser and are often suffered to remain in this state during the whole of their life'.

He wrote further *that:*

> …the daughters of the Arabs, Ababde and Djaafere, who are of Arabian origin, and inhabit the western bank of the Nile from Thebes, and generally those of all the people to the south of Kenne as far as Sennar, undergo circumcision, or rather excision (*excisionclitoridis), at the age of from three to six years. Girls thus treated, are also called Mukhayaet'. (61)

Burckhardt mentioned that piles was very common amongst the 'country people' and less so amongst the 'slaves'. He stated that he first saw genuine Guinea worm in Shendy and remarked that it was very common 'in Soudan', where people call it '*the fertit*' (The name may have originated from Fertit, which was the name used for the south-western frontiers of Darfur). Interestingly enough, he remarked that 'the worm does not attach itself exclusively to the leg; I have seen it issuing from the arm, the breast, and the knees, though its favourite place seems to be the calf of the leg' (62). He made some epidemiological remarks, saying that it is rarer in people from Shendy than in those from Kordofan. He also described the few cases of 'ophthalmia' he saw, stating that venereal disease was commonly seen, and he made the interesting observation that its consequences tended to be less fatal than in Egypt, and that he himself never saw any of the those 'with ulcerated faces' (likely referring to the facial mutilation in the aftermath of tertiary syphilis) which he had seen frequently in Egypt. During his one-month stay at Shendy (63), the most important trading post in Central Sudan, Burckhardt wrote about various medicines used by the native medical practitioners, stating that 'grocers and druggists are the most frequented of any' and those sell various herbs and native medicine imported from either India, Egypt, or other parts of the Sudan like Sennar, Kordofan and Darfur' (64). Those items included substances like Fenugreek (called Helba), of which Burckhardt commented that local people of Shendy and elsewhere used it as tonic. antimony (local name: *Kohol*), *gerfa* (cinnamon shrub, which he remarked that it is used as a stringent to treat fever and dysentery), Sembil, Mehalab, and a fruit called '*tamr el-Berr*', imported from Kordofan, which is used to treat flatulence, on which Burckhardt commented that 'it is believed here to be a remedy for flatulencey (sic), of which many people here complain' (65).

The diarrhoeal illness that Burckhardt developed while in Medina in 1815 became chronic and eventually led to his demise in October of 1817. Is not clear whether it was a form of parasitic dysentery, tuberculous enteritis, or some form of inflammatory bowel disease. One can only speculate.

Endnotes

1 today, the market town of Gedaref. Teawa in Bruce's writings probably refers to the small hill outside Gedaref spelled by the native as Towawa

2 Wed Agieb or Wad Ageeb ('Wed Agib') was probably Agieb Almanjuluk, or one of his descendants, the Abdallabi king at Halfaya.

3 *Simoum*: an Arabic word meaning intense heat waves typical of Sudanese summer.

4 *Daif* (adj): Arabic for guest.

5 *Suffair* (slang) is a very common word used by most Sudanese people to refer to the illness stemming from liver derangement.

6 Probably referring to *brucea dysenterica,* the emetic substance used by James Bruce.

7 Sukkot: a subgroup of the northern Sudanese Nubian tribes.

8 Mahass is a major subgroup of the northern Sudanese Nubian tribe. They became highly dispersed in the modern Sudanese central regions. To this group belongs many of famous religious scholars and holy men of modern Sudanese history.

9 Goz Rajab is a famous Sudanese market town on the Atbara River in the eastern province of Sudan

10 The inoculation of smallpox.

11 Meyrafab; a subfaction of the Jaalyyien tribe, who mainly reside in Berber region.

12 Siout was the word used by Burckhardt to refer to the southern Egyptian town of Assiout.

13 Synonym: female genital mutilation. It commonly used by Sudanese people to refer to that extreme version of female circumcision.

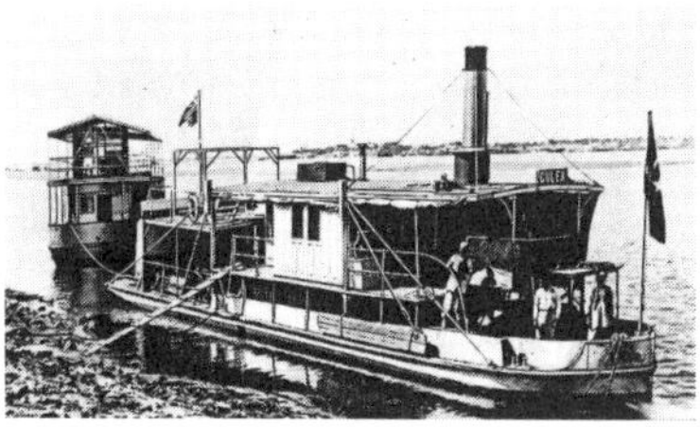

Chapter 2
Medicine & European Medical Encounters during the Era of the Turco-Egyptian Sudan (1820-1884)

Muhammad Ali Pasha and Antoine Clot Bey[I]: Early Milestones of Modern Medicine in Egypt

Following the conquest of the various Sudanese Kinglets and Kingdoms and the establishment of what came to be known as the Turco-Egyptian Sudan in 1821, the government of the newly conquered territories began setting the foundation of the new state. This took time, as the first few years were full of turmoil following the assassination of Ismail Pasha and his entourage by Mek Nimer[2], the Ja'aliyyien Sheik (66, 67). From the scanty sources that could be traced, the kind of public services created were more or less rudimentary. Further, it was provided within a very narrow sphere. The new order was mainly concerned with exploitation of resources to fuel its expanding order in Egypt, and to meet the imperial aspiration of the new master, Muhammad Ali. The quest to secure slave soldiers, treasures from the gold mines of 'Fazougli'[3], and iron ores in Kordofan seemed to be the main objectives of the Egyptian Viceroy.

So, the evidence was compelling against any form of planning for public services that was not on the agenda of the new masters. However, whatever came up later as a form of public services took several decades to take shape and remained substantially backward compared with what was set up in Egypt. We have not yet come across many documents highlighting the shape and scope of the health services during this era, which lasted just over sixty years. What is known from the available records is that Muhammad Ali and his successors put some plans in place for a state structure that, more or less, has given rise to the modern Sudan which came out into the international scene following the conquest by Lord Kitchener and his troops in the dying years of the nineteenth century. Much more research is needed to unravel the scale and scope of public services during the era of the Turco-Egyptian rule in the Sudan.

The sources that give us at least some picture of the health services during that era were primarily obtained from the records and writings of several European travellers and officials in the Sudan. Muhammad Ali was preoccupied with recruiting European professionals from across a range of various disciplines. The Egyptian Viceroy, an admirer of Napoleon Bonaparte, who was allegedly his role model, set off in recruiting mainly French technocrats to establish his new modern Egyptian state. He also utilized the expertise of several European military 'freelance' cadres to fill in the rank and file of the armies he dispatched to build up his own empire and to muscle the Porte. The French were predominant among those European professionals who were recruited to fuel *'el-Nizam el-Jadeed*[4]*'*. Indeed, the credit of establishing the modern health services in Egypt goes to the Frenchman Antoine-Barthleme Clot 'Bey'. Clot was born in Grenoble in 1793, studied medicine at Montpellier, and then started his career as a physician in Marseilles. While he was a 'nobody' in France, Clot ascended to fame and fortune in Egypt. Clot, who was recruited initially to help organise the military corps of Muhammad Ali, was shortly taken as a private physician to the Pasha, together with an Italian physician, Dr. Gaetani. The Frenchman soon became his favourite; the Pasha could see his ingenious potential, and he would exploit this to the maximum. During the late 1820s, Muhammad Ali was expanding his army and he could see the need for medical personnel to support this venture. Further, epidemics of plague and cholera continued to ravage his new state. In 1824 an epidemic of plague claimed the lives of 400,000 of the poor Egyptian fellaheen. Clot oversaw the building of the new military hospital at Abu Zabalin in 1827, which he designed to host between 800 and 1,000 patients staffed by 150 foreign doctors (68). The Pasha assigned his French genius to found the first medical school in Egypt. Probably, the Viceroy's motives were primarily to support his expanding army. According to Amira El-Azhari Sonbol, the motives of Clot Bey were broader—primarily as a tool of modernization (69). Clot made great efforts to establish a model medical school which had other components that included a veterinary section, a pharmacy, and a midwifery services, a true feat of its kind (70). He faced tremendous difficulties in establishing his school in nineteenth-century Egypt. He recruited his first teachers from amongst professors in France, Germany, and Italy. He solved the dilemma of the language barriers by hiring interpreters and even made some of them medical students, who later became instructors. He was also faced by religious fanaticism from the group of religious leaders known as the 'Ulema'[5]. He even made some of his students from those Ulema. On the other hand, the firmly held beliefs and cultural taboos in the contemporary society of nineteenth century Egypt made it very difficult to establish medical teachings. Clot solved that dilemma by recruiting black and Abyssinian female slaves into the midwifery school. Clot succeeded against all odds, and the teaching of medicine in Egypt in his day was not inferior to that in Europe (71). Clot, during his early days in Egypt, supervised the hiring of many European doctors for the services he was building. When he first came to Egypt, in January of 1825, from Marseilles, on board the ship he had 20 physicians from different European nations recruited to work under his direction as Surgeon-in-Chief of the Armies (72). They were mainly from France, with some Swiss, German, and Italian doctors. Many of them were later transferred to work in the Turco-Egyptian Sudan. In 1837, Clot Bey established Qasr el-Aini Hospital, which later hosted the old medical school of Abu Zabal. Clot Bey trained many Egyptian doctors who served in both Egypt and the Turco-Egyptian Sudan (73, 74, 75).

The Early Medical Services in the Turco-Egyptian Sudan

Following the conquest of 1820, the exact structure and shape of the health service destined for the natives of the Sudan was not clear. The first hospital to be established in the Turco-Egyptian Sudan was built at Wad Medani after Ismail Pasha decided to move his capital from Sennar, the old capital of the Fung Sultanate. Sennar, which he made his first capital, proved to be unhealthy for his troops, with as many as six hundred of his soldiers succumbing and two thousand becoming invalids due to malaria and dysentery (76). According to the earlier Sudanese historian, a veteran of both the Fung and the Turco-Egyptian administrations, Ahmed bin Alhaj Ali, known as *'Kattib Alshouna'*[6], Muhammad Ali commissioned a group of European physicians to go to Sennar and other towns in his new territories to decide on the suitability of one of these towns to be its new capital after Sennar proved to be unhealthy for his invading troops. They decided the new capital would be either at Wad Medani in the Gezira peninsula or at Shendi, the famous medieval market town north of present-day Khartoum. The decision was based upon geo-political and health grounds, but the Egyptian Viceroy chose Wad Medani (77). Ismail moved his capital there in October of 1821 and he built a palace, officers' quarters, barracks for the troops, and a hospital (78). However, the new capital proved again to be unsuitable from a health perspective, as epidemics of malaria and other illnesses continued to ravage his troops. Ismail decided yet again to move the capital to the second-choice site, Shendi (79). But Shendi, once Ismail moved there, proved to be his nemesis, as he was tragically burnt alive there in November of 1823. When the capital was then moved to Khartoum, a military hospital was built there during the reign of Ali Khurshid Aga[7] early in 1826 (80, 81). The service was primarily destined for the troops and the ruling elite. Even for the military troops the service was selective and discriminatory (82). A blurred picture could be drawn from the excellent panoramic accounts given by Ignatius Pallme, a Bohemian trader to Kordofan in the late 1830s. From his writings, the health services were very much rudimentary and backward, and possibly reflected the overall medical care in the conquering country, Egypt (83). The army medical personnel were permitted to open private clinics, where they could even employ their subordinates, to boost their income (84). So, the health service destined for the natives was delivered by proxy, rather than being a dedicated service provided by the ruling regime. The natives primarily sought treatment from their traditional healers, the '*Faqih*' or '*Fagir*', who used traditional methods and superstitions. A vivid description of the methods used by natives for healing was provided by several European travellers like Ignatius Pallme, Dr. Holroyd, and Samuel Baker. This is covered in the appropriate chapter.

At the beginning of the Turco-Egyptian era, the bulk of the doctors and other healthcare professionals who were serving in the Sudan were mainly Italians, with some French, a few Greeks, and other nationalities. Worth mentioning is that, for the most part of the nineteenth century, the commercial *lingua franca* of the Europeans in Egypt and the Sudan was Italian. The dominance of French (in Egypt proper) would come later, after the Suez Canal was constructed and more French dominance would take place in other aspects of professional life. The heading on the stationary of the Austrian Vice-Consul in Khartoum was in Italian, not German (85). Recruitment of various professionals to work in the newly acquired territory of the Turco-Egyptian Sudan began with the Conquest. Ismail Pasha had several Europeans in his invading army (see Chapter2, Section 2). Amongst them, there were scientists, geology experts, architects, and doctors. Mention was made of G. B. Brocchi, a distinguished Italian scientist who died in Sennar in 1826 (86). Ismail Pasha had in his entourage his own personal physician, *his protomedicio,* the Italian D. Bozzari, and Dr. Andrea Gentili, an Italian physician and dispenser, who was also present during the earlier campaigns against the Wahabites in Arabia. Gentili perished at Merowe around the time of the skirmishes with the Shaigiyyia, and he was thought to have been poisoned by Bozzari (87). Dr. Bozzari would be amongst those burnt alive with Ismail Pasha at Shendi in November of 1822. The eldest son and regent of Muhammad Ali, Ibrahim Pasha *'el-Wali'*, later joined his youngest brother, Ismail Kamil Pasha, in having his private physician, Dr. Antonio Agostino Scotto, an Italian, who later died in Sennar from what was described as 'black water fever' (88). Dr. Agricola Dumont, a French physician and apothecary from Marseilles, was in Ismail Pasha's army as an army doctor. Dumont subsequently settled in Wad Medani and was thought to have died there in 1843 (89). The principal physician at Wad Medani during the visit by Lord Prudhoe in 1829 was Dr. M. de La Font and his apothecary was a Maltese by the name of Zemeet (90). Dr. Guiseppe Ferlini, who was born in and qualified from Bologna, was also in Ismail's army. He worked at Sennar in 1830 and was transferred to Kordofan in 1832. In 1833 he was in Khartoum, where he obtained permission from Ali Khurshid Pasha, then Governor General of the Sudan, to conduct some archaeological work in the area north of Khartoum. He was later discovered to have plundered the pyramids at Merowe and did a lot of damage to their archaeology while looking for gold (91).

The French cult, Saint-Simonianism, which was a religio-sociological cult founded by Claude Henri Comte de Saint-Simon, played a crucial role in the technical administration and the civil services of Egypt and the Turco-Egyptian Sudan. Bartheleme Prosper Enfantin, who was a leading figure of the sect, came to Egypt to join the service of the Pasha and through him many other members were recruited. Several physicians from the cult worked in the military hospitals established in various parts of the country. Many of them were mentioned in the journal of Reboul, a French trader and a Saint-Simonian, who first came to Sudan as a clerk with Georges Thibaut, a well-versed French merchant, during the early years of the Turco-Egyptian rule. Thibaut, who was also a live game hunter, once procured giraffes for the London Zoo from Kordofan. Reboul joined Thibaut during that venture in 1834, and he wrote a journal which was translated later by Santi & Hill (1980) (92). In this journal, several European doctors were mentioned to have been in the employment of the Egyptian military service in the Sudan. Dr. M. Gallina, an Italian doctor who worked in Kordofan, was also mentioned by Pallme as being lucky to survive a day when he became lost on travel between Dongola and el-Obeid. He survived after he resorted to drinking the urine of his camel (93). He was reported to have died eventually at Galabat near Gedaref, on the Abyssinian border in 1838. Others included Dr. M. Drouart, a Frenchman who was the military medical officer stationed at Dongola; Saint-André, a military pharmacist who accompanied the French traveller Edmund Combes to Dongola in 1833; and Dr. M. Landini, the Senior Medical Officer at El-Obeid Military Hospital. Also, in the same journal, there was mention of Mr Lascari, a Greek, who was senior pharmacist, and Mr Tiran, a French pharmacist at the same hospital.

From Lord Prudhoe, a British notable who visited the Turco-Egyptian Sudan in 1829, we could make interesting inferences. Prudhoe, who apparently spent several weeks touring Khartoum and the Gezira with the intention of visiting Kordofan, which apparently did not materialize, wrote some interesting remarks about the few medics he met during his stay in Sudan. On arrival at Khartoum, he seemed to have been welcomed by a French or Italian physician by the name of Dr. Ronnie, who could well had been the private doctor of the Governor of the Anglo-Egyptian Sudan, Khourshid Pasha. During his brief stay at Wad Medani,[8] which he spelled 'Wellid Medani', he made interesting remarks about a young French physician, Dr. M. de La Font, whom he met there. Prudhoe mentioned that the young Frenchman had been in the service of the 'Pacha' (sic) for around three years, and that he gained much credit with the Turkish colonel…

> …by the extent of his cure; for one day the regiment was ill and took them into hospital. In four days, he discharged the whole of them, in sound health. If the invalid does not know his complaint, the doctor says very naturally 'how should I know it'. (94)

Possibly Prudhoe was not impressed by the young doctor's attitude, as he went on to state:

> …found we were in repose, he addressed himself to Mohamet, first begging his pardon for taking him for a Turk, and then making as many excuses for not taking him for a Turk, rattling away in half French, half Italian and going off humming his French air in the same thoughtless manner as if he had been at Paris'. (95)

In 1838, the Austrian Bohemian trader Ignatius Pallme came to Kordofan. In his writings, he described its capital, 'el-Obeid', as an amalgamation of several villages similar in appearance to each other. Those included 'Wady Naghele' and 'el-Orta' (also called 'the town of the Turks') and a few others. In the former resided mainly the native traders, principally the Danaqla and other Riverain Sudanese. El-Orta later harboured the various government buildings, military barracks, officers' quarters, and a hospital (96). A first-hand description of the health services in the late 1830s could be taken from Pallme's writings. Despite the fact that his observations were exclusively on Kordofan, one may postulate that this could be generally extrapolated to the rest of the Sudan, despite this being far from scientific. At Kordofan, Pallme was not a simple passer-by, as he stayed there for eleven months, so was probably well-versed to give a more or less true and candid picture of the days and ways of life in Kordofan of that era. He described the diseases and health services as he saw them, and you could sense that he was quite passionate about what he witnessed. Describing the buildings and amenities of the hospital at el-Obeid, he wrote:

> The hospital consists of a few hovels of clay covered with a straw roofing; they are ill-ventilated, and, in the wet season, the rain beats in upon the sick soldiers through the narrow windows, as they are not furnished with glass; the cold nights, moreover, proves very severe trials, especially to those who are suffering from smallpox. The invalid lies on an angareb and is left to his fate. (97)

Pallme went further and described some of the diseases he saw among the natives in Kordofan. He mentioned that the two main ailments were fever and dysentery. The description he gave of 'fever' is typical of malaria as he related its peak incidence to the rainy season, and that it usually proved fatal within days once the Europeans and Turks fell victim to it. He also mentioned that other significant diseases were smallpox, skin diseases, 'dropsy' (= oedema), jiggers (parasitic infestation), lues (same as syphilis), and abscesses about the neck. The latter may be akin to 'cold abscesses' due to glandular tuberculosis. Dropsy, he described, may be generalised odema related to liver or renal failure, or may be malnutrition or cardiac failure. Pallme made sound comments on the unhealthy drinking water which was consumed in Kordofan and he incriminated it as the main culprit for dysentery. He also observed that syphilis was 'totally unknown in these regions during the preceding century, and the natives have only been inoculated within recent years, through the intermediation (sic) of the Egyptian troops quartered in the province' (98). He stated that the natives used a special type of earth called '*traiba*' which they brought from near Shendy or the White Nile and they used it in a specific technique to treat syphilis (99).

Mansfield Parkyns, a British traveller who landed in Suakin in 1840, described the incident of a Syrian doctor who came to Suakin with the intention of setting up a practice and how his life ended tragically following treatment of one of the local natives of the 'Beja tribe' who had been wounded in a battle. The patient died and his family, blaming the poor Syrian for his death, took the doctor to the outskirts of Suakin and cut him into pieces (100). Dr. Guiseppe Toscanelli, a Sardinian, was reported to have been killed in Khartoum in 1841 when his house collapsed on him during an unusually high flood of the Blue Nile. Dr. J. B. Gand, a French physician (c. 1790-1839), was initially the personal physician to Abbas Hilmi I and was then attached to Ahmed Pasha Shamli 'Abu Widan', during the campaigns of Muhammad Ali's troops in Arabia. He later became personal physician to Abu Widan during his tenure in the Sudan. Gand was reported to have died near Abu Hamad in 1839 while on his way to Egypt (101). The Hikmidar, Abu Widan, then appointed a German Physician, Dr. J. Werne, as senior medical officer and surgeon for the military hospital as well as private physician for himself and his family (102). Father Luigi Montuori, who established the first Catholic Church and school in Khartoum in 1842, described the city as having a population of 13,000 natives, 200 Copts, and a few Catholics and Algerian Arabs. He mentioned a few amenities in the city, including a hospital and a medical storehouse (103).

Possibly in the early 1840s, when the graduates of Abu Zabal Medical School began to fill the ranks, some of them were employed by the Egyptian Army and then posted to the Sudan. According to Alsafi, in his treatise on traditional Sudanese medicine, the grandfather of Dr. Sobhi Al-Hakim, an obstetrician from a notable Sudanese family, Dr. Ahmed Yusuf Al-Hakim, came to Sudan in the early 1840s as a medical officer in the Egyptian Army (104). It transpired that Dr. Ahmed Al-Hakim, whose original name is Ahmed Yusuf

Al-Siddig Al-Hahiawi, was born in Hahiya, a town in the Shargiyia Province in the eastern Egyptian Delta in 1802. He studied medicine at Abu Zabal Medical College and graduated in 1828 as part of the second batch. He was posted to France and specialized in surgery. He appears to have been appointed as medical officer in charge of Dongola and Berber Hospitals. He practiced medicine and surgery and performed surgical operations, including removal of renal stones, tumour excision, limb amputations, and even tooth extractions. He died in Sudan in 1893 (105).

The Medical Service in the Post-Muhammad Ali Era

By 1850s there was further recruitment of European professionals to work in the Sudan, but to a far lesser extent than to Egypt. Dr. Alfred Peney, a Savoyard, who was born at Saint-Genix-Sur-Guirs, graduated from Monteplier and Paris and moved to Egypt, where he became secretary to Clot Bey (106). Peney later moved to Khartoum, in 1851, and at the time of the visit of Andre Melly he was Chief Medical Officer to the Egyptian troops in the Sudan (107). Dr. Peney married an Abyssinian slave girl, Marie, shortly after he was appointed to the post in Khartoum. He became much preoccupied with the dream of discovering the source of the Nile, and in pursuit of that dream he travelled into southern Sudan and Uganda, accompanying the Maltese trader, de Bono. Peney made a significant contribution to the understanding of the geography of central Africa in the nineteenth century by traversing the area west of Yei, in western Equatoria in southern Sudan, and he made very useful maps (108). During these travels, Peney became very sick and perished at Gondokoro in 1861, before reaching Khartoum (109). Marie, his wife, was noted to be sobbing passionately at his funeral in Khartoum. She later remarried, to Adolfo Antognoli, who was accompanying her husband at the time of his mortal adventure. When he died in 1874, she married his business partner, Flaminio Finzi Margini, a Ferrarese Jew. She died in Cairo in 1891 (110). A Sicilian named Onofori Abbate, was the medical attendant at the court of Mohamed Sai'd Pasha, son and successor of Muhammad Ali. When the Egyptian Viceroy visited the Sudan in 1856-1857, Abbate was in his company, and he thereafter wrote an account of that visit. He later authored some scientific treatise on the Sudan concerned with improving the sanitation of Khartoum (111). When Prince Mohamed Abdel Halim became Governor General in 1856, he appointed Dr. Elia 'Bey' Rossi (1816-1892) as medical officer in Khartoum. Dr. Rossi worked in Khartoum till 1865, and he published a book on his experience in the Sudan: *La Nubia edil Sudan* (Constantinople, 1858) (112).

During the tenure of the Armenian, Arak Bey el-Armani, Governor of Khartoum and Sennar (kin to Nobar Pasha Bogos, the famous Egyptian Prime Minister in the late 1800s), a prolific Italian physician, Leopoldo Ori, was recruited as Medical Officer of Health of Khartoum. Ori, who was born at Gascia, Tuscany in 1830 and graduated from Florence in 1854, first joined the Egyptian Health Service in 1856. He was transferred to the Sudan in 1858 and later took up the post of Chief Military Officer for the Egyptian troops on the death of Dr. Alfred Peney in 1861. Ori made significant achievements by setting up a sanitary system for Khartoum, building a wall along the bank of the Blue Nile, setting up a drainage system, and organizing an efficient vaccination service (113). When Arak Bey died at Khartoum, his successor, Musa Pasha Hamdi, appointed a Christian Syrian in place of Ori before the appointment of Dr. Gheorgios Demitrios Douloglu, a Greek physician, to the post. Douloghlu, who belonged to a Greek family that had long domiciled in Egypt, studied medicine at Cairo and qualified in 1850. He was sent thereafter to get further medical studies at University of Pisa. From 1857 onward, he worked at Qasr el-Aini, and in 1863 was transferred to the service of Musa Pasha Hamdi, Governor General of the Sudan. He also worked for some time in Kassala. He became Surgeon General (Chief MO) to the troops in the Sudan. He was killed at Shaikan on the eve of the Mahdiyyia uprising in 1883 (114). Others included Dr. Joseph Biron, of Chambery, who was Medical Officer at the Military Hospital in Khartoum, and Dr. Antonio Figari, who was also concerned with the health sector and published his observations in one of the Italian medical journals (115). Also, a notable physician was Dr. Perron, a Frenchman, who had a special interest in anthropology, who also translated into French the magnificent treatise of the Tunisian traveller, Muhammad bin Umar el-Tunisi (116). Others who worked during the 1850s and 1860s were Dr. Cunny, who compiled important information about Kodofan, its people, and its conditions, and Dr. Castelli (117).

In 1862, the first Egyptian physician to be appointed to a senior medical post in the Sudan was Dr. Hassan Bey Hashim (1825-1879). Dr. Hashim, who initially studied pharmacy in the Pharmaceutical School at Cairo, was sent to France in 1847 for further studies in Pharmacy, but instead he took studies in medicine and went on to specialise in obstetrics. On his return to Egypt in 1862, he took up the post of Assistant Director of the Egyptian School of Medicine. He was sent on several missions to the Sudan, and in 1863 he was appointed Chief MO at Khartoum during the tenure of the Sudanese notable, Sheikh Ahmed Bey Awad Alkariem Abu Sinn, Governor of Khartoum and Sennar. Gaafar Mazhar Pasha, Governor General of the Turco-Egyptian Sudan (?1865-1871) during the reign of Ismail Pasha, was likely the first advocate of training of Sudanese in medicine during that era. He was reported to have recruited twenty Sudanese elementary school pupils to learn the rudiments of medicine and dispensing under the guidance of the Principal Medical Officer of the Sudan, the Egyptian Dr. Hassan Bey Hashim. However, and intriguingly enough, the Viceroy forbade the training of Sudanese assistant doctors in Khartoum, which prompted Mazhar Pasha to request more doctors from Cairo. This gave rise to exchange of correspondence between the centre and the periphery, and Mazhar Pasha was demanded to justify his claims. Here we quote Richard Hill:

> ...in a sobering report, pointed out the drastic limitation of the country, with only one senior doctor at each province headquarter there could be neither general vaccination nor registration of births and deaths. (118, 119)

During the tenure of Gaafar Mazhar Pasha, the health service would reach its zenith. There was a total of six hospitals in the whole of the country, with a total capacity of 438 beds. These were divided as follows: Dongola Hospital 15 beds, Kassala 38, Berber 20, Kordofan 35, Khartoum 270, and Sennar 60 beds. However, the service very much remained exclusive to the military and the ruling Turkish and Egyptian elite. Native Sudanese were not privileged to use the service and they kept consulting their local healers, the *Fakis* and the *Bassirs*[9].

Sir Samuel W. Baker, who came to the Turco-Egyptian Sudan in 1861 and travelled extensively along both the Blue and White Nile regions till 1865, also made some remarks about some diseases he witnessed. Baker possibly unwittingly made one of the earliest descriptions of what sounded like viral haemorrhagic fever that inflicted several of his men (120). He described the epidemic to which he referred as an epidemic typhus (sic), that swept across the 4,000 black troops, who were stationed at Khartoum, and left only 400 of them alive (121). By the early 1870s, there was a hospital in each of the main provinces, '*Mudeiriyyia*', of the Turco-Egyptian Sudan. The 1873 official report of the Governor General at Khartoum stated that there were hospitals in Dongola, Berber, Khartoum, Fung, Kordofan, Taka, and Suakin. In the same year, two more hospitals were opened in the southern part of the country, at Fashoda, and the Lado in Equatoria (122). These brought the total number of hospital beds from 438 to 519 (*vide supra*). Each one of these hospitals was staffed by at least one doctor. Although these hospitals were generally small, the one at Khartoum had 270 beds, and the Principal Medical Officer was stationed there (123). By then, the medical staff were a mixture of Egyptian and European doctors. The details of those hospitals, their bed capacities, and level of staffing, etc., is not known. Some scattered notes of some staff can be found in a few books covering the era. Dr. Abramo Ambron, an Italian doctor, who studied at the Universities of Pisa and Florence, served in the Sudan in the late 1870s. He moved to Cairo and set up a private practice at the onset of the Mahdist uprising. Richard Hill remarked that his talents brought recognition (124). During the 1870s, there were many European doctors practicing at Khartoum, some of them privately (125).

Epidemics & Public Health

From a public health perspective, outbreak of epidemics was a regular occurrence in the Sudan during the Turco-Egyptian era. Waves of cholera epidemics kept sweeping through the Sudan, primarily from Mecca or from Egypt, where it was well documented that a total of nine cholera epidemics ravaged through the country in the nineteenth century (126, 127). Following the efforts of Gaafar (or Ja'afar) Mazahr Pasha (r. 1865-1869) to improve public health and sanitation in Sudan, vaccination was given routinely at the quarantine stations that had been established earlier in Suakin and Mussawa (Mussawa was then part of the Turco-Egyptian Sudan). It seems likely that most of those epidemics spread south from Upper Egypt into 'Nubia' and Sudan. In 1831, an epidemic of cholera struck the city during the reign of Ali Khurshid Pasha. This epidemic was thought to have originated from Mecca and to have spread with the pilgrims to Syria, Palestine, then Egypt, and eventually to Sudan via Suakin (128). An outbreak of smallpox took place early after the Turco-Egyptian conquest in 1826 and took many lives, amongst them was the founder of Khartoum and Governor of Sudan, Uthman Bey Jerkis al-Bringi. An account of some of those epidemics was found by the British traveller Mansfield Parkyns, who visited the Sudan in 1845-1848. Parkyns presented a manuscript detailing those epidemics, and the writer seems to be an Italian doctor or pharmacist who was likely in the service of the Turco-Egyptian administration. These accounts were translated by Whitehead (129), and later by Richard Hill (1995) (130). A Sudanese writer, Ahmed bin Alhaj Abu Ali, who authored a manuscript dealing with the history of the Fung Sultanate and the first decade of the Turco-Egyptian regime, mentioned this epidemic, which he stated was preceded by a famine. He gave vivid description of the cholera which the native used to call the 'yellow wind', or a local synonym, '*Haida*'. He gave descriptions of those affected, with the typical symptoms of dehydration, hypovolaemic shock, sunken eyes, and cold extremities (131).

The British traveller/explorer, Mr (later Sir) Samuel W. Baker, who first came to Khartoum in 1861, witnessed an outbreak of smallpox that took a large toll of death among the natives. He described that his own servant died from what sounded like typhus fever (132). Baker mentioned another epidemic of smallpox in Khartoum, on his return journey, when he stated that over 15,000 natives perished[10]*. Baker's companion in his travels, the Hungarian slave girl, Florence, whom he later married, was mentioned to have done some basic nursing while in Sudan (133). Probably in recognition of that role, the first hospital ship in Sudan, 'Lady Baker', which was launched in 1922, was named after her. Baker, when he came again to the Sudan in 1869, this time as Governor of the Equatorial Province of the Nile Basin, with a mandate to curb the slave trade, had Dr. Joseph Gedge, a British doctor, as his personal physician. Dr. Gedge earlier was a registrar at Addenbrooks Hospital, as well as a demonstrator of Histology at Cambridge University Medical School (134). He later fell ill at Bahr el-Zaraf, when the expedition was on its way to Godokoro, and was sent back to Khartoum, where he later died. In his book, *Ismailia*, which he wrote several years later following completion of his mission to Sudan and Central Africa, Baker described some of the health conditions of the natives. He wrote:

> On the White Nile districts smallpox is prevalent, but cholera rarely attacks the country, but it is known. Dysentery is very common in the White Nile district but is rare in the highlands. This complaint is generally fatal at Godokoro. Great caution should be used, and impure water avoided. Marsh fever is the general complaint of the low ground but is rare in the highlands of Fatiko and Unyoro. I have never met with typhoid fevers in central Africa although they are common at Khartoum. Measles, whooping cough, scarlatina, croup, diphtheria are quite unknown. (135)

Baker went on to make some interesting observations. He quoted that 'blindness is only the result of extreme age'[11] and that 'he never met a person with a psychiatric illness' (136). He also observed that tooth decay is rarely ever seen (after examining a great number of skulls!!). He also reported that dwarfism was extremely rare. He mentioned that:

> I saw only two dwarfs, one had been described by John Speke, he is since had died. We measured this little fellow, who was exactly three feet and half an inch in height, at the age of about eighteen years. (137)

Epidemics of smallpox, meningitis, and cholera continued to ravage the country. Occasionally, typhus, which could well have been endemic amongst Egyptian and Sudanese soldiers, may have had spells of epidemic outbreak. One epidemic was reported to have occurred among the soldiers in eastern Sudan who were dispatched into Ethiopia under the command of Rateb Pasha in 1876 (138). Epidemics of smallpox were rife during the last two decades of the Turco-Egyptian rule. Those were mentioned by the Italian Gaetano Casati, who stayed in Sudan for many years, including ten years in Bahr-el-Ghazal and Equatoria with Emin Pasha (*vide infra*). Casati, in his treatise, *Ten Years in Equatoria* (published first in Italian in 1891 and later translated to English by Clay and Randol in 1898), gave a good account of the contemporary history of the 'Soudan' following the Turco-Egyptian conquest in 1821 (139). Casati came to Sudan in January 1880, travelling from Genoa to Suakin. He stayed for few months in Khartoum and then left for the south. He mentioned several epidemics, including the one in 1863 that broke out in Kassala during the expedition in which Musa Pasha Hamdi waged against the King of Abyssinia. That expedition had to be abandoned upon the news of the death of Mohamed Sai'd Pasha, the Egyptian Viceroy. However, following the return of Musa Hamdi Pasha to Khartoum, a second wave of the epidemic broke out there and took many victims, the Governor himself being amongst them (140). Casati also wrote about the cholera epidemic that drove the son of Muhammad Ali, Prince Abdul Halim, to abandon his visit to the Sudan in 1847 and return to Egypt via Berber (141).

There were contradicting statements about the public health of Khartoum encountered in the writings of various explorers or others who passed through or lived in the city. Samuel Baker described Khartoum blatantly as follows: 'I arrived at Khartum, the capital of Soudan, a more miserable, filthy and unhealthy spot' (142). Others, such as the American traveller Bayard Taylor, who visited Khartoum in the early 1850s (just under ten years before Baker), made some statements about the health and sanitation of Khartoum. In his book *A Journey to Central Africa,* published in 1856, he wrote a rather different account and made favourable comments about Khartoum (143). He described it as a cosmopolitan city, with many of its houses extending over a mile on the bank of the Nile embowered in gardens of palm, acacia, orange, and tamarind trees. He wrote about the native quarter, the Coptic quarter, European consulates, the Catholic Church and school, the military barracks, and the hospital. Here are some extracts from his descriptions : 'We entered a tolerable street, cleanly swept, and soon came to a coffee shop….'; he was obviously impressed by the variety of the people he met there, which included 'various Europeans, Syrian merchants, Egyptian physicians and an Ethiopian Princess and every tribe between Darfur and the Red Sea' (144). Bayard went on to assert that 'it will be a lucky day for Rome and Florence when their streets exhibit no more filth than those of this African city' (145). Father Luigui Montouri, the first Catholic missionary who lived in Khartoum for several years (1842-1848), was reported as being entranced by Khartoum. In a letter that he appeared to have written to a fellow priest, Montouri asserts that 'There cannot be a more pleasing or interesting spot in every way than that of this city….' (146).

The 'miserable and the unhealthy' Khartoum, as seen by Baker in the 1860s, was to witness a remarkable transformation when Charles Gordon took office as Governor General of the Turco-Egyptian Sudan in 1877-1880. Dr. Robert William Felkin, a medical member of the English Church Missionary Society, made comments on the improved sanitary condition of Khartoum following his repeated visits to the area around this time (147). It transpired that he was asked to conduct an inspection of the hospital by Charles Gordon when he became Governor General of the Sudan in 1877. Felkin, who was born in Nottinghamshire and qualified from Edinburgh and Marburg Universities, travelled in the Sudan with his missionary fellows on their way to Uganda. In another contradictory statement in 1877-1878, the Khartoum Hospital was visited by the Italian physician explorer, Dr. Pellegrino Matteucci, who described the situation there 'as horrible' (148). Gordon, soon after he assumed office, tried to make reforms and improvement in health and education. However, he was preoccupied by other political matters, which were his prime tasks, and into which he put most of his energies (149). Gordon, in his efforts to re-organise the service, appointed the Greek physician, Gheorgios Demitrios Doulglou, as the 'Chief Inspector' of public health, with a mandate to improve the health and sanitation of the country (150). As Douloghlou failed to deliver, Gordon next turned to his fellow British native, Dr. David Lowe, who was in Cairo at the time. He persuaded Lowe to take the post of chief medical officer for the army in Sudan, which he accepted in 1779. However, Lowe spent most of his time touring the provinces and he himself suffered from prolonged ill health, which forced him eventually to resign and return to Egypt in 1880 (151). Gaetano Casati even referred to an enterprise by Gordon of establishing a 'pharmaceutical school' during his tenure as Governor of the Sudan in 1877-1879. In his descriptive account of Khartoum as he saw it in the prelude to the Mahdiyya, Casati wrote: 'among the government establishments, the arsenal, the military school, and the printing-office deserves to be mentioned; the two latter (sic) were founded by General Gordon; the Pharmaceutical School was very short-lived' (152). During the reign of Charles Gordon, the hospital in Khartoum witnessed the first European nurses, the Verona Sisters, the Catholic nuns who were attached to the Catholic Mission in Khartoum. Indeed, Gordon requested Daniel Comboni to help to staff the other hospitals in the provinces with more nuns to be recruited from Italy (153). The request was passed by Comboni to his superiors in Rome; however, the Verona Sisters already in Sudan suffered chronic ill health, so the dream to staff more hospitals with nuns remained unfulfilled (154).

In 1777, an outbreak of smallpox killed many in Dongola Province, and in 1878 a major malaria epidemic took its toll in the country after a high flood season; the year was called 'The Mosquito Year'. In 1878, an epidemic of cholera erupted at Al-Hudayda, the old port of Yemen, and there was a real threat of spreading the disease to the Sudan through Suakin. However, following some strict regulation on the movement of passengers and ships to and from Alhudayda at the Suakin Quarantine, the spread of the epidemic to Sudan was curtailed (155). In 1874, when Gordon succeeded Samuel Baker as Governor of Equatoria, he was joined in 1876 by Dr. Edward Carl Oscar Theodore Schnitzer, a German doctor of Jewish origin. Schneitzer, who later became known in history as Emin Pasha, had an interesting life and career. He studied medicine in Vienna, but it transpired that he never took his finals. Instead, he drifted into private practice before qualifying. He then travelled extensively in Europe, aiming to be a ship surgeon before eventually reaching Turkey. There, he befriended the Pasha of the Turkish port of Antivari and obtained the post of a district surgeon and quarantine officer. Following the death of his sponsor, and for some years thereafter, Schneitzer looked after his wife. It was a strange relationship, maybe platonic, maybe not. Schneitzer eventually got to Khartoum in 1875, after spending some time in Cairo. Friends helped him to set up a private practice in Khartoum. In 1876 he joined Gordon at Equatoria and, since then he was known as Emin Pasha; having adopted the name of his predecessor, Dr. Alias Emin Pasha, an Egyptian doctor. Emin Pasha became an administrator at the Egyptian Headquarters in Gondokoro rather than a physician. He eventually gave up medical practice and became a soldier/administrator. When Gordon was appointed Governor General of the 'Soudan' in 1877, he appointed Emin as his successor in the post of governor of 'Equatorial Province of the Nile Basin' (currently the region that includes the area of most of southern Sudan plus northern Uganda). Shortly after Emin Pasha took up his post, he was joined by a Jewish pharmaceutical dispenser named Vita Hassan, who was a son of the dragoman[12] at the Sardinian consulate in Tunis (156). Hassan wrote an account of his adventures with Emin Pasha and he also assisted Casati in the compilation of comparative tables of southern Sudanese languages published in Casati's book. The rise of Mahdiyya spread south and, after the fall of Khartoum in 1885, Emin became entrenched and then besieged by the Mahdist troops led by the Mahdist Emir Fadlallah Arabi in 1888. He was forced to go further south, where he became lost in the hinterlands of central Africa. Here history repeats itself, the *New York Herald* came again to the forefront to orchestrate a rescue expedition. There was no one more versed than Henry Morton Stanley to lead the adventure in the same way he had led the famous one several years before to find David Livingstone. The operation became a *'cause celebre'*. Eventually the rescued and the rescuer reached Mombasa, where a large party was organized. Emin Pasha had been only a nominal hero of the whole enterprise. As he was only partially sighted (quoted to have developed severe short sightedness), he fell from the balcony of the hotel where the party was hosted, and it took him long time to recover. Emin refused emphatically to leave Africa and returned again to the Congo Basin, where he was murdered in 1892 in a place that bore his name. Lieutenant Surgeon Hazel Parke, an English doctor in the RAMC who was amongst the famous 'Emin Pasha Relief Expedition' wrote extensively about the medical encounters during that expedition (157).

Few British doctors came to the Sudan during the Turco-Egyptian era. Like other Europeans, they were mostly travellers/explorers. Amongst them was Dr. Arthur Todd Holroyd. Holroyd was born in London in 1806, and at age 18 studied medicine at Winchester and Webb Street School of Anatomy, Southwark. He later qualified from Edinburgh in 1830, and Cambridge (1832). He practiced as a physician in London but became fascinated by travels. In 1837 he came to Egypt and then travelled to Khartoum from el-Dabba, becoming the first European to cross the Bayouda Desert. He had a brief stay in Khartoum and went thereafter to Kordofan. During those travels in the Sudan, Holroyd acquired first-hand information about the slave trade, a very hot topic in Britain at the time. He published those observations in the *Journal of the Royal Geographical Society* in 1839 (158). He also helped Dr. John Bowring, the slave trade abolitionist, with useful data that was used to forge the slave trade abolition treaty with Egypt in 1840 (159). Dr. Holroyd later migrated to Australia and he practiced law rather than medicine. In Australia, he published his observations on his Sudan experience shortly before his death in 1887 (160). In that treatise, which he wrote primarily for the Australian troops that were sent to Suakin and resided there for some time as part of the Gordon Relief Expedition (161). Holroyd described his few medical encounters, including his first-hand experience with the Sudanese traditional medicine in its heyday, having been a patient himself treated by a traditional healer when he had fallen sick to a febrile illness (see next section). Holroyd revealed or concealed his status as a physician according to the circumstances. He realised early on that he might easily and quickly run out of the medicines stock in his 'Medicine Chest' if he continued to reveal that he was actually 'Hakim-Bashi*'[13] (162). He volunteered at Berber to reveal his status to Abbas Agha, governor of Berber 'al-Mekhirif'[14], and treated him with a mixture of Epsom Salt and rhubarb. He also gave some complimentary medicines to the Coptic scribe of the Turkish Governor of 'Alkhandak', a town near Dongola (163)

The two British physicians on record to have practiced in the Turco-Egyptian Sudan were both Scotsmen. The first, Dr. James

Murie, came to the Sudan employed by the British Acting Consul, John Petherick. Murie was a prominent naturalist and a physician who earlier had been pathologist to Glasgow Royal Infirmary. He was especially fascinated by studies of zoology in the upper Nile when he accompanied Petherick during his treks there. Murie was in company of Pethrick at Gondokorro when the latter met Speke and Grant on their way back to Khartoum in 1864 after they discovered the source of the Nile. Thereafter, Murie devoted his life to a splendid career in medical practice and zoology and wrote several papers to the Proceedings of the Zoological Society, London. He died in Rochford, Essex, in 1925 (164). The second was Dr. David Lowe, who was mentioned earlier. Lowe, also a Scotsman, was born at Skene in Aberdeenshire in 1849 and qualified from there as a physician before he moved to Egypt in 1872 as an assistant in a private medical firm. He subsequently entered the Egyptian Government service and was commissioned as the Medical Officer during the initial phase of building a railway line at Wadi Halfa in 1875. In the same year, he joined a group of surveyors to plan the building of a railway line from Al-Dabba on the Nile, to el-Fashir, in Darfur. In 1876 he was appointed by Ismail Pasha Ayyub, then Governor General of the Sudan, to the post of the Chief Medical Officer of the Sudan. Lowe later worked under Charles Gordon, who appointed him Inspector General of Hospitals. In 1880 he moved back to Egypt, where he worked as Medical Inspector of the Sanitary Board of Alexandria (165).

The early 1880s saw the beginning of the Mahdist revolution, so little attention was paid to further improving the health services. Dr. John Bloss, of the Sudan Medical Service, personally interviewed Dr. Hassan Effendi Zaki, one of the few remaining doctors from the Turco-Egyptian era (166). Zaki stated that during the final years of the Turco-Egyptian Sudan, there was a large 'Egyptian Hospital' in Khartoum that was staffed by several doctors. The senior doctor in Khartoum during the final chapter of the crumbling state was Dr. Nessib Salim, who was assisted by Dr. Hassan Effendi Zaki. Zaki was to play an important role in the medical history of the Sudan in years to come. Dr. Nessib Salim was renowned during his time there as a physician and surgeon of repute, operating on bladder stones,

Madura foot, abscesses, and wounds. Chloroform was available as anaesthetic. During the siege, it was recorded that 'Gordon would visit the hospital daily bestowing materials and morals on the inmates'. Syphilis, dysentery, trachoma, and 'bilharziosis' (sic) were the main scourge. Measles was particularly fatal among children, with a mortality of about 10% (167). Following the success of the Mahdiyyia, the only surviving/remaining of the Egyptian and other doctors on record at Khartoum, was Dr. Hassan Effendi Zaki, who was taken initially as captive and then became the Mahdi's private physician. Following the untimely death of the Mahdi after a very short rule, Dr. Zaki became the private physician of his successor, Khalifa Abdullahi el-Taishi (see next chapter).

Endnotes

1 *Bey*: a Turkish title.

2 *Mak* or *Mek:* a Sudanese word, possibly an abbreviation of the word '*Malaik*' (Arabic = king; see Richard Hill, *Biographical Dictionary of Sudan*). However, Alfred Wallis Budge argues that it is a title of honour rather than one for a king (refrences above).

3 A border Sudanese district on the south-east region adjacent to Ehiopia.

4 Nizam eljadeed: Arabic – used by the Egyptian Viceroy Muhammad Ali Pasha to refer to his 'New Order'.

5 Ulemma (Pl.), Arabic learned men

6 Sudanese: the clerk of the treasury.

7 Aga: a Turkish title of honour.

8 The major Sudanese city on the Blue Nile in the Gezira district.

9 *Faki* and *Bassir* were titles of local Sudanese healers. *Faki* is a title also for a learned man in religious matters.

10 Possibly this was an exaggerated figure taking into account the total number of the native population of Khartoum at that time was estimated at 30,000

11 author: cataract, ?senile macular degeneration

12 A dragoman was an interpreter, translator, and official guide between Turkish-, Arabic-, and Persian-speaking countries and polities of the Middle East and European embassies, consulates, vice-consulates, and trading posts (Wikipedia).

13 *Hakim bashi*: Turkish for medical doctor.

14 al-Mikheirif was part of Berber town, which, in the nineteenth century, used to be an amalgamation of several villages.

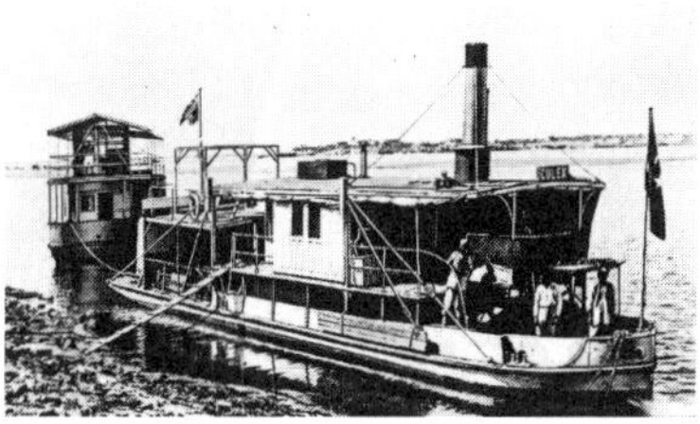

Chapter 3

Medicine & Medical Practices during the Mahdiyya (1885-1898)

Despite the era of the Mahdiyya succeeding the Turco-Egyptian period, the new order elected not to inherit the already rudimentary public services that existed in the country, regardless, whether backward or not. Indeed, the revolution ushered in a new order; with a system of administration and services different from the pre-existing one during the rule of the 'Turks'. During the 'First Turkiyya' (the term used by the Sudanese to denote the Turco-Egyptian era), the ruling elite in Cairo attempted, particularly in its last thirty years or so, to provide a health service that was more or less a miniature copy of some of the services running at the time in Egypt *proper*, especially for the military. Once again, due to the difficulty of tracing proper records for the health services during the Turco-Egyptian era, the researcher will face an equally, or even more difficult task when attempting to construct a clear picture of the scope and shape of health services during the Mahdiyya. Some piecemeal details could be found amongst a few writings. Writings covering the era of the Mahdiyya very much lagged behind, following the colonial reconquest of the country by Lord Kitchener in 1898. It is to the credit of Richard Hill and Peter Holt, two eminent scholars of modern Sudanese history, in conducting some of the early research and producing some balanced and objective writings about the reign of the Mahdiyya. Earlier writings about the Mahdiyyia, including those by Rudolph von Slatin, Reginald Wingate, and Father Joseph Ohrwalder, were largely influenced by the prevailing atmosphere of war propaganda and could be considered biased in terms of scientific analysis (1, 2, 3). However, on the other hand, one may find difficulty in dismissing some facts and disputing some of the events cited in their writings.

The years 1881 to 1885 saw the beginnings of the revolt of the Mahdi and his rise to supreme power. Those years were marked by anarchy and turmoil, so it was no surprise that whatever simple public services existed during the Turco-Egyptian rule suffered and crumbled in the wake of the revolution. As mentioned already in the previous chapter, on the eve of the Mahdiyya there was a hospital in each province (or Mudeiriyya) in the country. These 'Mudeiryyras' were ten in number and they included Khartoum, Dongola, Berber, Kordofan, Takka, Suakin, Sennar, Darfur, Fashoda, and the Nile Basin Province of Equatoria. As most, if not all, of these hospitals were *de facto* military hospitals, they suffered greatly in the wake of the ultimate defeat of the Turco-Egyptian regime. Taking the military nature of those hospitals, the revolt would have left far-reaching effects and resulted in significant damage inflicted upon them. The details of the fate and destiny of the staff are scarce, and little became known about the fate of the staff of these hospitals. Some rudimentary records that filtered out about those who were in Khartoum following the decisive victory in the early hours of January 26, 1885 gave a more or less blurred picture. The 'military' hospital in Khartoum was possibly abandoned after the transfer of the capital to Omdurman. However, Khartoum did not become a ghost city, as portrayed in the writings of Slatin and Ohrwalder (4, 5). Contradicting his own allegations, Slatin had produced a detailed map of Khartoum and Omdurman, to be used by the military intelligence section of the Egyptian army. In that map there was the obvious presence of a military hospital in Khartoum. Recent writings of some contemporary scholars have revealed new evidence on the days and ways of Omdurman during the Mahdiyyia, which has contested the accuracy and impartiality of the earlier writings of Wingate, Slatin, and Ohrwalder (6).

During and following the siege and fall of Khartoum and death of Gordon, those who were delivering the medical services in general were either captured or killed. Following his capture, one of the medical officers of Khartoum during the siege, Dr. Hassan Effendi Zaki, an Egyptian doctor, was taken by the Mahdi as his private physician. Within few months and in June of 1885, the Mahdi succumbed to a brief illness and was succeeded by Khalifa Abdullahi bin Mohamed, widely known as Khalifa Abdullahi el-Tai'shi, after his tribe, a clan of the Baggara of western Sudan. Zaki then became the physician to Khalifa Abdullahi al-Tai'shi. Omdurman developed into a sprawling city, as it was not only the troops that came. It was the sheikhs and notables of different tribes from different parts of the Sudan flocking to show their allegiance. They came, not alone, but with their families and retinue of slaves. The facilities of the town struggled to satisfy such huge numbers of newcomers. It was barely capable of sustaining its original dwellers. There were no facilities for sanitation and the resources of the arable land were barely enough for its own people. Thus, epidemics soon broke out. An early epidemic of smallpox took place shortly after the fall of Khartoum. The Mahdi ordered a search for all physicians in Khartoum and Omdurman and the recruitment of everyone who had medical experience in a campaign of vaccination. Dr. Zaki was put in charge of this campaign. He later wrote that 'we were able to vaccinate nearly one 1000 subject every day till everybody was vaccinated. The Khalifa issued an edict for similar vaccination campaigns to take place in other parts of the country' (7). Thus, it seems very likely that the only surviving physician from the old order was Dr. Zaki. Dr. Musa Abdellah Hamid, in his short account of the history of Omdurman Hospital, quoted some writings of Dr. Hassan Effendi Zaki (8). Zaki asserted that he was ordered by the Mahdi to move from Khartoum and to settle in Omdurman. He was given a house in Hillat Fangar, which used to lie between Hayi Al-Umaraa and Khor Abu Anga, both being suburbs in the old Omdurman (possibly part of the current Mourada and Abbassia suburbs of modern Omdurman). He was also instructed by the Khalifa to establish two clinics, one in Alshuhada (in the centre of the city) and the other was in Al-Shajaraa (famously known as Suk-al-Shajaraa)[1]. (9). In the first few months after the Mahdi's victory, further epidemics continued to ravage Omdurman and the country. One such epidemic swept the city in June of 1885, taking many victims, including the Mahdi himself. The exact cause of that lethal epidemic was not clear. According to Dr. Zaki, it was cerebrospinal meningitis, but others thought it could well have been an epidemic of typhus (10).

From the various writings about the reign of the Mahdiyya, no details were mentioned about the medical services and medical staff practicing in the Sudan. P.M. Holt, in his documentary, *The Mahdist State 1881-1898*, made little mention, if any, of how the medical services were organized (11). He may not have found any documents covering the subject, as he has given some accounts of the administrative, judicial, and financial services. Few manuscripts gave some rudimentary accounts of the shape and scope of medicine during the Mahdiyyia. Kraemer, in his recent treatise on Omdurman, has offered some previously missing insights into the scope and structure of the public services and the 'administrative order' of the Mahdiyya (12). According to him, following the death of the Mahdi and the ascendancy of Abdullahi al-Tai'shi, the latter set about establishing the new Mahdiyya order. He organized his administrative and judicial systems. The highest organ of administration during the Khalifa rule was 'Bayt al-Mal' (the Treasury) (13). 'Bayt al- Ma'l' had under its authority what would be considered in modern day the various ministries and government departments, as it effectively controlled both the revenue and expenditure. Its director, Amin-bayt al-Mal, could be regarded in modern terms as the person combining the posts of prime minister and chancellor of the exchequer or finance minister, the most important executive in the state. Bayt al-Mal, during the Khalifa's rule, encompassed a soap factory, telegraph employees, an ammunition store, a pharmacy, and a hospital (14). All employees running those departments were under direct responsibility of Amin Bit al-Mal. Dr. Hassan Zaki was employed at Bayt al-Mal and, under instructions from the Khalifa, he was effectively the 'Chief Medical Officer' of Omdurman and indeed of the whole of the Sudan (15).

On the other hand, an important department of Bayt al-Mal was 'Musliheen al-Suk' (market regulators). They were a force of irregular police who were under direct command of a former Turco-Egyptian official, Mohamed Wahbi wad Hussein Aday. Wahbi was born in Berber to Ja'ali and Ababdi parents, and from 1886 till 1895 was in charge of this important section of the administration during the Mahdiyya. He held several titles, including 'Sheikh al-Suk' (market director), 'Amir Alshurta' (Police Director), and others (16). He had 25 irregular police under his command, delivering the various tasks and duties assigned to them. An important part of their duties could well be considered the sheer work of public health and sanitation by today's standards. That included inspection of meat, vegetables, and other various commodities (17). One could argue that some of their duties also included what we regard today's as general matters of 'health and safety'. That included disposal of carcasses of animals, garbage, and control of street congestion. In the words of Kramer, they 'discouraged forms of antisocial behaviour prohibited by the Mahdi and Khalifa; e.g., verbal and physical abuse, public urination and defecation…' (18). An important aspect of the Mahdiyya's teachings placed special emphasis on core Islamic values and principles that exhort cleanliness in person, place of residence, and place of work. The Khalifa used his weekly Friday prayer sermons to address the people of Omdurman. After his ascendancy to power, he made attendance at Friday prayers compulsory for all Omdurman residents. In these sermons, the Khalifa kept emphasising to his subjects the need to keep their neighbourhoods clean and streets unobstructed (19). Another aspect of law and order during the Mahdiyya was the ban imposed on alcohol and tobacco; both considered (in the Mahdi's jurisdiction) to be violations of the teachings of the Mahdiyya and of Islam. Muslihien al-suk, as a department, was not only confined to Omdurman. They were also employed in various towns and cities of the country, including Dongola, Rufa'a, Wad Medani, Gedaref, and Massalamiya (20).

An account of medicine and the medical practices during the Mahdiyya was written by Dr. Hassan Effendi Zaki with a supplementary report by Rudolph Slatin, and these were published in the *Third Report of the Wellcome Laboratory* in 1908 (21, 22). These primarily painted an image of 'native medical practices and superstitions', rather than an account of any true medical services. Further, they had given the impression that there were no true medical services (by the standards of that era). One may take it for granted that the article argues against the presence of any true medical practice, compared to the preceding era of Turco-Egyptian rule. Such an argument stems from the fact that during the preceding rule of the 'Turco-Egyptian Government', there was a hospital in every provincial town (23). According to Dr. Hassan Effendi Zaki, in an article written in Arabic, translated by Dr. Andrew Balfour and published in the *Third Wellcome Report* in 1908, there were others associated with him during the siege of Khartoum. No records could be traced about those 'others'. Possibly they were all killed or fled. Dr. Zaki stated that there were others during the Mahdiyya who were dispensers, especially some Greek merchants who possessed drugs, some Austrian priests like Father Joseph Ohrwalder (and Father Bonomi, the other captive), in addition to some nurses (the two nuns who were also captives with the Austrian priests, Sisters Elizabetta Venturini and Catterina Chincarini) (24). Dr. Zaki asserted that in addition to himself (as the only doctor who possessed Western medical knowledge), the medical hierarchy in the Mahdiyya was composed of the El-Bassir (pl., *Bussara*), the barber surgeon, and the native midwives (called *Daya*[2]). He went on to state in detail:

> The Bassir was considered the wise physician and was entrusted with the compounding of medicines. Very often he possessed considerable knowledge, but he took care to secure his fee before prescribing, and too often his 'cures' were a mixture of savage quackery and charlatan tricks. The Hallag, who did not possess any special technical knowledge, was nevertheless regarded as a practical workman and was a familiar figure with his razor, bleeding horn and circumcision clamp. It was the fashion to be bled once every six weeks, so that the barber surgeon was kept busily employed. (25)

From that article, which to my knowledge was the only document that shed light on the structure of the medical services during the whole period of the Mahdiyya, one could infer that there were no other doctors practicing Western medicine throughout that period except Dr. Zaki himself. Hence, following the collapse of the old order, the medical services were relegated again to lag behind the contemporary medical practice in the last quarter of the nineteenth century. As stated above, at the top of the hierarchy there was the Bassir and the one next to him was the Hallag or barber-surgeon. The native midwife or '*Daya*' dealt with midwifery and she was the one who also performed female circumcision.

Dr. Zaki in that article gave a detailed account of the surgical procedures carried out during the Mahdiyya era. This is important, as the period was rife with wars in various parts of the Sudan as well as against enemies in the eastern front (the Abyssinians), the northern front (the Egyptians and the British), and the south (the remnants of the Turco-Egyptian regime represented by Emin Pasha and his troops in the Equatoria region). The surgical procedures were conducted in primitive ways and, unsurprisingly the mortality and morbidity were very high, especially gangrene. When a person became injured by gunfire, sword, or spear, the wound would be washed with water and ground coffee, then pressure would be applied to stop bleeding. If there was no bleeding, native butter (from cow's or goat's milk) would be applied. Dressing was then applied daily after the wound was bandaged and left to dry by air. No medication would be applied, as it was possible none was available. If fractures ensued, this would be stabilised by '*jareed*' (ribs of compound palms leaves) used as splints. Simple fractures were managed in a similar way and left for forty days to knit. Following healing, the part was massaged with ostrich fat (26). According to Dr. Zaki, the technique to deal with wounds in the wake of more advanced weapons was modified. He cited the accounts of one certain Bassir, Mohamed Nur-El-Barudi, who was at the Battle of Toshki, the one which took place in February of 1889 and saw the decisive defeat of the Mahdist army led by Abdel-Rahman Wad El-Nejumi. In that battle the wounds were treated with beeswax and sesame oil and covered with cotton linen (*damoor*). Perforated parts of the body caused by bullets were covered by honey (27). Amputations were carried out without anaesthetics and the part to be severed would be passed through a hole in the wall of a room or through the window. The stump was immediately plunged into boiling oil so that haemorrhage would be immediately arrested. The wound would then be bandaged and dressed with butter, usually after three days. Patients with fractures were advised to eat plenty of dates, which were thought to promote healing (28).

Various medical conditions were treated by native doctors (the Basurra), according to specific recipes. For instance, syphilis, as stated in the paper by Rudolph von Slatin (aided by a local '*hakim*'), was treated with a mixture of various substances and foods mixed in certain proportions. This included milk with natron mixed with a type of earth called *turaiba* (29). Headaches were treated by snuffing goat's butter, which was then rubbed over the head and some sugar taken with water. If the headache was felt to be caused by excessive exposure to the sun, or by a flu illness, a special salt brought from the region of Dongola in the north, called '*al-Kab* salt', was melted in red vinegar and placed on the head after shaving the hair (30). Dysentery was treated by a recipe made of wheat, milk, and *helba* mixed together. Gonorrhoea was managed by submerging into a bath of water mixed with *helba* (31). The latter is possibly a type of legumes very much commonly used in Sudan to the present day in traditional remedies (32). Mention was also made in Slatin's paper of the disease called '*Dabas*', which is a lay term used by Sudanese, especially the riverain tribes in rural and semirural areas, to describe this illness, which could well be an allergic reaction, as it commonly causes swelling of lips, throat, and face. Slatin's paper mentioned that the illness was treated by snuffing the fat of fox and rubbing the skin with it, or making a paste from the bark of the Arak tree (*Salvadora persica*) and applying it to the swollen part (33). On a similar encounter, Dr. Zaki in his paper also elaborated on the various remedies used by the native doctors to treat various medical conditions. Colic was usually treated with Hargal (*Solemnostemma Argel*), which should be used boiled with native bread (*kisra*), given in a single or repeated dose. Diarrhoea was treated with Karad (fruit of *Acacia Albida*), or Aradeeb, Tamarind (*Tamarindus indicus*), sometimes given together. The treatment used for gonorrhoea was made from the roots of the Rabah plant (*Trianethema pentandra*), which was said to grow in Tuti Island. In a dried form, the plant was made into powder, then mixed with the locally brewed beer, *marrissa*. The stuff taken as a drink would cause inflammation of the genitourinary tract. The treatment was said to result in cure of some cases, but in others retention of urine might prove fatal if not adequately relieved (34). Dr. Andrew Balfour of WTRL noted the use of the quill of the turkey feather as a urinary catheter after being seared with fat and carefully passed into the urethra. Other native doctors treat gonorrhoea by natron, known in the local Sudanese slang as '*Atrun*'. It acts as a strong purgative and a diuretic. Respiratory diseases like bronchitis and cough were treated by '*Galiya*', which was a ground millet prepared like coffee. Another substance used was the flowers of Karkade (*Hibscuss abdriffa*). These were made into a liquid with the addition of sugar and served to those affected, usually as a hot drink. Often, venesection was used to treat those with pneumonia (35). Other contagious conditions like chickenpox, which has since been called '*El-Burgum*', was treated by senna burge and application of mud to the vesicles, and no bath was allowed till one week after the end of the disease. Smallpox was very much dreaded and those affected were taken several miles away and isolated and nursed by someone who had had the disease before. Snake and scorpion bites were treated by cutting the site of the bite or cupping it or burn it and then applying a specific powder called '*Erg-Aldabeeb*' or '*Erg-El-Agarb*', for the snake and the scorpion respectively. It is noteworthy that most of these methods used by the native doctors during the Mahdiyya era were still in vogue several decades later, well into the twentieth century (see section on traditional medicine, Appendix 4. Also see Ahmed Alsafi, *Traditional Sudanese Medicine*).

Both Slatin and Zaki lived and were parts of both eras. It was unlikely that there was any other remaining doctor from the Turco-Egyptian era who survived the Mahdist revolution except Dr. Zaki. Records mentioned none, which so far have been traced by the author. Taking into account that Zaki was a practicing doctor during the whole period of the Mahdiyya, he only shed light on the medical practices of the native doctors and local healers. It was intriguing that both Zaki and Slatin did not give any account of the events that affected the health system following the collapse of the old order. Dr. Zaki in his paper covered some specific aspects. In that paper, Zaki elaborated well on what could be a first-hand account of the native medical practices and superstitions of the era. Much of what he wrote about is still practiced to this very day in many parts of the

Sudan (36). The supplementary notes by Rudolph von Slatin also stemmed from first-hand experiences during the years he spent in the Sudan between 1874 and 1896. Like Zaki, he had good insight into the trepidations of indigenous Sudanese medicine during the last quarter of the nineteenth century. Apparently, the native methods of healing and various health superstitions persisted and were rampant throughout the Anglo-Egyptian rule, despite the fact that they were not well researched except during the first decade following the Reconquest (37, 38).

The one and a half decades of the *Mahdiyya* were marred with internal strife and conflicts on several fronts. This reached a climax in 1896, when the country was faced with the menace of the Reconquest campaigns waged by Lord Kitchener and his troops. The accession of Khalifa Abdullahi to supreme power following the short rule of the Mahdi was the beginning of a militant and autocratic state that focused primarily on military and state expansion. This allowed little opportunity for establishing the foundations of a modern state with sound public services. Furthermore, the Khalifa's rule was also preoccupied with internal conflicts. He faced the threat of being deposed by the nepotism gathered around the late Mahdi's family, who were then called 'the *Ashraf*'. The Ashraf Revolt was not the only internal threat to the rule of the Khalifa. Several tribes mutinied, including the Rezaigat, the *Kababbish,* and the *Fur* Sultans in the west, and the *Ja'aliyyien* in the north.

Over the thirteen-year span of the Mahdist State, several epidemics and famines broke out. The most remembered was the brutal famine of the years 1888-1889 (H 1306), known in the public memory as 'The Famine of Sanat Sitta[3]' (39). Vivid descriptions of the horrific maladies of that famine that struck most of the Sudan were narrated mainly in the two books, *Fire & Sword in the Sudan* and *Ten Years of Captivity in the Mahdi's Camp* (40, 41). Some useful descriptions were also made by Yusuf Michaeil, a Copt, who was a clerk and confidante to the Khalifa (42). Between 1885 and 1890, several epidemics of cholera broke out, primarily through the pilgrims returning from Mecca. As essentially no quarantine methods were employed nor any modern medical means or medical staff were available to deal with such epidemics, the outcome was devastating.

In 1896, a major cholera epidemic broke out during the Dongola Expedition and took the lives of many men of the invading army led by Lord Kitchener. The epidemic began in Egypt and, as per the energetic movement of the troops, it travelled very quickly from Aswan to Wadi Halfa, appearing in Aswan on June 29, 1896, and in Wadi Halfaon the 30th, reaching Dongola in July after sweeping through Suarda and the remaining outposts along the Nile (43). The British Army instigated quick measures to curtail the outbreak by moving the troops away from the Nile, imposing stringent quarantine and sanitary measures. The death toll from the epidemic surpassed that from combat, with a total of 1,000 cases, of whom 800 died (44). The mortality was very high among the Sudanese troops and their families, with a total of 406 cases of whom 260 were left dead (45). The Xth Sudanese Battalion bore the brunt of the death toll, with 50 soldiers left dead, representing 6% of its total manpower (46).

A disease that became deeply entrenched in the Sudan before, during, and after the Mahdiyya was smallpox. Earlier on, the process of 'pocking the pox', a means of primitive vaccination, was described by both James Bruce and John Lewis Burckhardt. It is not clear whether this process continued to be practiced in the country during the Mahdiyya, as there is a dearth of records. Several outbreaks of smallpox took place during the era of the Mahdiyya. As early as 1885 a major outbreak of smallpox, witnessed by Dr. Hassan Zaki, swept through Omdurman, leaving over fifteen thousand dead (47). Ohrwalder, another eyewitness of that era, stated that; following the fall of Khartoum in January 1885,

> The enormous multitudes around Khartum (sic) had been engaged during the whole of the winter season in war, consequently cultivation was neglected, and had it not been for the quantities of the cattle available, a disastrous famine must have occurred.... In addition to fever and dysentery, smallpox, which in Sudan is endemic, increased with fearful rapidity. In Omdurman hundreds died, and the principal business of the beit el mal was distributing *'kafans'*. (48)

Another outbreak in the south-eastern region of Kordofan, helped Hamdan Abu Anja, one of the most able military leaders, to subdue the uprising of the Mak of Tagali Kingdom of the Nuba Mountains in 1886 (49). Another outbreak early in the 1889 rescued the Mahdiyya from the menace of the Abu Jummayza revolt that destabilised the rule of the Mahdiyya in western Sudan in 1888-1889. The epidemic took the life of Abu Jummayza himself and helped to defeat the rebel forces in February 1889 (50).

On the eve of the Reconquest, there were only four hospitals in the Sudan, one of them at Omdurman. The location of the other three hospitals awaits further research. It is possible that this hospital was located at the site of the current Omdurman Hospital, which was built in the 1920s (51, 52). The author, so far, has not found any details about the other three hospitals or their exact locations. The hospital at Omdurman was run by Dr. Hassan Effendi Zaki. The hospital at Khartoum, which was built around 1826, during the Turco-Egyptian era, was deserted following the fall of Khartoum and death of Gordon in 1885 (53). However, its building was still existing at the time of the flight of Rudolph Slatin, who created a detailed map to be used by the intelligence section of the Egyptian Army directed by Colonel F.R. Wingate. This map showed the location of that hospital. Following the Reconquest, Dr. Hassan Zaki was re-instated in the Egyptian army, given a military rank, and appointed as medical superintendent of Omdurman, with the mandate of treating the wounded Mahdist soldiers (54).

Endnotes

1 Al-Mourada, Alshuhada, Abbassia and Souk Alshagra, are Omdurman suburbs.

2 *Daya* is the Sudanese slang word for 'midwife'.

3 *Sanat Sitta* = year six (referring to the 1306 H, circa 1888/1889), a very famous year in modern Sudanese history of a famine that is deeply imprinted in the Sudanese people's memory.

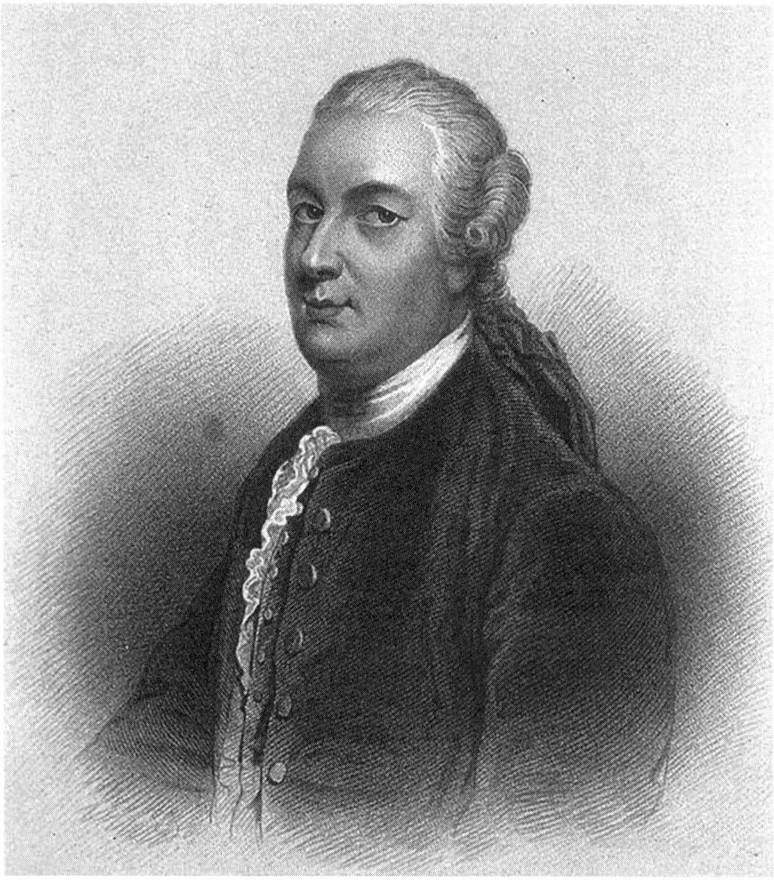

James Bruce of Kinniard
(Courtesy of Wikipedia)

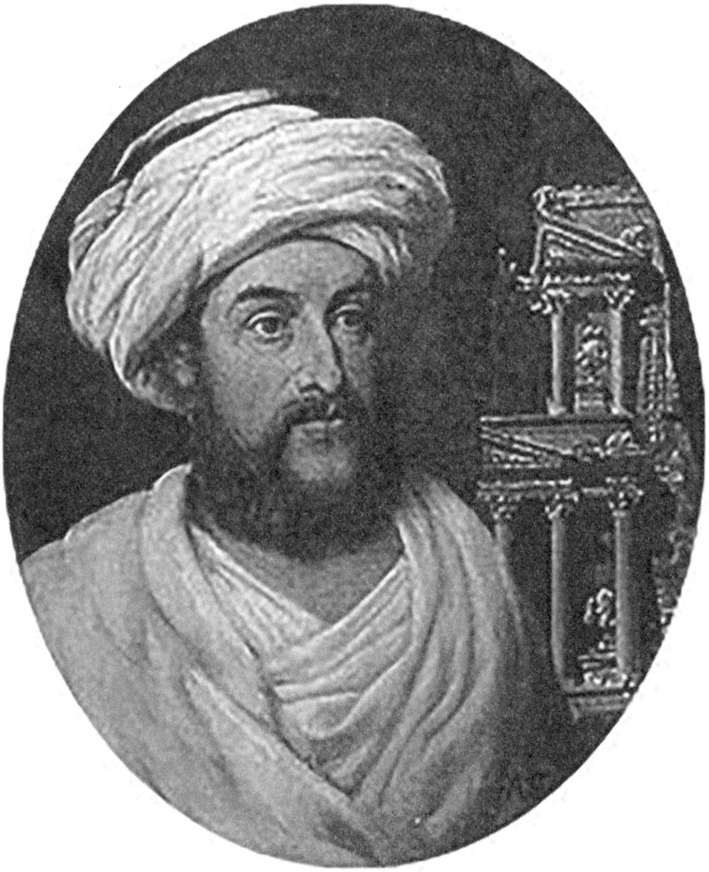

John Lewis Burckhardt
(Courtesy of Wikipedia)

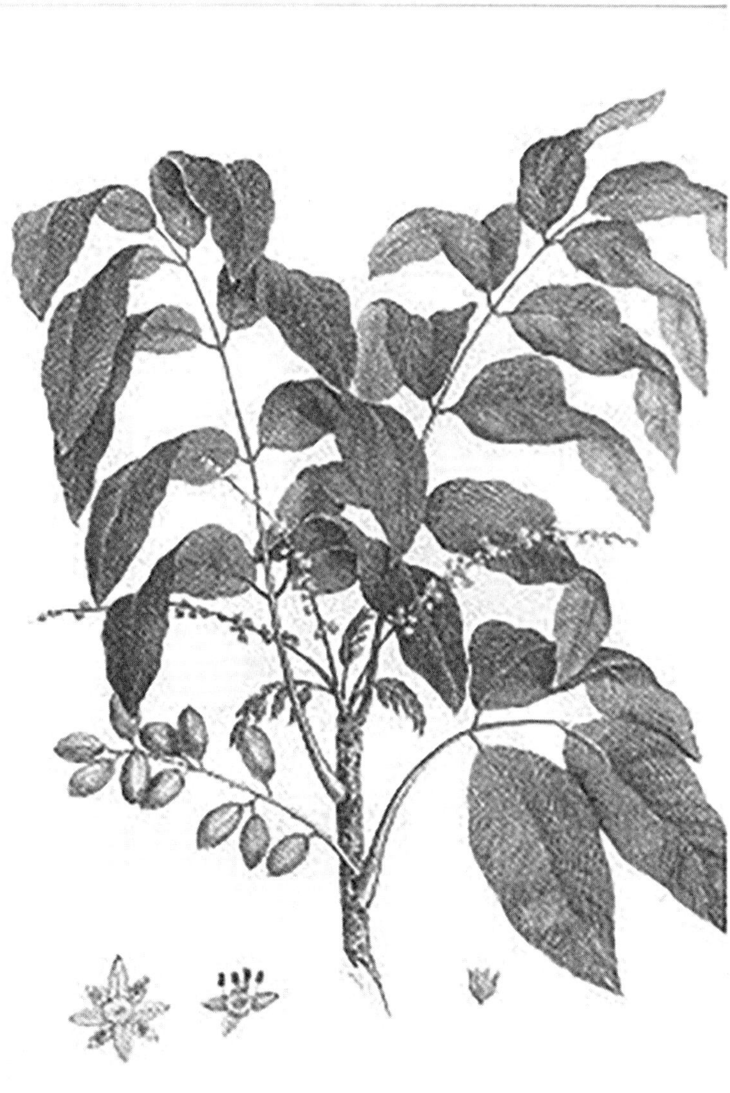

Brucea anti-dysentrica
(Courtesy of Wikipedia)

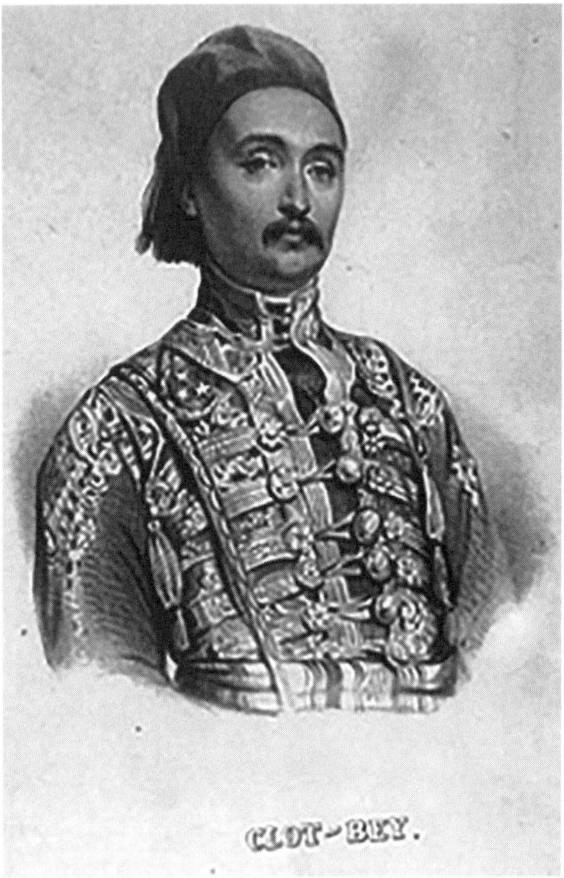

Antoine Clot Bey
(Courtesy of Wikipedia)

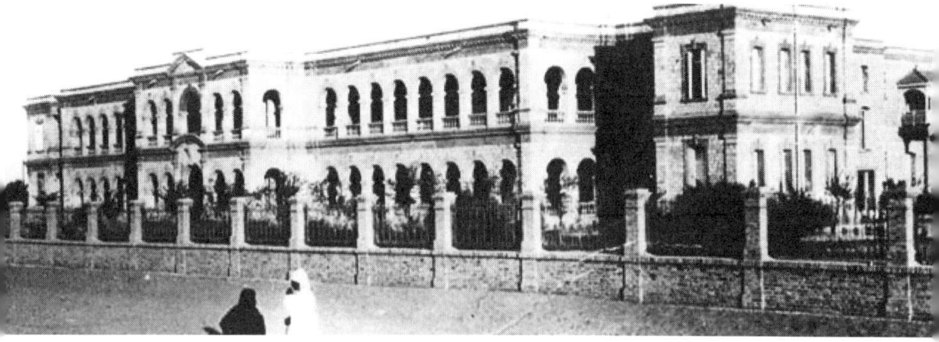

PART 3

THE EARLIEST FOUNDATION OF MODERN MEDICINE IN THE ANGLO-EGYPTIAN SUDAN

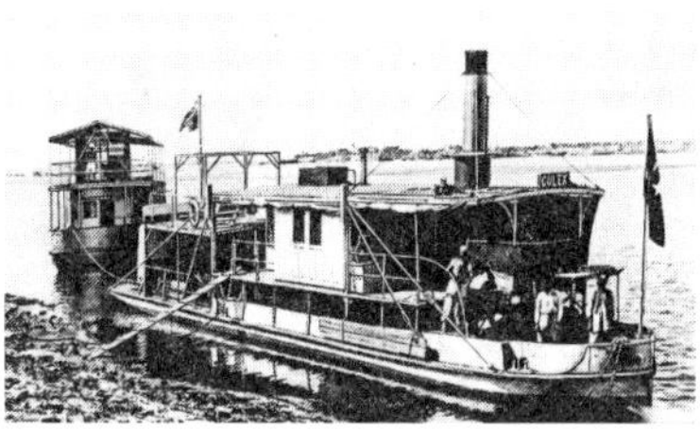

Chapter I

The Earliest Footsteps of Modern Medicine:
The Re-Conquest & the Royal Army Medical Corps

In the early 1900s, the grab for Africa was in full swing and colonialism was not yet a dirty word. For the control of Sudan, the hypothetical question might be: 'If not the British, who? King Leopold of the Belgians, the Egyptians again, the French, the Italian, the Turks?'

–Ann Crichton-Harris, *Poison in Small Measure*, 2009

Section I:

Early Days: Suakin Military Garrison & Its Medical Encounters

The Royal Army Medical Corps (RAMC) was an essential component of the British forces participating in operations to relieve General Gordon. Some of the troops were primarily stationed in the Red Sea Port of Suakin (or Suakim, as it appears in the British and European writings of the nineteenth century) and its adjacent hills, others in the Nile border port of Wadi Halfa, which remained under control of the Turco-Egyptian forces. These were the only two major cities in the Sudan that did not fall under the Mahdist control and remained throughout under the control of the urco-Egyptian forces The details of those medics in the RAMC were either sketchy or difficult to trace. Despite the fact that their role was particularly restricted to the care of the soldiers and the army personnel, some notable figures went on to make landmark contributions to the medical profession in general. Indeed some of them formed the core of the early structure of the future medical services, serving the invading troops as well as the native citizens. During the Mahdist siege of 1884-5, two relief expeditions were sent via Suakin. The first was in 1884, known as the 'First Suakin Expeditionary Force'. The second followed in 1885, and both failed to provide any crucial support to the besieged Gordon in Khartoum. The Red Sea port of Suakin, in addition to the border Nile port of Wadi Halfa, were the only two major cities in the Sudan that did not to fall under the Mahdists' control.

Dr. James Howard Thornton, an English doctor who qualified from King's College and University of London in 1855, was enrolled with the Indian Medical Services as a deputy army surgeon, working primarily in Bombay, and at the time of the Mahdists' uprising had had earlier experience working in Egypt during the Urabi Revolution. In a treatise titled 'Memories of Seven Campaigns', which was published after he retired from service in 1895, he included his medical experiences in Suakin (1). The Foreword being written by Egmont Hake, author of *The Story of Chinese Gordon* and editor of *General Gordon Journals at Khartum*. His interest in the events in the Turco-Egyptian Sudan began earlier when Colonel Hicks Pasha was ordered to lead an expedition to curb the Mahdists' revolt. At the time, Thornton thought of volunteering, as he had been an acquaintance of Hicks Pasha during his service in India. In the aforementioned treatise he writes: 'On hearing of this I was at first much inclined to apply for employment there on the strength of my previous war services and Egyptian experience. After mature consideration, however, I refrained from doing so, and gave up the idea' (2). Thornton later heard of the news of the Hicks forces being routed and massacred at Kasgil (Shaikan) outside el-Obeid in October of 1883. Destiny, however, would later take Thornton over to Sudan and he would witness the several battles against the Mahdist Emir Osman Digna around Suakin. A mixed force of British and Indian troops was then sent to Suakin in February 1885, as the news of Gordon's death filtered out, and Thornton was assigned to be the Principal Medical Officer of the Indian troops, with a mandate to establish two field hospitals in the build-up to the offensives against Emir Osman Digna and his Hadendewa warriors (Fuzzy Wuzzies). Thornton was responsible for the 3,250 Indian officers and soldiers in addition to a sizeable number of camp followers. After landing there in March of 1885, he established two field hospitals, with 100 beds each. He was assisted by a few other British medical officers, including Brigade-Surgeon Morice next in command (3).

Thornton, in his accounts, gave ample description of the city of Suakin, which was considered one of the jewels of the Old-World ports during medieval times and beyond. Thornton also had considerable artistic skills and illustrated his book with fine drawings of the buildings, the inhabitants, and the harbour of Suakin. He described the city and its inhabitants:

> The town of Suakin is situated to the west of the Red Sea coast, about half way between Suez and Aden.....the town is on an island in the harbour; it contains many large houses several stories high, build on blocks of white coral, and numerous shops , both European and native, with ample supplies of all kinds. There is considerable trade with Jeddah and other places on the Red Sea littoral, and with the interior also in peaceful times. The space

> in the harbour is still further diminished by another island of considerable size called Quarantine Island, which was occupied during our expedition by detachment of British troops and the Madras Sappers and Miners. These islands are both connected with the mainland by causeways; that of quarantine Island leading to the fortified position then known as H Redoubt, while the Suakin causeway leads to the extensive suburb called El Kaf, inhabited chiefly by Arabs of the Bishareen and Hadendowa tribes, who are at times of peace are carriers of goods from the interior to Suakin......The inhabitants are very mixed community, comprising of Europeans of several nationalities (chiefly Italians and Greeks), Egyptians, Levantines, and Arabs of various tribes....). (4)

Thornton established his two field hospitals as well as '*Czarevitc'*, a military ship that was converted to a floating hospital of 125 beds (5). In between the Battles of Hashin (Hasheen), el-Tebb, and Tamai, few skirmishes took place. Thereafter, Thornton was appointed principal medical officer (PMO) of Suakin Garrison. He undertook the task of improving the sanitation of Suakin and 'its environs' (sic). Dead animals were either left unburied or buried in the town. Refuse, filth, and the decomposing animals were dumped on the shore, and flies and mosquitoes were rampant. For the sake of good public health, he obtained an order that burials of dead animals were to be carried out two miles outside the town. A number of labourers were employed to clean the worst parts and the area close to the harbour, where a lot of filth and debris had been thrown and dumped, was covered by sand brought by trucks from outside the town. Pools of foul stagnant and smelly water were buried, and several places were reclaimed from the sea and converted into firm dry ground where dead animals and filthy refuse could be burnt (6). When the summer of 1885 arrived, the heat became so intense that several members of the garrison, especially British troops, were found dead from 'heat apoplexy' and others succumbed to enteric fever (7). The former only affected British troops when the ice ship *Bulimba* departed from Suakin. Indian troops were least affected by these. Thornton described other illnesses that inflicted the British and Indian troops to be mainly '*ague fever*' (the old name for malaria), which in some proved fatal. However, the prevailing diseases, especially among the

Indian troops, were dysentery and scurvy. By November 1885, Dr Thornton returned to India with some of his Indian troops. A garrison of Indian and British troops remained in the city. Regular skirmishes were the norm between the forces and those of Emir Osman Digna. The climate of Suakin and the Red Sea region of the Sudan in most parts of the year were very unhealthy for the British and Indian troops. At Suakin, there was a base hospital on the mainland and several small ones in the approach to the harbour. The cemetery of the British troops in Suakin was the major sign of how death and disease played a major part during the expedition of 1885. Questions were asked in the Commons and the *Lancet* commented that in May 1885, 14% of the troops were invalided home, with the figure rising to 16% in July of that year (8).

Another notable from the RAMC **Sir Alexander Ogston**, who was an Aberdeen graduate and held the chair of surgery at Aberdeen before volunteering for the military expedition planning to relieve General Gordon. He was also involved in the battle of Hasheen (Hashin). He landed at the Red Sea ports of Trinikitat and Suakin and played a crucial role in setting up the field hospitals for several of the skirmishes between the troops of Sir Gerald Graham and the Mahdist warriors of Osman Digna; the 'Fuzzy Wuzzy'. Sir Ogston became a pioneer of military surgery, and he is considered to be the architect of the Royal Army Medical Corps, founded in 1898 (the same year as the Battle of Omdurman). **Sir Alexander Ogston** was one of the most distinguished doctors of his time, having discovered and named the bacterium 'staphylococcus'. Some of the novel technique he implemented during the battles around Suakin, in particular the Battle of Hasheen, went on to become novel methods of care adopted later by military doctors elsewhere. Sir Ogston could be considered one of the key doctors who laid down the foundation of military medicine, and he was one of the few notable military doctors who convinced Lord Landsdowne to establish the Royal Army Medical Corps in its modern form in July1898 (9, 10).

Up to 1898, there were four hospital ships in Suakin harbour, and three Nightingale nurses were sent from the Guard's Hospital in London (11). The main water supply was outside the city and it was guarded heavily by military and civilian police. Inspection for venereal diseases, conducted by the Army medical doctors, was carried out weekly on civilian police and prostitutes. Taxes for sanitary and electric services were levied on all. Several sanitary workers were employed. In 1889, the worst famine in Sudanese memory broke out in most of the regions of the country and it spread fast with many deaths (12). The famine spread to the Red Sea littoral. The Suakin authorities organized famine relief for the allied and enemy troops alike. The 'Dervish' forces who were a constant presence outside Suakin benefited equally from these relief efforts. During the same year, Cholera broke out and in 1892 the Russian/Asiatic influenza pandemic swept across the littoral, affecting many troops (13).

Dongola Expedition 1896, Nile Expedition &the Battle of Omdurman

Cholera again broke out and during the Dongola Expedition; many died, including Egyptian, Sudanese, and British soldiers and among them was Captain Roddy Owen, an amateur jockey who had won a Grand National. The battle of Atbara sealed the fate of the Khalifa. The battle of Omdurman lasted only a matter of hours, and by mid-day the Mahdist's troops were either slain, captured, or in retreat. Among those killed were several of the leading officers of the Khalifa's army, including his son, Osman 'Sheik el-Dien'. In the 'Sudan Despatches' by Lord Kitchener, he mentioned that there were 27 members of his army at the 'Battle of Omdurman' who were members of the RAMC. Among them were Lt-Colonel AT Sloggett, Lt SL Cummins, Major Bray, Captain Penton, and Major HB Mathias. Some of these RAMC doctors would remain in the Sudan and later would hold key positions in the health services after the process of the Reconquest came to an end (*vide infra*). The Khalifa retreated to Omdurman, which became subject to heavy bombardment that destroyed several key buildings, including the Tomb of the Mahdi. Then quietly the Khalifa slipped away, heading southwest to Kordofan to prepare himself for a second round with Kitchener. Members of the RAMC were heavily involved in the medical care of the wounded. Military correspondence during the campaign of 1896-1898 mentions several doctors who were actively involved in the campaign. In correspondence from Lord Kitchener to the War Office of Great Britain, in what later been known as 'The Sudan Despatches', he reported on the progress of the operations in 'the Soudan' subsequent to the defeat of the Khalifa at Omdurman. In one of these documents; Kitchener praised the courage of his fighting men, and particularly 'Captain Fleming' of the RAMC whose 'medical care of the troops was a decisive factor in the victory over Ahmed Fedail in fighting at Gedarif in December 1898'. In the same document, Kitchener went on to mention 'the officers who have distinguished themselves during the recent operations in the Sudan; a list containing three members of the RAMC, Lieutenant-Colonel J. A. Clery, Major G. D. Hunter, and Captain C. C. Fleming (14).

The material relating to the health of the nation in the immediate aftermath of Battle of Omdurman and in the following years was scarce. Some extracts from the entries of the Principal Medical Officer of the Egyptian Army, included as part of the Military Intelligence Reports (MIRs) and also in the 'Governor General Report', afford some insight into the development of the medical services by the RAMC. In the MIR 1898 & 1899, Colonel H. S. Penton, PMO of the Egyptian Army, wrote:

> To attempt the medical treatment of so vast a country is a daunting task' Following the Battle of Omdurman 4,000 of the Khalifa's Army surrendered. The number of those who were wounded or maimed was several thousand. In one record there were 1222 wounded who were later been given medical aid and treatment. Arrangement to aid those wounded were made initially in the first military field hospital which was established at Khor Shambat. (15)

Dr. Hassan effendi Zaki, the former prisoner and private physician of the Khalifa, was appointed medical superintendent of Omdurman, with a mandate to organise the attention paid to the wounded. The army facilitated Dr. Zaki's task by providing a large stock of dressings and surgical appliances needed for the wounded in Omdurman, who were present in every house there:

> ...upwards of 400 of the worst cases were tended; a large number of outpatients attended daily to have their wounds dressed; in

addition to the above many of the wounded were tended in their houses and every effort was made to alleviate their sufferings. All possible assistance was rendered by the Egyptian Army Medical Department by whom surgical appliances, fields dressings etc were freely provided and the efforts made to treat the wounded elicited their gratitude and surprise, affording a very agreeable contrast to the manner in which they were accustomed to be treated under the Khalifa rule. (16)

Section II:

The Pre-Civilian Medical Services:

Beyond Kerri: 'Medical Despatches' of the Military Intelligence Reports

Following the Battle of Omdurman (also known as the 'Battle of Karrari'), special attention was paid to sanitation. (Karari: is an area of low hills to the north of Omdurman. The battle of Omdurman is known to the Sudanese as the 'Battle of Karrari'). In the 1899 Governor General Annual Report, Major Penton, the PMO of the Egyptian army, wrote: 'Vast improvement[s] in sanitation have been effected in the town of Omdurman since its occupation by the Egyptian army. Its condition was such as to render it quite unfit for human habitation' (17). Other public health measures were related to vaccination against the menace of several illnesses, including smallpox. Since the nineteenth century, wave after wave of smallpox and cerebrospinal meningitis epidemics took place. Vaccinations against smallpox and meningitis were started immediately following the Reconquest, especially in Omdurman and Khartoum (18). In 1899, there was a serious outbreak of cerebrospinal meningitis outside Omdurman, but the town itself was not affected. Around 131 cases were diagnosed inside the town and those were traced to infections acquired outside the city. Colonel Penton referred to this epidemic in a subsequent report, stating that it has 'great mortality' outside Omdurman, but with the improvement of sanitation inside the town 'that there are grounds for believing it will, in the future, no longer be a cause of anxiety under the present improved conditions of sanitation' (19).

Some insight into the state of health and medical services in the period immediately after the Reconquest and beyond, until the formation of the civil medical department in 1904, could bc gained from the Sections of MIRs of the Egyptian Army dealing with medical matters. Those are usually written by the PMO of the Egyptian Army (EA) or by one of his subordinates from the military hierarchy. Those reports were usually meant for the Governor General, Lord Kitchener, and thereafter his successor, Sir Reginald Wingate.

In the first few reports, the focus was mainly if not exclusively on the 'health of the troops', although there is some evidence to show some health services being provided to the native Sudanese. Every part of the newly conquered territories was penetrated by the RAMC. These extracts give some insight into some of the problems encountered and into the health of the Sudanese people at the time. In these reports, the services of the RAMC, although intended primarily for the troops, was also tendered readily and willingly to the natives. Indeed, the medical service was used as a lever for 'pacifying the natives'. In the MIR of 1899, Major Hill Smith, RAMC, who accompanied the Sobat Expedition up the Sobat River in southern Sudan, wrote about how a hospital was established at Nasser and how the natives were still unfriendly. However, Kaim-makam* Maxe (Kaim-makam: Turkish military rank equal to Lt-Colonel) was in charge of a party that went up the Pibor (a tributary of the Sobat River) to the town of Waratong. He wrote:

> ...after this I offered medical treatment to the sick as I had brought a medical officer and a pannier for the purpose. Syphiltic ulcers, fevers, abscesses and infant mortality are the prevailing complaint' 'The medical officer was soon surrounded by an eager throng and the general effect of the visit was good. (20)

Bimbashi J. McArdle, Senior Medical Officer at El-Obeid, had one Egyptian Medical Officer. He stated that they established a field hospital under a canvas. He went on to request permission to establish a hospital of 'five beds' and introduce a wagon transport. He reported that guinea worms are common in the area (21). Lt-Colonel Penton, PMO, wrote in the MIR of 1900:

> ...there has been increase in sickness this year amongst the troops serving in the Sudan due to exceeding prevalence of 'malarial fever'. The rainfall was excessive throughout the Sudan, including Kordofan, White and Blue Nile and Kassala districts. During and immediately after the rains, the sick rate steadily rose, reaching its maximum in September and then slowly declined. The increase in sickness this year is certainly related to malarial fever both remittent and intermittent. (22)

By 1901, small civilian hospitals were built at Omdurman, Khartoum, Wadi Halfa, Berber, Dongola, Suakin, and Kassala (23). The incidence of 'infectious diseases' was reported to have decreased significantly among the civilian population, such that only 25 cases of smallpox occurred in the districts around Khartoum (probably reflecting easiness of reporting those) as compared to 131 cases in 1900. On sanitary measures, Colonel Penton stated:

> The Moudirieh* towns are kept clean. Surface cleaning is thoroughly carried out. The main difficulty is the disposal of sewage. In these towns, improvement[s] are yearly noticeable. Sanitary regulations cannot be rigidly reinforced in the Sudan. It is found impossible to control outlaying districts in the vast extent of the country, owing to the want of the government staff. (24)

Many of those who surrendered from the Khalifa army and taken prisoners were later used as a labour force in several ventures, including that of the 'Sudd Expedition' to clear the Sudd Swamp, which hinders navigation up the White Nile. The following extract gives insight into the state of medical care and the various health problems that were seen during that period, which witnessed continuous campaigns either to open more territories (e.g., Kordofan and the southern provinces) or to conduct special projects like the opening of the Sudd Swamp for navigation in the Upper Nile. In the medical report of the 'Sudd Cutting Expedition', the following entries appear:

> ....the Sudd Cutting Expedition under Major Peake, Kaimkam Dunn Bey SMO, with Selim Effendi Talhouk, Ibrahim Effendi Haddad and later Ibrahim Effendi Huzni (Syrian doctors). A section field hospital and medical orderlies accompanied the steamer south. Base camp hospital at Gabat al-Maghahid 7 miles north of junction of White Nile with Zeraf and separate hospitals for Dervish and military sick. On the journey up several cases of smallpox occurred and all women and children were vaccinated with poor results. Owing to the semi starvation of the Dervish prisoners when first taken there were numerous cases of sickness and five cases of deaths occurred on the journey besides others subsequently at the base camp. Dysentery, ulcers, and other diseases results of starvation were rife at first but the health of the

> prisoners under a three 'rotl*' daily issue of dura supplemented by meat when available. A small epidemic of smallpox followed by cerebrospinal meningitis took place but neither spread under the precautions taken. When rain commence in March fever increased, but at base camp fever not very great but reports from Fashoda says it was hot bed of fever. (rotl: Arabic=just over half a litre). 50 sick returned to Khartoum by Gayassa*. Parties working in the Sudd suffered from ulcers on legs and feet. Quinine was used prophylactically apparently with good results. Military hospital had 36 admissions and civilian 207, average daily sick military 2.63 and civilian 22.8. 35 deaths occurred among the civilians none in military. Diseases in civilian hospital; chickenpox 20, smallpox 3, wounds ulcers 53, malaria 23, dysentery 33, gangrene of legs 1, embolism 1, guinea worms 5, burns 8, syphilis 5, pneumonia 18, C.S.M. 7. Civilian death exhaustion 2, drowned 4, asphyxia 1, C.S.M 1, gangrene lung, 1, dysentery 13, chickenpox 2, embolism 1, pneumonia 4, malaria 2, rheumatic fever 1. (25)

By 1902, more sanitary work with significant improvement in sanitation was achieved in large towns. Vaccination campaigns against smallpox, which continued to be a major threat, had made a good start with positive effect, diminishing the number of cases. At Wadi Halfa a different outbreak occurred, caused by cholera, where nine cases were reported. It was assumed that the source of the cases could be traced to travellers coming from Egypt. During this outbreak, Mr James Currie, Director of Education, was temporarily in charge of the province and efforts to keep the outbreak at bay were successful. 'The natives' were having more confidence in the civil hospitals, which were providing services. This was reflected in the number of outpatient cases seen (26,591) and those who were managed as in-patients (2,396). In the MIRs of 1901 and 1902, mention of the need of more funds and more 'government staff' was made to reflect the 'ambition' to cover more territory and provide more services (26). In 1903, significant public health measures were carried out in the major cities of Khartoum, Kassala, el-Obeid, and the Blue and White Nile and Bahr el-Ghazal districts. This is best exemplified in the following extract:

> ...the destruction of mosquitoes and their larvae, draining operations and other measures in connection with the plan of

> campaign are being energetically carried out.....It is too early to expect any very striking improvements in the records of sickness , but already there are encouraging signs of the success of the system, and when thoroughly developed, I am confident that, in the larger and more important stations, there will be a marked diminution in the prevalence of fevers, which cause so much sickness amongst the troops and the civil population. (27)

By 1904, there were 10 hospitals, located at Omdurman, Khartoum, Berber, Halfa, Dongola, Suakin, Kassala, Wad Medani, Kodok, and el-Obeid. During that year, another hospital was under construction at Meroe (Dongola Province). Outdoor relief was given to civilians in stations where there was a military hospital (e.g., Gedaref). In that year the number of in-patients was increased to 967, compared to those recorded for 1903. For outpatients the number increased to 3,867. In that year, Lt-Colonel Penton pointed out the need to consider building a large hospital in Khartoum. Public health measures which spanned several towns in the country coincided with those carried out by Dr. Andrew Balfour, the Director of the 'Wellcome Tropical Research Laboratory', who was appointed as Medical Officer of Health of Khartoum. He worked totally independent from the military personnel. As early as 1903, efforts to eradicate mosquitoes and curb the menace of 'malarial fever' (sic) had begun. 'Mosquito Brigades' were formed in several large towns, including el-Obeid and Kassala, in addition to Khartoum and other towns in the Blue and White Nile provinces (28). Efforts to conduct regular drainage of rainwater with 'improvement of the drainage that have been of the greatest value and productive of excellent results', as quoted in the the preceding text (29). Vaccination against smallpox was introduced earlier, in 1902, to try to curb the outbreak of those epidemics, which had been the norm for several decades in the Sudan. The available vaccine against smallpox, utilizing 'calf lymph' (the old vaccine against smallpox), was brought from Cairo, but transport and ensuring the 'cold chain', proved difficult resulting in significant loss of potency. In 1904, vaccination campaigns yielded better results, with successful vaccination of 11,929 subjects after arrangements were made to obtain 'calf lymph' packed in ice from Cairo . To improve the yield of vaccination and boost the number of people vaccinated, local barbers were trained to carry out this task, from 1903, and with their help regular vaccination campaigns continued to be conducted in the principal towns in the North. By 1904, vaccination campaigns were extended to Bahr el-Ghazal in Southern Sudan. However, smallpox was reported to be still a major communicable disease in Sudan. In 1905, a total of 49,000 were vaccinated as compared to 12,000 in 1904 and 7,000 in 1907, but Smallpox was still reported to be a major communicable disease in Sudan (30).

Another major communicable disease in addition to malaria and smallpox was venereal diseases, which had a high prevalence. In 1904, Colonel Penton writes: 'I regret to say that VD shows no sign of abatement. This is the prevailing course of the Sudan, and efforts in attempting to combat it are prodigious' (31). In 1905, a total of 5 provinces were reported to be free of malaria, and these included Khartoum (mainly due to the efforts of Dr. Balfour and his Mosquito Brigade; see Part V), Berber, Dongola, Halfa, and Suakin. Registration for 'Births and Deaths' began in 1904, and this was initially conducted by 'barbers' trained to carry to carry out this job, along with vaccination, but it was stated that, due to insufficient staff, this was found to be unreliable (32).

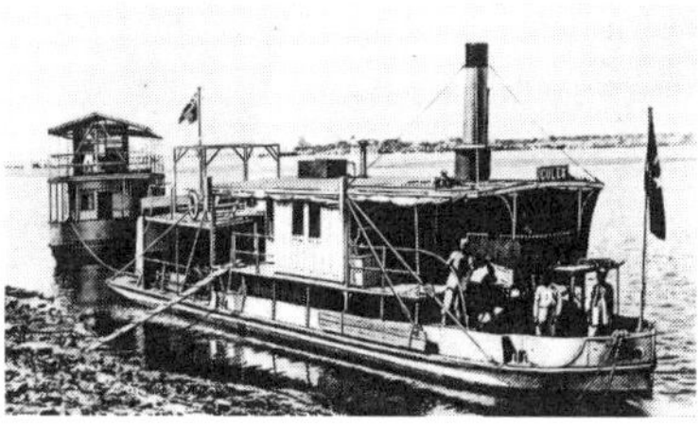

Chapter 2

The Forgotten Pioneers: Egyptians & Syrians in Service

In the period that immediately followed the Battle of Omdurman, the number of medical doctors in the RAMC who were seconded to the Egyptian Army, seeing active medical service in the Sudan, were quite few. With the policy of 'pacification of the natives' and the opening of the rest of the provinces of the old Turco-Egyptian Sudan, and with the subsequent expansion of the service, there was a need for more human resources to meet the challenges that lay ahead. For various reasons, the Egyptian military doctors were reluctant to work in the Sudan. Such a trend was not new. Since the era of Turco-Egyptian rule, service in the Sudan was considered a punishment and exile by most if not all of the Egyptian professionals and military personnel. By then, compared to Egypt, the country was backward and diseases that could be lethal were rife. These facts were deeply embedded in the subconscious of the Egyptian people. The newly inaugurated government of the Anglo-Egyptian Sudan was faced with the demand to man the outlaying stations with doctors, an obligation that it found difficult to fulfill. Faced by the paucity of the British and the reluctance of the Egyptians, it had to look elsewhere for recruitment. The market that proved to be vital to satisfy the need of the medical services turned out to be in the 'old Syrian' medical schools (33). The Syrian doctors that were recruited were, like their British counterparts, employed by the Egyptian Army and then seconded to the Sudan Government. All were given a military rank and were sent to man the peripheral small hospitals established in various provinces. Further, they became of special help serving in southern Sudan, where the military medical personnel continued to deliver services in solo, with no role for the civil medical personnel to play till the late 1920s. The only exception was the services foiled by the hospital ship, 'Lady Baker', manned by civilian medical personnel, which was introduced in the early 1920s to cover the areas of southern Sudan, which could only be circumnavigated.

For many years to follow, funding of the health service in the vast wilderness of the Sudan was a real dilemma. The British, at the core of their administrative policy, were not inclined to spend much on public services. Whatever was available was run on a 'shoestring budget'. Here I am quoting Heather Bell in her treatise, 'Frontiers of Medicine in the Anglo-Egyptian Sudan' (34). Under the heading o 'Medical & Sanitary Department', the following is extracted from the MIR of 1904:

> Wants of funds has hitherto prevented any establishment of British Medical officers for the civil medical requirement of the Sudan, but from the beginning 1904 two British Inspectors, Doctors Christopherson and Crispin were appointed. The former as Senior Inspector at Khartoum, and the later at Wadi Halfa. This beginning of the civil medical organization has already been productive of great benefit, and in the coming year it is hoped that the staff may be further increased. At out stations the civil work is still supervised by the AMCs. The recent journey of PMO, Lt-Col Penton to Beyrouth, will, it is anticipated, be productive of good results in this respect. (35)

The Syrian doctors were recruited from the graduates of two medical schools in Beirut. The first was the Syrian Protestant College, which later became part of the American University of Beirut. The second was the French Medical School in Beirut (36). At the inception of the SMD in 1904, there were only a few Egyptian doctors working in Khartoum under the guidance of Dr. J.B. Christopherson, its first director. Their number increased in January 1905 by 4 more doctors, who were freshly recruited from Beirut (see Part IV, SMD). By 1908, the number of those Syrian doctors reached more than 30, as compared to only 6 British doctors (37). It was an irony that the Egyptian doctors were quite few in comparison with the Syrians, despite the disapproving 'hum hum' that continued to echo from Cairo.

> As complaints are sometimes made in Egypt about the number of the Syrians who are employed in the Sudan, I may mention that every endeavour has been made to attract Egyptian doctors to that country, but without success. The result is that, the Government of the Sudan has been obliged to fall back upon the Syrian supply. (38)

By 1905, the first wave of those recurits were in the service of the SMD. These were Drs Mohamed Bey Nikhlawi, Selim Yusuf Atiyeh, Selim Taniuos Ghusun, and Mikhaiel Sughayur. They were followed by Yuzbashi Suliman Eff. Salibi (recruited in March 1905), Dr. Selim Eff. Sagh (recruited in May 1905), and finally, in the same year, Dr. Khalil Effendi. Magid Khouri was the last one to join, on December 24, 1905 (39). In general, the records related to those Syrian doctors are meager and, if found, very much rudimentary. You may find nothing except names, dates of appointment, dispension (*sic*), or resignation. From the limited information obtained, those doctors were recruited as early as 1899. Before the establishment of the SMD, all these Syrians were recruited to the military medical services, Egyptian Army Medical Corps, given a military rank as Yuzbashi (Turkish military title equivalent to Captain), and then appointed to the rank of medical officer (MO). They were almost always subordinate to the British medical doctors (who were, as a rule, appointed as Senior Medical Officers (SMOs). They would then be seconded to the service of the Sudan Government. Further, as a general rule, each British medical officer was assisted by one or more of the Syrian MOs, depending upon the size of the hospital and how large the province under his domain was. Large stations were staffed by one British doctor and several Syrian assistants (40). The small stations in the provinces would only be staffed by one or more Syrian doctors, depending on the size of the station and the load of work. Even sometimes the presence of a military and a civilian hospital would be under one Syrian doctor as in the case of the town of Gedaref in 1909-1910 (41). Such arrangements appeared to have been rather arbitrary and depended very much upon the availability of enough medical staff, which was a sticky issue. The British MOs had the task of conducting inspection visits on regular basis. Captain William Byam, Senior military MO at Kassala (1908-1911), like his predecessor Captain Leonard Bousfield (1905-1908), was the only British military doctor in the whole of Kassala Province. In his autobiography, he wrote about the frequent inspection visits he conducted to the stations under his responsibility at Gedaref, Gallabat, and Mefaza (42). In 1909, when he went out to inspect the station at Gallabat, he had one Syrian subordinate, Dr. Anton Hanna, who manned the hospital there. When Dr. Byam established the first leper colony in Sudan at Galabat during that visit, Dr. Hanna was left to look after both the hospital and the leper colony.

At the inception of the SMD, the position of the Syrian doctors remained the same. The Principal MO of the Egyptian Army Medical Corps (EAMC) continued to have the responsibility of recruiting and interviewing the Syrian doctors for both the civil and the military sectors of the service. That was usually conducted at Beirut. Those selected for the civilian service, the SMD, would continue to be subordinates to the British doctors, as stated earlier. However, it was not clear what governed the working relationship between the two. The author also found no records of their exact number and the locations where they worked. A few names filtered out in various documents. After more robust records began in the 1920s, appointment lists were usually a routine enclosure of the annual reports of the SMD and its successor, the SMS. According to Paul Squires, by 1908 the total number of Syrian doctors reached thirty (43). Between 1908 and 1922, the accountability and administrative 'umbrella' of those Syrian doctors were less clear. However, one has to remember the fact that, following the firing of Dr. Christopherson, the first director of the SMD, in 1908, the military doctors were very much in control of the service. This status quo continued until 1917, when re-organization of the service took place and the 'civilian SMD was reborn'. Between 1904 and the first wave of expansion and recruitment of more British doctors in 1919 and beyond, the Syrian doctors outnumbered their British counterparts. One could argue that the health service in the Sudan (both in the civilian and the military sections) was practically carried out by those Syrian doctors. Most of the military doctors who were manning the small hospitals of the 'Borders Region' (Kassala, Darfur) and the whole of the southern provinces (Mongalla, Bahr el-Ghazal, and Upper Nile) was composed primarily, if not exclusively, of Syrians. Furthermore, the core of the doctors on the Sleeping Sickness Commission (established in 1905) also comprised mainly Syrians (see Part VI). One of them, Dr. Derwish Baz, went on to be a leading expert in the field of sleeping sickness. Further, of special note, he was the first to hold the post of Senior Medical Officer among the Syrians. In recognition of his contribution to the service, he was awarded an MBE in the 1930s (44). The Annual Report of the SMD of 1923 included an announcement of the new medical staff who had been appointed in 1922 and 1923. These included the medical officers, Dr. Daud Eff. Salman and Dr. Ibrahim Eff. Malhama, as well as the resignation and the discharge of Drs Habib Bey Khalil, Marcos Eff. Butros, and Bishara Eff. Asaad Moutran. From that year till the late 1930s, similar announcements were regularly posted in the Annual Reports of the Sudan Medical Services (45).

The quality of those Syrian doctors was variable. This is well represented in the statement of Dr. William Byam, a British military doctor who worked in Sudan from 1908 to 1914. He writes in his autobiography: 'The Syrian doctors who had served under me varied greatly in ability and character. Some, like Ibrahim Abu Haider, were capable and trustworthy. By contrast, Musa Zacharia was a scoundrel, who knew I knew he was a scamp' (46).

Following the assassination of Sir Lee Stack in Cairo by an Egyptian nationalist, the Egyptian troops were expelled in November 1924. In that year, a pure Sudanese battalion was formed. That battalion metamorphosed into the future Sudan Defense Force (SDF). The 'old' Egyptian Army Medical Corps in the Sudan became the SDF Medical Corps in 1924. Beyond 1924, the Syrian military doctors who worked in Egypt continued to form part of the cadre of the SDF Medical Corps. By the mid to late 1930s, when the Sudanese graduates of the Kitchener School of Medicine were coming up through the ranks, the recruitment of Syrian doctors ceased. Most of the Syrian doctors went back home; however, a few stayed behind and embraced the Sudan as their adopted country. Of these we can trace a few names. Dr. Selim Bey Yusuf Atiyah and Dr. Rene Malouf. Dr. Selim Bey Yususf Attiya was a Syrian physician who was educated at Syrian Protestant College (later American University of Beirut) and in the USA. He later served in the Egyptian Army Medical Corps till 1904. He then transferred to the Sudan Government Service. He worked as MO in charge of hospitals at Wadi Halfa and Omdurman from 1905 to 1920. His brother, Samwil Bey Atiyah, a graduate of the same College in Beirut, was among the first to serve in the Intelligence Department of the Sudan Government in 1899. He was succeeded by his nephew, Edward Atiyah (son of Salim Atiyah). Edward was educated at Victoria College, Alexandria (a prestigious school in that day) and Oxford, later became a teacher at GMC, and mentored the prolific Sudanese writer, Muawia Nur. He wrote two books, *An Arab Tells His Story* (47), and *The Black Vanguard* (48). Edward later in his life moved to England where he died in 1964. His son, Michael Atiyah, became one the most celebrated mathematicians of his time. He became the Principal of Trinity College, Cambridge (1990-1999) and was later knighted (50).

Like doctors, other healthcare professionals were also recruited from Syria, especially dispensers (pharmacists). Here one must mention a notable Syrian, George Morhig. Morhig came to Sudan as an officer in the Egyptian Army. He was attached to the GMC, where he was trained by Dr. Andrew Balfour as a dispenser. With Dr. Balfour's support, Morhig studied pharmacy in London. He subsequently established the first modern pharmacy in the Sudan, in 1907. Further, he was also running the pharmacy of Khartoum Civil Hospital and was involved in the famous dispute between Dr. Christopherson and the ruling hierarchy (51). The 'Morhig Pharmacy' at Khartoum, in its heyday, was second to none in the whole of Africa and the Middle East. It continued to be a model of private pharmacies in the Sudan till the 1970s, when, following the *coup de ètat* by Colonel Gaafer Numerie, the pharmacy and business of George Morhig's family were confiscated to satisfy the slogans of the communist propaganda adopted by the dictator's regime and his junta. George's son, Alfred Morhig, and the rest of his family left Sudan once and for all to settle initially in the UK, and later in New York (52) (Hadi Stambolia, personal communication) (53).

'Dr. Christopherson's Brigade'

Dr. Hassan Effendi Zaki was in the service of the Turco-Egyptian government before the Mahdiyya uprising. When Charles Gordon became Governor General of Sudan in 1883-1885, Zaki was chosen as his physician. He remained in Khartoum during the siege and, following the fall of Khartoum, he was captured and was later taken as private physician of the Mahdi. He nursed the Mahdi during his mortal illness and probably he was the one who had most of the knowledge of the exact cause of the short illness that led the Mahdi's demise. Zaki thereafter became physician to the Khalifa. He was the sole physician at Omdurman Hospital during the regime of the Mahdiyya, 1885-1898. Dr. Musa Abdalla Hamid and Dr. Kamal Salih, in their 'Omdurman Hospital chronicle, *Omdurman Teaching Hospital: Past, Present and Future*, published in 1986 in Arabic, stated that:

> Dr. Hassan Zaki, an Egyptian doctor was formerly private physician to Gordon Pasha and then he was private physician to The Mahdi. Dr.. Zaki asserts: 'I was physician to the Khalifa and I was very close to him. After the fall of Khartoum, the Khalifa ordered me to move to Omdurman, and I obeyed. I was given a house at 'Hillat Fanger' a suburb which lies between Khor Abu Anga and Alumarra neighborhood. The Khalifa organized two clinics where patients used to come and consult me. One clinic was in Alshuhadaa and the other was at Alshajarra suburb'. Following the Reconquest by Kitchener he was re-instated in the Egyptian Army Medical Corps and was assigned to re-open the hospital at Khartoum. He was the 'Hakim-Bashi'of the hospital from 1900 to 1908. (54)

At Khartoum Hospital, Zaki was a close friend and confidante of Dr. John Brian Christopherson.

At Khartoum Civil Hospital, there were other Syrian and Egyptian doctors who worked under Dr. Christopherson. We don't have much information about those doctors, at best only names and a few personal details. From a circular letter sent from Dr.Christopherson, to around 20 Syrian and Egyptian medical officers who were working in various districts of the Sudan early in 1908, we could find only names and place of employment, but no other details. Dr. Christopherson was apparently requesting information on various subjects, including native remedies, tribal markings, and circumcision of female children, as well tribal customs (55). The replies included letters from several of them. Names included a few doctors who were working in the northern Riverain districts, including Dr. Habib Suaadi, MO at Wadi Halfa; Dr. W. B. Haddad, MO at Dongola; Dr. J. Maschariff, MO at Merowe; and finally, Dr. Nicola K. Malouf, MO at Atbara. Replies from MOs who were working in the Blue Nile Province came from several of Dr. Christopherson's subordinates. Those included Dr. Tawfik Rasi, MO at Singa; Dr. Dr. Asaad Qamar, MO at Wad Medani; and Dr. M Zughayar, MO at el-Obeid. Some other MOs' locations could not be ascertained. Names included Dr. H. M. Khoury, Dr. Ghosa, and Dr. Salim Saigh. The list also included Drs Hassan Jehr and Dr. Jamal, from Khartoum Civil Hospital (56).

Colonel William Byam, one of the most prominent RAMC doctors, who worked at Kassala and then at Khartoum Military Hospital, performed impressive public health work at Kassala in 1908. In his quest to control malaria in the town, he was assisted greatly by his Syrian MO, Dr. Asad Malouf (57). In a rather different encounter at Qalabat, a small town on the border with Ethiopia, Byam established the first leper colony in the Sudan with a generous donation from his mother. After establishing that colony, Byam assigned his Syrian subordinate, stationed at Qalabat, Dr. Anton Hanna, to continue to look after patients there (58). When Byam was assigned to accompany a military patrol to punish the Anuak tribe in 1912, he established a small hospital in Akobo Post (which later grew into an important town in that part of southern Sudan). He was assisted there by a Syrian MO, 'Yuzbashi' Ibrahim Abu Haider (59). Following that mission, Byam became seriously sick, was later rescued and treated back at Khartoum Military Hospital, and was nursed during his recovery from severe pneumonia by an Egyptian doctor called Rushdi (60).

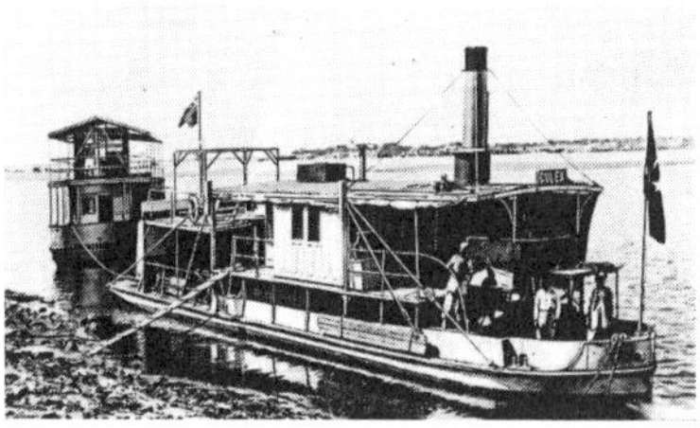

Chapter 3

The Beginnings of the Civilian Medical Services: The Sudan Medical Department, 1904-1924

Section I:

Christopherson, Crispin & the Sudan Medical Department: 1904-1909

The story of how the Sudan Medical Department came into existence is rather blurred. Surfing through the detailed records of Sir Reginald Wingate, the Sirdar and Governor General of the Sudan, kept at the Sudan Archives in Durham, gives no specific correspondence in dealing with the early foundation of the SMD. The country was *de facto* under military rule. It was another irony that it took over six years after the Reconquest of the Sudan for the SMD to come into existence. However, it should be remembered that the medical department was the first governmental department to pass to the civilian control. As mentioned earlier, the medical services in the interim were delivered mainly by the members of the Royal Army Medical Corps who were normally seconded to the EAMC and then employed by the Sudan Government. However, another crucial factor was the fact that Sudan was run on a very tight budget throughout the first two decades of the Condominium rule. Very little money was allocated to health, education, and other public services (1,2). Heather Bell (1999) in her excellent thesis stated that 'conquest and administration including services was done with little resources and few staff and run with 'shoestring' budgets' (3). The administrative system started as military and continued as such for several years. Even when civilians assumed responsibility, the military control continued, for various reasons. Furthermore, the civilian control, which was more or less limited, didn't last long and the military personnel continued to run the business following professional feuds and personality clashes.

The well documented evidence for the earlier foundation of the SMD was related to the 'appointment blunder' that accompanied its birth and the bitter personal feud that followed between Dr. Edward Crispin and Dr. John Brian Christopherson (4,5). The term 'appointment blunder' was used by Ann Crichton-Harris, who carried out painstaking research while writing the biography of her great uncle, Dr. John Brian Christopherson (6, 7). The story as recorded initially by Dr. Squires and later by Ms. Crichton-Harris, centred on the fact that the same post of the director of the newly established SMD was offered to both Dr. Christopherson and his colleague and later adversary Dr. Crispin. That created a rivalry which went on to engulf the newly established department. It transpired that the post of the director of the SMD was offered to Dr. Christopherson by Dr. Theodore Dyk Acland, who was the medical advisor to the Governor General, Sir Francis Reginald Wingate. Acland was then the Principal of the EAMC. At the same time, the same post was offered to Dr. Crispin by the Principal of the EAMC in the Sudan, Colonel Penton, who also accepted the offer. Eventually it was decided that Christopherson was more suitable for the post. Crispin, obviously resentful, threatened to resign in protest, but he was persuaded to take the post of a senior medical officer at Port Sudan (which by then was under construction) (8). According to Daly, the first director of the civil SMD was Colonel C. D. Hunter Bey, who became the director from March 1905, and Christopherson 'was fobbed off with the distinction of 'Physician to H. E. the Governor General in Khartoum'. Christopherson became officially the Director from January 1907 (9). One could argue that that 'appointment blunder' was the key factor in delaying the potential of the SMD to have 'springboard' beginnings, as it crippled its efficiency and led eventually to the department being placed under the control of military doctors of the RAMC until 1917.

According to Squires (10) and Robert Kirk (11), the first Civilian British doctors to join the Sudan were three. They were all recruited, primarily by Dr. Theodore Dyck Acland in 1901. The first of them was Dr. E. A. Gates, OBE, who was placed initially at Omdurman and then worked at Kassala. He left after one year and later established himself in a first-class West End practice in London. He also acted as a member of the Egyptian Medical Board in London (12). The second was Dr. Webb Jones, who stayed for only few months at Wadi Halfa, and returned to take the post of a surgeon at Alexandria. The third was Dr. Edward Smyth Crispin, who joined the service on January 13, 1901, followed by Dr. John Brian Christopherson, who joined on June 10, 1902 (13). Shortly after, in January 1903, Dr. Andrew Balfour took up his post as the first Director of the WTRL (see Part IV). Balfour, when he agreed to take up this post, was to set up, with Henry Wellcome, an agreement with the Sudan Government that the laboratory was to be administered separately from the rest of the medical services, so he was never under the domain of the military or the subsequent civil medical administrations. In fact, WTRL was placed under nominal administration by Mr (later Sir) James Currie, Director of the Department of Education (14). That arrangement was probably made because there was no civilian medical department at the time. Further, the laboratory was physically hosted on the premises of GMC. James Currie was the first Principal of GMC. Ann Crichton-Harris and Patrick D'Arcy would argue that Balfour may have sensed some troubles looming on the horizon (15, 16). Despite Balfour's being appointed as Khartoum Medical Officer of Health (Public Health Physician), he continued to function completely independently from his other colleagues in Khartoum (see Part IV). When he left in 1913, the job was passed to his friend and 'confidante', Dr. Leonard Bousfield, of the RAMC. Such an appointment may not have been arbitrary in view what occurred in the 'state of the relationship' between Christopherson and Balfour beyond 1908. The public health services in Khartoum would continue under the directorship of Dr. Bousfield until his retirement in 1922. Following this, the post moved under civilian control following establishment of the Sudan Medical Services in 1924 (17).

The civilian SMD first came into existence in March 1904. As mentioned earlier, some sources suggested that Christopherson was only 'acting director' and did not become full director until late in 1905. It was argued that the first director of SMD was not Dr. Christopherson, but Colonel G. D. Hunter, who was the Principal of EAMC. It was possible that Colonel Hunter took over from Lt-Col Penton, the first PMO of the Egyptian Army in Sudan. At its inauguration, the SMD had only three civilian doctors (Christopherson, Crispin, and Hodson), nine or ten Syrian and Egyptian doctors, a few clerks and other employees, and a total of ten hospitals. Khartoum, Port Sudan and Berber Hospitals were under the civilian SMD, and the remaining seven hospitals were under the military doctors of the RAMC (*vide infra*). The work of the medical services in the capital, Khartoum, was shared between Dr. Christopherson and the rest of the military doctors of the RAMC. The information relating to those military doctors is scarce and piecemeal. Limited information could be found about only a handful of them. Among the names that could be traced were Dr. Stevenson Lyle Cummins, who was Senior MO of Khartoum in 1903 (18), and Dr. Penton, who was the first PMO of the EA in the Anglo-Egyptian Sudan. Penton was succeeded by Colonel Hunter Bey, possibly late in 1904. In later years they had Drs Leonard Bousfield (who moved from Kassala to Khartoum in 1908), Dr. Gaymeor Anderson, and Dr. William Byam (who also moved from Kassala to Khartoum, in 1911). However, the main support for Dr. Christopeherson was his 'loyal bandits', the veteran Egyptian, Syrian, and Lebanese doctors. Those were Drs Hassan Zaki, Hassan Lebib, Nikhlawi, Nicola Malouf, Sasson, Izzaldien, Abdelateef, and others (Christopherson & staff at Khartoum Civil Hospital, 1912) (see List of Illustrations).

At the birth of the SMD, there were already several small hospitals, which were established in 1900-1901 at Khartoum, Omudurman, Wadi Halfa, Berber, Dongola, Suakin, and Kassala. The bulk of these hospitals were staffed and run by the military for years to come according to a specific agreement (19, 20). The bed capacity of these hospitals was very limited, mostly around 40-50 beds per hospital. By 1904, more hospitals were opened, at Wad Medani, El-Obeid, and Kodok, and another one later at Merowe. By 1906 the number of the British doctors rose to six and the Syrian/Egyptian doctors rose to 20 in addition to three pharmacists (21). Dr. Vincent S. Hodson was the only civilian doctor north of Khartoum, assuming full responsibility for 'Berber Province'. He was based at Atbara. Hodson joined SMD on October 22, 1903. Later he was to replace Dr. Christopherson as the Director of Khartoum Civil Hospital (*vide infra*). In 1905 Dr. Norman E. Waterfield joined the service and, after spending the period up to 1908 at Khartoum working alongside Dr. Christopherson, he was posted to Port Sudan to replace Edward Crispin, who moved to Khartoum as Senior Medical Inspector and then Assistant Director to Colonel Mathias. This followed the dispute between Dr. Christopherson and the military administrative hierarchy, which resulted in his dismissal. Waterfield remained at Port Sudan until he retired from the Sudan service in 1922. In 1905, Dr. Oliver Francis Atkey was recruited, and in 1908 Dr. Herbert Chavasse (Paul) Squires joined in to fill the vacant post of Dr. Nedwell, who had spent only one year at Kassala and then left for Britain. The last of the British doctors to be recruited was Dr. George R. Footner, who joined the service in 1909, employed primarily by the Sudan Government Railways during the extension of the railway line to Kosti and then to El-Obeid. Footner went on to join the SMD formally in 1911. By 1909 there were only six civilian British doctors and the number of the Syrian/Egyptian doctors rose to 30 (22). Those continued to run the service till after the First World War, when more funds became available and more doctors were recruited to meet the demands of the expansion of the health services. By 1904, the building of a new port for the Sudan had just begun, financed by a loan from the Egyptian Government. The hospitals at Dongola, Wadi Halfa, Suakin, and Kassala were all staffed by Syrian doctors. Dr. Selim Bey Atiyeh was the doctor responsible for Wadi Halfa Hospital (23). Dr. Oliver Francis Atkey joined the service in 1905, and he assumed responsibility as senior medical inspector of the Blue Nile Province based at Wad Medani. The hospital there was built in 1904.

The headquarters of the SMD was stationed at Khedive Square (later named the Khartoum Central Bus Station). The structure, scope, and hierarchy of the SMD at its beginnings was not clear. From the limited information available it appears that the service was rather rudimentary in scope and had very limited resources. Furthermore, its hierarchy was very much overshadowed by the military medical personnel (who were running the show in most of the country). The resources allocated to this newly created civil department were smaller than those allocated to the military medical department of the EA. Even those allocated to the latter were meager and its PMO continued to complain about lack of resources and 'wants of funds and staff' in his annual reports (24). On the other hand, the exact relationship and interface between the newly formed civil department and that of the military medical department is difficult to tease out from the available records. However, we do know about the territorial responsibility of each department. The major responsibility for health seems to lie within the military department, and this is supported by some scattered records. Annual reports written by the PMO of the EA in the first few years following the Reconquest shed some light on the 'public health and sanitation' of the Anglo-Egyptian Sudan. At the beginning, at least, Dr. Christopherson, the Director, appeared to have enjoyed a somewhat good relationship with Colonel Penton, PMO of the EA. The annual reports written by the latter continued to include statements of praise for the 'efforts of… and ...the most indefatigable energy and skills of Dr. Christopherson, who with the small means at his disposal has produced excellent results and has gone far to gain the confidence of the inhabitants' (25). Also, it seems that the official records of the civil department were placed under the umbrella of the military department, probably because the 'regime was still a military one of an occupying force'. On the other hand, the annual reports of the PMO continued to make references to the reports/statement of the activities of the director of the SMD, Dr. Christopherson. There were no separate reports or supplements by the director of the SMD in those MIRs. In 1905, the PMO Annual Report contained the following statement:

> Dr. Christopherson, the Head of the Civil MD writes hopefully about public health: (It is possible to strike a cheerful chord this year. The Sudan is not the fever-stricken, smallpox ravaged country, into which the 'Egyptian' diseases {ophthalmia, bilharzia and ankylostoma} are rapidly being introduced, while sleeping sickness is advancing , cholera and plague threatening Port Sudan and leprosy creeping in from the west. (26)

In the beginning, the civilian doctors were given a military rank and were under the umbrella of the military administration until the creation of the civil department. They initially enjoyed 'partial autonomy', but this didn't last for long. The policy of delivering the health service by way of 'pacification of the natives' seems to have been the mindset of the administration (27). The 1905 Annual Report contained the following statement:

> ...two areas still not easy to pacify the natives via providing medical services. Bahr el-Ghazal, where it is still difficult to get to the custom of the people, and the Eastern Sudan where people there are still timid and suspicious.

On the other hand, and by way of a corollary, a native correspondent of the *Sudan Times* asserted:

> ...a few years back, the arrival of the medical officer in the village meant a general alarm; everybody sought a hiding place. Now things have changed in 'such a manner that native patients flocked to the hospital to be treated. (28)

In the first few years, however, well before the establishment of the SMD, there were no formal nurses in various hospitals, and hospital orderlies, especially males, were used as attendants. They were taught by apprenticeship and no formal courses were given (see section on nurses training). Even recruitment of these hospital orderlies was a painstaking task; only a few illiterate men were provided in the first few years and only after much persuasion by the first Director, Dr. Christopherson (29). Overall, few female hospital orderlies were employed, due to a variety of reasons, especially the cultural and the conservative Islamic traditions of the Sudanese natives at the time. Some female orderlies were employed as early as 1903 in the old Khartoum Civil Hospital, which was stationed in a rented house of the Greek merchant Ortolani. They were few in number and were also used to sort problems stemming from cultural misconceptions about medical treatment held by Sudanese female patients. They were called '*Hakeema*' by the natives (30). The recruitment of proper nurses took some time, and formal training of nurses in the Sudan did not begin until 1925. By 1907, the volume of work in the civil hospitals had grown enormously, and during that year the first British nurse, Miss Maria Pye Moore, joined the SMD (31). The PMO Annual Report for 1906 contained the interesting remarks by Dr. Christopherson:

> Sudanese have been drinking too much of the local liquor called Merissa. This is very considerable. Some measureS were to be implemented to control the 'merissa shops' has been sought of by the Governor General!! Dr. Christopherson stated that Sudanese drinks very little of the imported liquor. (32)

In that year, a total of 94,051 patients were seen as outpatients and those seen as inpatients reached 7,266. In that year also, the first case of 'Malta fever' in the Sudan was reported, from Kassala, due to 'goat's milk' consumption. A total of nearly 50,000 patients were vaccinated against smallpox and at Suakin, the port of exit and entry for pilgrims, every effort was made to prevent the entry of cholera from '*Hedjaz*' (sic). In 1908, Dr. Christopherson, the Director, reported minor outbreaks of cerebrospinal meningitis (CSM), infectious pneumonia, smallpox, chickenpox, diphtheria, dengue fever, and some sporadic cases of Kala-azar, 'black water fever', and Malta Fever. At Khartoum, Dr. Christopherson treated five cases of Kala-azar; however, an outbreak of several cases occurred in Kassala, and a medical officer was sent there to investigate this outbreak (33). The number of those seen as outpatients reached 121,214 and those seen as inpatients rose to 7,000. In that year, Dr. Herbert Chavasse (Paul) Squires joined the services of the SMD and was initially based at Khartoum. In that year, Captain William Byam, RAMC, joined the service, replacing Dr. Leonard Bousfield at Kassala. In the same year, the second British nurse, Miss Jones, joined the service of the

SMD. She had received her training at St Thomas's Hospital in London (34). In Dr. Christopherson's view, however, 'so far they have been a failure as regards training for nurses is concerned, they are indolent, incapable of learning and quite unfit to be left in charge' (35). During that year, the work of building new hospitals that had begun earlier in Khartoum, Atbara, and Port Sudan was nearly completed.

It worth noting that, from the available records, the exact duties of the director of the SMD and the scope and limitations of his authority were unclear. His influence was rather restricted, and he was more or less under the umbrella of the military hierarchy. Furthermore, his relationship with his subordinates, only a few of whom were British, but many were Syrian and Egyptian, was not clear. The extent to which he had a free hand to plan for healthcare delivery was also unclear. Possibly in view of all these limitations, plus other confounding factors dealing with personality clashes, personal feuds, and the personality makeup of Dr. Christopherson himself, and following intense dispute with the supreme military hierarchies, in 1908 he was dismissed from his post as Director of SMD (36). Christopherson was replaced by Colonel H. B. Mathias, the Principal MO of the EAMC. Christopherson was transferred to the post of Director of Khartoum & Omdurman Hospitals. Dr. Edward Crispin was appointed as Assistant Director to Colonel Mathias.

The way doctors were recruited to the service was rather interesting. It began as a rudimentary process in the first few years, stemming from the fact that the service, at its inception, was very limited. As the military personnel had the upper hand in running affairs, the recruitment was mainly through the military establishment. That continued till the inter-war period, when more autonomy for the civil department began to take shape. Indeed, immediately after the Reconquest, the principal person in charge of the recruitment process of the British medical staff was Dr. Theodore Dyck Acland. Acland, through his personal relationship with the Governor General, Sir Francis Reginald Wingate, was in full charge of this process. However, it seems that the PMO of the EA also had some delegated authority to recruit staff for the service in Sudan, but that could have been primarily in the military. Dr. Byam, in his autobiography, *The Road to Harley Street*, mentioned the way he was recruited to the service via Colonel Lyle Cummins, then the acting PMO of the EA (37). On the other hand, the 'appointment blunder' incident, mentioned earlier, reflects the lack of clarity of that process in the first five years. After 1911, Acland became the official representative of the Sudan Government in London, and he quite possibly remained the one, and the only one, through whom any recruitment of staff occurred until 1928, when he was succeeded by Dr. Vincent Hodson (38). Simon Mullan, in his interesting research of the subject, advocated the hypothesis of the 'Gentlemanly Order' proposed by Cain and Hopkins when they examined the British Imperial workforce (39, 40). That process was primarily linked to 'networking' and 'personal recommendations' that persisted well into the 1940s. The notable urologist, Dr. Kenneth Owen, who worked in the SMS from 1945 to 1948, went to Sudan through the influence of his mentor and his network. In a personal interview with the author, the late Dr. Owen stated that he was mainly tempted by one of his mentors who had links with Dr. Finlay Mayne, the Senior Surgeon of the SMS in the inter-war period. Dr. Owen has also alluded to this in his personal memoir of his life and times in the Sudan. In his article 'Sudan Interlude' he writes:

> It is hard to recall the factors influencing a decision to join the Sudan Medical Service. Dickson Wright* was encouraging, having heard something of the service from Finlay Mayne* who had been the senior surgeon in Khartoum.... It had a high reputation and was said in its earlier days to be 'the most highly qualified in the world. This judgment unlike the claim by recent ministers that the NHS is the best in the world, was factually based, the Sudan Medical Service having the highest number of doctors with higher qualifications. (41) (See Volume 2.)

On the other hand, the recruitment of the non-British staff, primarily Syrians and Egyptians, was directly under the domain of the PMO of the EA. Worth noting is that British doctors, when recruited, were generally young and at the beginning of their careers. That was also applicable to those who were recruited to work not under the umbrella of the military medical services at the time, like Andrew Balfour (see Part IV). According to Mollan (2002), from a total number of seventy-three doctors recruited between 1899 and 1938, forty-three were recruited during the first seven years of their career. Further, most of the recruits, like the rest of the British 'Sudan Political Service' staff, were generally graduates of Cambridge or Oxford in addition to London University, especially St Thomas' (42). It was the influence of Acland and later Squires that encouraged graduates of St Thomas' Medical School. Dr. Acland himself was a St. Thomas' graduate, and he became one of the staff there late in his career. Dr. Squires spent part of his career as medical registrar at St Thomas'. Mollan had pointed out that around 42% of the recruits during 1899-1938 came from the triangle of Cambridge/Oxford/London. Even for nurses, special preference had been given to St. Thomas', St. Bartholomew's, and other graduates of London hospitals (43).

The number of civil hospitals began to increase gradually. By 1909, in Kassala Province, for instance, there were already four civil hospitals. The major one was in Kassala, and there were three small hospitals in Gedaref, Galabat, and Mafaza, respectively (44). There were two military hospitals, one in Kassala and the other in Gedaref. The administration of these hospitals was under the direction of the Senior British MO, who was normally stationed at the main provincial military hospital at Kassala. This British Senior MO would usually carry out inspection every few months or so, touring the small hospitals under his responsibility, and during such inspection tours he would see patients in villages and refer cases needing hospital care to the nearest hospital (45). The smaller military hospitals and the civil hospitals would be under a Syrian MO, who was considered a subordinate to the British SMO. The hospitals at Wadi Halfa, Suakin, Merowe, and Dongola at the beginning were staffed by non-British medical staff. That system apparently continued till the expansion years in the early and mid-1920s, when availability of funds allowed for recruiting more British civilian doctors. In the 1930s, the Syrian MOs were gradually replaced by the Sudanese graduates from KSM and more British doctors recruited from the UK.

Special mention must be made of the fact that licenses for private medical practitioners were open since the early days of the Anglo-Egyptian administration. As early as 1901, five private medical doctors were mentioned to be practicing at Khartoum. Those were three Greeks, one Briton, and one American (46), and the first private dentist service was advertised in the *Sudan Gazette* in February of 1905 (47).

Section II:

The Annual Health Reports: The Scope and Level of Service and Staff, 1909-1915

In 1909, the new Khartoum Civil Hospital was opened, as well as two other new civil hospitals, in Atbara and Port Sudan. From the Annual Health Reports of the SMD one may be able to draw some picture of the level and scope of the health service after the dismissal of its first civil director, Dr. John Chrsitopherson in 1908 and the end of the First World War. From information that could be extracted from these reports, the number of outpatients reached 140,000 and that of inpatients remained at 7,000. There were no major epidemics apart from few cases of smallpox and what has been described as 'the mysterious fatal disease, *Kala azar*'. Kala-azar first appeared in Kassala and Blue Nile Provinces, and many cases proved fatal. That led the government to set up a special commission known as 'The Kala-azar Commission' (*vide infra*). This was dispatched along the Blue Nile on board the 'Floating Laboratory' of the WTRL at Khartoum to begin a special investigation of what was described as a 'mysterious disease'. The other major epidemiological survey in that year was that of the Sleeping Sickness Commission (SSC) in the Lado Enclave and Bahr el-Ghazal (see section on health commissions, Part VI). During 1909, the number of those vaccinated against smallpox reached 41,000 subjects, as compared to 19,000 in the previous year. In the 1910 Report, there was a statement referring to the lack of subsidiary hospital buildings, lack of properly qualified attendants, and a significant increase in outpatient activity but little increase in inpatient activity (48). That represented the trend over the preceding few years. During that year, there was a minor epidemic of diphtheria that broke out south of the town of Dueim in the White Nile Province, and the first cases of sleeping sickness made their appearance in the Sudan. Two cases were discovered at Raga, near the French Congo border, in addition to a disputed third case in Wau, Bahr el-Ghazal. No case of sleeping sickness had hitherto been identified in the Sudan. Colonel Mathias, Director of the SMD, who was also president of the SSC, wrote that the officers of the SSC succeeded in confining the disease to certain definite areas in the Lado Enclave (which has just been regained from the Belgian Congo following the death of King Leopold II) (see Map 5). During that year, research and investigation into the outbreak of many cases of Kala-azar in Kassala and Blue Nile provinces continued. Also, some routine vaccination tours were made in various provinces, including Berber, Dongola, and Halfa.

In early 1911, an epidemic of pneumonia broke out at Zaidab, in Berber Province, but it was quickly stamped out. Further, there was a small outbreak of chickenpox and measles at Omdurman, Khartoum, Khartoum North and some of the provinces in the south. The 'Public Health' section of the MIR for that year contained a note stating 'absence of any place for isolating cases of infectious diseases which has again proved most embarrassing and the provision of small infectious hospital and means of isolating contacts is one of the most pressing for Khartoum from a public health point of view at the present time' (49). During that year, arrangements were made to ensure that appropriate sanitary and public health measures were implemented during the beginning of the experimental irrigation scheme at Tayiba. (This scheme was possibly one of the first pilot schemes to study the feasibility of growing cotton at Gezira.) The housing of the working men and their families, the closeness of their villages to the irrigation canals, and measures to prevent the breeding of mosquitoes were carefully examined and pointed out. The provision of a 'trained sanitary inspector' was advocated, and all these were to report to the Central Sanitary Board at Khartoum. These preliminary measures proved to be vital, as, during the subsequent year, the irrigation schemes at Zaidab, Kadaru, and Izergab suffered heavy outbreaks of malaria, and the mosquito breeding was very troublesome, but the scheme at Tayiba remained free of such problems. That was attributed to the 'excellent collaboration between the 'traveling sanitary officer and the resident engineer of the scheme'. In 1911, the quality of water supply to Khartoum was felt to be excellent and it was planned that, with more funds available, the water supply was to be extended to the remaining parts of Khartoum and later to Khartoum North. During that year a special committee visited Atbara and examined its water supply and made its recommendations to install mechanical filters. Funds for these filters were sanctioned by the Director of Railways. A similar committee looked into the problem of water supply at Port Sudan and decided on the temporary measures of sinking some wells in the area around the town, pending a proper scheme for water provision. There were some frustrating remarks on 'understaffing' and it was mentioned that 'it has been impossible to find money for the rebuilding and completion of the civil hospitals in out-stations'. During that year, Dr. Robert Footner, a surgeon by training, after his tenure with Sudan Government Railways had expired, became the last British doctor to join the SMD till after the First World War.

In June 1912, Colonel H. B. Mathias, Director of the SMD, died suddenly in Khartoum and Major H. A. Bray took over as Director. There was a troublesome outbreak of malaria cases in the pilot irrigation schemes at Zaidab, Kadro, and Izergab; otherwise that year was free from serious epidemics. In the same year, a 'Nursing Fund' was established by private subscriptions and nurses were recruited from the 'free-lance pool' of nurses available at Cairo. That fund was meant primarily to satisfy the needs of the 'British Expats' and their families (50, 51). The Fund was later opened for others. The Government helped this scheme by providing suitable accommodation for the nurses on the premises of the KCH. The report for that year, however, highlighted the ongoing problems of lack of 'Hospital Attendants'. Their number remained small, and there was a need for providing training, as those who were already in post were insufficiently trained. During that year, there were some plans to oversee the work of the 'Sanitary Barbers' who were assigned the work of 'Births & Deaths Registration' in addition to conducting vaccination. There were also some proposed plans to establish dispensaries at Kosti, Tokar, Sinkat, and Mongalla. The major area affected by sleeping sickness in the country remained the Lado Enclave, with some fears of the spread of the disease to the Moru District. On the other hand, kala-azar cases were confirmed not to be on the rise. In 1913, there were no serious epidemics and, apart from a minor smallpox epidemic at Gedaref and sporadic cases at Dongola, Halfa, and el-Obeid, there were no other major concerns. Malaria was less prevalent, thanks to scanty rainfall and more stringent measures to control mosquito breeding. There were also some isolated cases of enteric fever that reached a total of 22 in different regions. A single case of bubonic plague at Suakin, imported from Messauwa, was reported. There were also reports of some sporadic cases of CSM at Mongala, Rejaf, el-Obeid, Kodok, and Suakin. In addition, there was a small outbreak at Khartoum and Omdurman. The infant mortality for that year was stated to be excessive, but no actual figure was given. The total number of subjects who were vaccinated was above 70,620 cases. During that year, the inhabitants of the western Kordofan town of Nuhud subscribed to building a small hospital. The number of inpatients rose in that year to 9,778, as compared to 9,454 in the previous year. Those seen as outpatients were 200,891, as compared to 172,138 in 1912. Research into Kala-azar was concluded during that year by Captain Marshall of the RAMC. He reported only 18 new cases. On the other hand, Captain Drew of the SSC reported 10 new sleeping-sickness cases in Deim Zubair and Raja, western Bahr el-Ghazal. The disease was also found in a larger area in western Mongalla Province, in addition to the original large area around the Yei River District. The number of cases of sleeping sickness in the camp was 398, as compared to 314 cases in the previous year (52). By contrast, during 1914 there was an outbreak of famine due to shortage of grains, as the rainy season in the previous year had been poor with resultant scanty harvest. Further, an epidemic of CSM broke out which was most serious in the Zaidab area, where 142 deaths were reported in April 1914 alone. Other outbreaks hit Khartoum, Omdurman, and Blue Nile Province, especially the area of Makwar. In the south an outbreak of smallpox occurred amongst the Anuak tribe of eastern Upper Nile, and a few sporadic cases were reported from Dabba and Khartoum. There was also an outbreak of typhus in 'Ginnis' near Wadi Halfa. Also, two cases of cholera from Omdurman were reported and an epidemic of dysentery in Bahr el-Ghazal, with high mortality. An investigation into the relative prevalence of malaria in the irrigated areas (Zaidab, Kadaru, Tayiba, and Izergab) confirmed the earlier report on the need to implement stringent measures of sanitation. The prevalence of malaria south of Khartoum was abundant, with the exception of Kassala and Nuhud, following heavy rains the year before. Infant mortality remained high and the recorded births were less by 1,257, and it was felt that the Registry of Births & Deaths was still imperfect. By 1914, more new hospitals were added at Atbara, Port Sudan, Merowe, and Dueim (53).

From the above extracts, it is obvious that the period from 1904 till 1915 saw the establishment of the civil medical department on a rudimentary basis, with scanty resources, and few staff, comprising mainly doctors from Syria and Egypt. However, despite nominal civilian status, the department continued to be under control of the military hierarchy. It was only after the onset of the First World War that the prospect of the re-birth of the civil department began to be a real possibility. This will be the theme of the next section.

Section III:

The Re-birth of the Sudan Civil Medical Department: The Re-Organization of 1915

By 1915, re-organization took place. The civil department was reborn as a separate department linked with but independent from the military medical department, and Dr. Edward Smyth Crispin was appointed Deputy Director. In the *Sudan Gazette* of September 11, 1915, it was announced that Captain H. A. Bray had ceased to be Director of the Medical Department, but no date for that decision was mentioned (54). Obviously, since that decision, Dr. Edward Crispin became acting director till he was formally appointed on December 7, 1916 (55). There were no individual reports for the years 1914-1919, and these were collectively lumped together in one report (56). This may be related to the war situation, where efforts were directed towards the military operations. Although the First World War was underway, the Sudan economy started to flourish, despite a few hiccups of looming famine due to shortage of grains in various provinces following a poor rainy season. In 1915, the Sudan Government was able to import some grains from India to close the gap (57). Posts of senior medical inspectors, which were not many anyway, were all filled by the existing British medical staffs. However, Dr. Crispin asserts in the above report that, despite the fact that more funds were allocated to meet new projects, 'considerable difficulty is still experienced in respect of both staff and hospital equipment. The advertisement for medical inspectors produced few replies and there has been similar difficulty in obtaining Syrian and Egyptian staff' (58). In 1916, however, funds became available to establish a 'Midwifery Training School', and buildings were already in progress by 1919. During this period a new system of 'Births & Deaths Registration' was introduced that resulted in better recording and an obvious increase in the number of registrations. The report included statements highlighting that the figures were still not very accurate, with the total population of Sudan in 1914 being estimated to be around 3.4 million. During this period, seven outbreaks of CSM occurred, but smallpox in northern Sudan had been substantially curbed by regular campaigns of vaccination. Only a single outbreak occurred in 1917 in Khartoum and Omdurman, but it was soon put under control. In 1919, there were occasional cases of smallpox seen in several districts, including Khartoum and Omdurman, but no major outbreak took place. In southern Sudan, however, smallpox was prevalent during that year in Mongalla and some parts of Upper Nile Province (59). Significant success with vaccination was achieved that year among the nomad Arabs, who were reported to have been 'much opposing to all attempts of vaccinations tours in the past'. An influenza epidemic made its appearance in the Sudan in September of 1918 and swept throughout the country, with considerable mortality. The worst district affected was Zaidab, in Berber Province, in February of 1918. However, the epidemic died away in April/May of that year. It was not possible to give more than an approximate estimate of the extent of the outbreak and consequent mortality. The SMO at Kassala estimated that nearly 1,600 out of a population of 6,000 in Gedaref alone contracted the illness, with 35 deaths. In 1918, the work of the SSC was considered complete. Its advisory role passed to the chairman of the Central Sanitary Board (60). In the period of 1915-1917 and then up to 1919, several patients with bilharziasis were treated with the antimony tartarte for the first time in the world. That was conducted by Dr. J. B. Christopherson, Director of Khartoum & Omdurman Hospitals (see Appendix 1). He was assisted by several of his subordinates, including Drs Ezzadin and Mr John Newlove, and at a later stage by Dr. Vincent Hodson. The Report of 1915-1919 mentioned that 'The pioneering work of Dr. Christopherson resulted in the discovery of a curative medicine for this "scourge" which inflicted many patients in the Nile Basin and in many parts of the world and witnessed a new chapter' (61). In June of 1919, Dr. Christopherson retired from Sudan service on pension.

Towards the end of the War, the Sudan economy began to show significant improvement, with doubling of exports and a revenue surplus totaling £E438,000 , for the first time. Sir Harold MacMichael commented that 'for the first time it became possible to find funds for social services' (62). This helped with the vision of expanding the health service, so a proposal to establish a native core of medical auxiliaries was put forward. According to that proposal, a school to train hospital orderlies as medical assistants was to be established. The father of that proposal was Dr. V. S. Hodson, Assistant Director of the SMD. In 1918, the school first began at Port Sudan. There were also some plans to extend the network of dispensaries to various villages and small towns. These dispensaries were planned to be manned by the new workforce of the health services, the especially trained hospital orderlies, the 'Hospital Assistants' (see Part VI). During this period, the 'Nursing Fund' was liquidated and the government took the responsibility of providing nurses, many of which actually came from among the wives of British governmental staff (63). However, the recruitment of more nurses was pursued more actively; funding to establish a midwifery training school was secured and building began by early 1919 (64). With more funds beginning to flow, recruitment of more British doctors began for the first time since 1909. Dr. J. C. N. Harris was recruited on June 6, 1919, and few months later, on October 30, 1919, Dr. Suleiman Amin Hajjar (a Syrian physician) was added to the staff of the SMD. More British medical staff was soon to join. Dr. J. P. Mitchell and Dr. Norman F. Smith both joined in April 1920, followed by Dr. C. Grantham Hill, who joined in 1920. Dr. Norman Smith was to be the first Registrar (Dean) of the Kitchener School of Medicine, in 1924. Bimbashi G. D. Rastrick Carr joined the SMD on March 1, 1920, followed by Bimbashi J. Mc. McKinnon in September, and in February and August 1920 Dr. Raji Selim Nasir and Dr. Farid Ali Talia, respectively, joined from Syria (65). (The last four likely were for the SSC.)

Early in 1920, a severe outbreak of smallpox occurred in all three southern provinces and the Nuba Mountains. As the natives there were not vaccinated, the epidemic spread rapidly and mortality was very high (66). The total number of subjects vaccinated was 156,378, as compared with 87,067 in 1919. In the same year an outbreak of CSM occurred at Mongalla, a mild influenza epidemic occurred in Kassala, and diphtheria was more prevalent than usual in Khartoum and Atbara. A site for a future leper colony was found along the Atbara River, and funds were applied for. During that year, in addition, the building of the Omdurman Midwifery Training School was completed, and by November 1920 its chosen Matron, Miss Mabel Elsie Wolff, arrived from Cairo (67). During that year new hospitals were under construction at Wadi Halfa, Kassala, Makwar, Hag Abdalla, and Gebel Awlia (the last 3 being connected with the irrigation schemes). Further, the newly trained hospital attendants, the medical assistants', began to come up through the ranks (68). They proved to be of considerable value: they manned the established dispensaries and helped to extend primary medical care to remote areas hitherto not covered by the medical officers. The number of civil patients seen as outpatients and as inpatients increased significantly relative to the previous year, both in civil and military hospitals. The Register of Births and Deaths was transferred from the district '*Mamurs*' (a Turkish title equivalent to district manager) to the medical staff of the hospitals and to the medical assistants in the dispensaries (69). Further, energetic measures were put in place towards the building of Makwar Dam (Makwar being the local name of that part of Sennar), and measures to recruit Egyptian labourers for the building process took place around that year (70). This would have serious public health consequences and would also place a burden on the health services, as quarantine measures to screen those labourers at Wadi Halfa had to be put in place. The following notice is taken from the Public Health Report for 1920:

> It has been considered necessary to enforce a more rigid examination of labourers from the Upper Egypt before their entry into the Sudan. This is being carried out at Halfa and it involved detention in the quarantine camp there for a period of 3 days. One hundred to one hundred and fifty men daily or between 600 and 900 a week, are medically examined, shaved, bathed, disinfected and treated with some vermifuge. The percentage up to date found infected with ankylsotomiasis is much lower than was anticipated and a degree of infection estimated by number of worms removed less. The cases of ankylostomiasis allowed in the Sudan will receive further treatment at their working destination. On the other hand, the the percentage of bilharziasosis (sic) is very much higher, and if all cases were rejected recruiting of 'Saidi' labour would be an impracticable proposition. For this reason and taking into consideration that bilharzias is already very widely distributed throughout Sudan, it has been decided to reject only severe cases of this disease and to allow others to be employed on the Gezira works until the canal system is much further advanced than at the

> present when the risk of spreading infection will be increased and, the question will have to receive further consideration. (71)

Obviously, that decision lacked both moral and scientific grounds and it received opposition from other doctors who had wide experience at the time with bilharzia in both Egypt and Sudan (see section on Byam's moral stand over the SudanAppendix 5).

On January 1, 1921, the Midwifery Training School (MTS) at Omdurman was officially opened. The School began with four student midwives, who attended the first class. The annual report of the SMD for that year mentioned that:

> the whole School was at first treated with suspicion. Later as they recognized the skill of the Matron, and value of training, numerous applications were received, and the succeeding class was easily filled, and extra accommodation had to be provided for an increased class. (72)

With more funds becoming available, and with the prospect of more expansion in the health services, more British doctors were recruited. Dr. Roy Mervyn Humphreys joined in early 1921 (73), and in the same year Lt-Col G. K. Maurice (for SSC) also joined (74). In that year, bubonic plague appeared for the first time since 1900 outside the Quarantine in Suakin. Three cases in that stting plus two cases among the sanitary staff were reported. All died. The epidemic of smallpox that was ravaging the Upper Nile Province showed signs of abating, and extensive vaccinations among Nuer, Shilluk, and Dinka (who were reported to have recognized the value of vaccination) were carried out (75). Further, bilharzia was reported to be on the rise in Nurei and Gurier in Dongola Province, and special staff were stationed out there (76). At the Red Sea Province, ten cases of heat stroke during the hot spell of July and August were reported, eight of which were reported to have died and two cases recovered. Cases were documented to have had temperatures reaching 109 °F (77). There was also a reported increase in the incidence of malaria cases in that year. Civil patients continued to be seen and treated at the Military Hospitals in areas where there were no civil hospitals (78). New hospitals were under construction at Kassala, WadiHalfa, and Malakal, and several dispensaries were opened at Debba, Argo,

Abri, Kosti, Um Ruaba, and Kariema. All these dispensaries were manned by *'Bash Tumourgi',* the Assistant Medical Officers. Reports of their work were stated to be distinctly encouraging (79). In that year, the steamer ship 'Atbara' was converted to a hospital ship to cover mainly the area of the Upper Nile (80). On the other hand, permanent buildings were being erected at the Wadi Halfa Quarantine. During that year a total of 14,068 labourers passed through that Quarantine and, of these, 9,120 received anti-bilharzia treatment. Up to 18% were found to be infected with ankylostoma and a further 19% with bilharziasis. Approximately 50% of them were reported to be carrying some worm infestation. Of the total number of those labourers, 2.9% were rejected and turned back to Egypt (81). The following remark was made in that year's Report: 'The value of this work was shown in the improved sick rate at Makwar. The % of labourers' daily sick rate from November to July varied from 0.5 to 1%, and in August to October it was 2%' (82).

The period from 1919 to 1922 saw the first period of expansion in the number of British doctors who were recruited from Britain. In addition to Dr. Humphreys, who joined early in 1921, Dr. J. C. N. Harris joined in summer of 1919, to subsequently spend many months in hospital after contracting Malta Fever. He was the first from the Service to be the Medical Officer of Health of Khartoum. Several others, including Dr. Norman Smith (who became the first Registrar of KSM), Dr. Grantham Hill, and Dr. E. A. H. Grylls, joined in 1920 and 1922, respectively (83)

Section IV:

Sudan Medical Department 1922-1924: The Reign of Oliver Francis Atkey

In 1922, Dr. Edward Smyth Crispin retired on pension, and Dr. Oliver Francis Hayne Atkey was appointed as the new Director. It transpired that the Directorship was initially offered to Dr. Vince Hodson, who turned the offer down. During 1922, the worthiest feature was successful training of more Assistant Medical Officers (AMOs), the 'Bash Tumurgis'. Two of them performed valuable work at Dongola where a severe epidemic of bilhariziasis broke out in connection with the pumping stations at Nourie and Gurier, and also to a lesser extent in the nearby Magall and Tangassi Island where they efficiently gave 5,478 injections of antimony to sufferers. Approximately 455 cases were reported to have been cured (84). In another area, five AMOs received a course of laboratory training, another feat of upgrading the knowledge and competence of those AMOs to execute a more elaborate work in supporting an expanding medical service with little medical manpower (85). During that year, the prevalence of malaria increased significantly due to heavy rains, especially in Khartoum and Omdurman, and smallpox epidemic broke out in Khartoum among recent immigrants from Kordofan (86). The epidemic spread both north and south. It reached up to Rosiers at the Blue Nile and Kosti on the White Nile, and into the Red Sea frontiers of Sinkat and Port Sudan, traversing through Atbara region north of Khartoum. Extensive vaccination was carried out, and here the efforts of the AMOs again proved to be invaluable. A total of 191,577 subjects were vaccinated, and the total number of those infected was 179, of whom 13 proved fatal (87). There was also an outbreak of CSM, though limited, among labourers at Wad el-Nu pumping station in the Gezira region, numbering 32 in all, of whom 28 proved fatal (88). In that year, another outbreak of bilharziasis took place in Dongola Province, and a survey of schools in that region showed that 20% of children were infected with bilharzias and 18.75% were infected with trachoma (Egyptian ophthalmia) (89).

On the other hand, a full school survey of students of GMC and Omdurman School was carried out for the first time. Similar surveys were also conducted, but less complete, among schools in Port Sudan, Atbara, and Wad Medani (90). The Report for that year stressed the need to continue annually with such surveys (91). In January 1922, a new system for 'Births & Deaths Registry' was started under the guidance of the medical staff in hospitals and dispensaries. A comment was made that the 'results of the return are now much more complete than it has been in any previous year' (92). Another important event during that year was the inauguration of the Lady Baker Hospital Ship, which was put into service on March 1, 1922. It was commissioned and handed over to the medical authorities at Khartoum (93). In that year, two more Syrian doctors, Drs Sami Fadlalla Hamada and Joseph Tannous Nasr, were recruited (94).

The year 1923 saw another wave of expansion in primary care endeavours, when 31 new dispensaries were opened and manned by 'native AMOs' (95). These dispensaries were chosen to be located in remote areas either densely populated or heavily infected with endemic diseases, like bilharziasis and malaria (96). Special arrangements were made to ensure that the 'camel-owning nomads' of northern Kordofan and the 'cattle-owning tribes' of southern Kordofan had a dispensary. Both had been beyond the reach of any doctor in the past (97). In that year's Report, the following was asserted:

> A concise elementary medical and surgical training is given to each AMO before appointment and it is desired in future to improve the standard still more and to increase the number of those qualified'. Another notable event was the completion of buildings of Kitchener School of Medicine and the plans to go ahead and take the first patch of prospective students from January 1924 were made. (98)

The number of patients seen as outpatients rose to 388,863 and those seen as inpatients rose to 18,172, with a noticeable increase in Malakal Hospital attributed to the activity of the Lady Baker Hospital Ship (99). There the number of treated as inpatients rose from 470 in 1921 to 901 in 1923, and outpatients increased from 8,432 to 19,301 (100). Recruitment of British doctors continued during this year when Drs E. A. H. Grylls and H. A. Crouch joined the service (101).

Dr. Grylls was later to succeed Dr. Norman Smith as Registrar of KSM (102), and Dr. Crouch was to accomplish significant medical work at the Lady Baker Hospital Ship, taking over from Mr Footner in 1926. He subsequently became Assistant Director of Public Health for many years (103). During December of 1922, a smallpox epidemic broke out in Tokkar District, Red Sea Province, and didn't subside until May of 1923 (104). A small outbreak of CSM, with a total of 17 cases, occurred at Makwar (105). The work against bilharzia in Dongola region had some success, with 935 cases reported as having been cured and a total of 1,405 cases receiving anti-bilharzia treatment with sodium antimony taratrate (106). Further, anti-bilharizia survey and measures began at the Um Rawaba and Abu Zabad regions of southern Kordofan. However, only limited success was achieved due to limited resources (107). During that year, two new snails were discovered by the team from WTRL in Khartoum, to be carriers of bilharziasis (108). The prevalence of malaria in that year underwent a decline attributed to better measures of malaria control, especially in Khartoum and Makkwar (109). A landmark event in that year was the installation of the first X-ray 'apparatus' at Khartoum Civil Hospital (110). The new hospital at Nuhud, which replaced the first one subscribed by the natives in 1913, was completed (111). A part of another new hospital at Malakal was also completed (112). Favourable progress was reported on the achievements of the Midwifery Training School at Omdurman (113).

By early 1924, the inauguration of the first medical school was imminent and more funds were funneled into the health services. A new era began when the SMD ceased to exist as it was replaced by the Sudan Medical Service (SMS), which was regarded as one of the most successful healthcare models in the whole of Colonial Britain. This will be the theme of a separate chapter (see Volume 2).

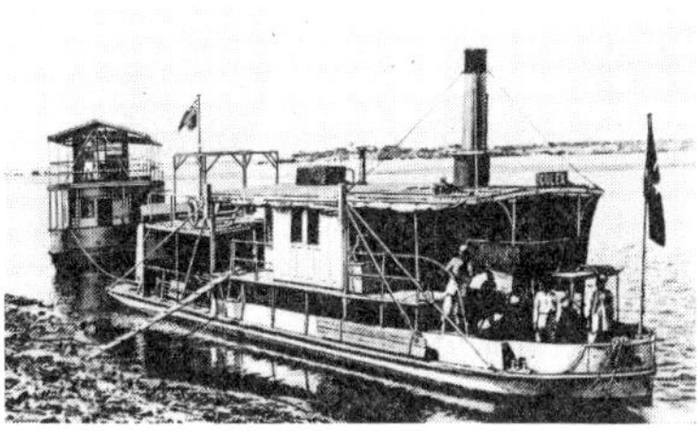

Chapter 4

The Sudan Medical Department: Other Records of Achievement

The achievements of the Sudan Medical Department were not confined to the area of curative medicine. The administration had input into other areas, primarily in the field of public health and the training of healthcare professionals. Some of these achievements continued to flourish as part of the expanding health services beyond the era of the SMD. These areas included what were known as the public health commissions; the training of the healthcare subordinates or 'medical assistants'; the establishment of the Midwifery Training School and later the Nursing School in Omdurmanin in the early and mid-1920s, respectively; and finally the building of big hospitals, especially Khartoum Civil Hospital. Some of these areas, as with the rest of the service, would continue to develop and expand with the expanding needs for the health service, especially following the formation of the Sudan Medical Service (SMS), the natural successor of the SMD. Hence, coverage of various areas in this section will not be restricted to the 'SMD' period which came to an end in 1924.

The Feat of Assistant Medical Officers & Early Primary Health Work

Dr. Vincent Hodson, Deputy Director of the SMD and one of the first few doctors who came to the country after the 'Reconquest', proposed the idea of training of a selected group of hospital male orderlies. The concept as laid out by Hodson was to provide these men with some intense training for one year in simple medical diagnosis and treatment of some of the common medical conditions. These medical subordinates were first called 'Assistant Medical Officers', a title that was later changed to 'Medical Assistants'. The central idea was to train these men and then send them to man the dispensaries that were planned to be established in villages and small towns in remote districts. The training of these men stressed clarity of instruction and a willingness to refer cases if they felt that hospital treatment was needed. This was probably one of the first primary healthcare enterprises in modern medical history in the whole of Africa. The first group of these men were trained at Port Sudan Civil Hospital in 1918, but the author found no further details about that. By 1921 a special school was opened at Omdurman to train them. That school was called the 'School of Medical Assistants' (1). On average, six male hospital orderlies were selected and then enrolled in the school beginning from 1921, the same year that formal training of midwives began in the same town of Omdurman. When the SMD ceased to exist and the SMS was established in 1924, the plan for expansion of health services into remote districts of the country was based on the maximum utilization of the MAs, who were indispensable members of the healthcare team. The training of MAs, however, became formal only in 1946 (2). A 'Board of Studies for Medical Assistants' was established around 1946 to oversee the training of MAs. The course was later designed to take one year and the intake was once every two years. The course was also designed to be as practical as possible and to run over 11 months, with the final month granted as a leave. The pre-requisite for admission was completion of at least four years of primary education (elementary school) in addition to at least six years as a dresser and being under 35 years of age. The period of study was to spend 10 months working in the hospital—surgical and medical wards, operating theatre, outpatient, pharmacy, and laboratory—and one month of house-to -house inspection. Practical activities were to be in the morning: the afternoon was devoted to lectures. Those lectures comprised 200 hours divided between the various subjects. An additional five hours a week were given over to English teaching.

The Province Medical Officer would make selection of suitable candidates and circulate notification of the available vacancies to them in advance. The selected candidates from the provinces would then undergo competition at Omdurman, where a final selection would be made for the prospective successful candidates. Those enrolled would receive their usual salaries plus an allowance proportionate to their dependents, clothing, boarding, etc. Prior to the start of formal training in the 1940s, refresher courses were given to the MAs once every two years. The course was for six months, with two admissions every year. The average number of MAs attending these courses was usually 12 (3). When formal training began in the 1940s, the South would host training of MAs in Juba. By 1942, around 12 MAs had graduated from Juba, and by 1944 seven more were added to those already trained. Candidates had to have completed their intermediate-school rather than just primary-school education (4).

Those MAs proved to be very invaluable staff in conducting other work, including vaccination, reporting of epidemics, and conducting surveys for schistosomiasis; especially in Dongola, Kordofan, and the Gezira regions. Dispensaries all over the country were built and were manned by those MAs. Extracts from the annual reports of the SMS state that the number of MAs trained by 1925 rose to 41. By 1933, the number totaled 200, and their average number rose from 70 in the 1920s to 270 during the period of 1930 to 1940. During the same period, the number of dispensaries rose from 146 to 327. It is worth noting that the number of hospitals by then had reached 40, with a total bed capacity of 5,900 (5). Between 1933 and 1939, on average, 15 MAs graduated annually (6). Those medical subordinates prove to be a crucial catalyst in delivering primary health care at minimum cost. Medical Britons who served in the Sudan in later years echoed their admiration for that enterprise. The late Dr. Kenneth Owen, a notable London urologist, in his memoirs wrote about his service in Sudan, expressing how impressed and fascinated he was by those MAs (7) (see also Volume 2).

The Public Health Commissions

A. The Kala Azar Commission

Leishmaniasis and its visceral form, termed '*Kala-azar*' (*Kala* = 'black' in *Hindustani*,; *azar* = 'disease' in *Persian and Hindustani*), is a tropical and subtropical parasitic disease that is prevalent in Central and South America, Africa, and several parts of Asia. By the turn of the twentieth century, Kala-azar was still a mysterious disease. The disease in its various forms, both visceral and cutaneous, was known to be caused by a parasite discovered by the distinguished Scottish pathologist, Colonel William Boog Leishman, of the RAMC, and later professor of pathology at the Royal Army Medical College, London. The parasite as it appears under the microscope was also noted around the same time by Dr. Charles Donovan of the Indian Medical Service. However, the life cycle and the vector of the disease were not known for a good number of years. The visceral form of the disease was first described in Sudan by the Wellcome Tropical Research Laboratory 'traveling pathologist', Dr. Sheffield Neave. Neave diagnosed the condition in a young Sudanese boy in Omdurman following a splenic puncture (8). Following the observation that several cases which exhibited the typical features of visceral leishmaniasis were reported to the WTRL, the Sudan Government, on the advice of Dr. Andrew Balfour, decided to set up a commission (known as the 'Sudan Kala Azar Commission') to investigate the disease in the eastern part of Sudan, close to the Abyssinian border. It was in those parts that most of the cases were reported. Bimbashi Leonard Bousfield, the military MO of Kassala Province, and Colonel Lyle Cummins were assigned to lead the Commission. Each would combine his clinical skills with his assigned role as an 'epidemiologist', to map out a visceral leishmaniasis profile in the eastern and south-eastern corners of Sudan. Bousfield led the team that was assigned to survey the Kassala and Blue Nile regions. The team trekked through the Atbara, Rahad, Dinder, and Blue Nile rivers close to the Abyssinian border. That Commission helped greatly to map out the prevalence of the disease in that part of the Sudan and added much to the current understanding of leishmaniasis in Sudan. Bousfiled published his findings in the Third Wellcome Reports in 1908. Stemming from a personal experience during the work of the Commission, Bousfield made the astute observation that there must be a vector/intermediate host for the Kala-azar parasite, but he never published it in a scientific journal. He only wrote that observation he made many years later in his autobiography, *Sudan Doctor*. It was only in 1925 that the vector was proven to be the sandfly, *Phlebotomus papatasi*. Bousfield, during the Commission's tenure, took a splenic puncture from a woman with suspected Kala-azar and, while handing the needle to one of his subordinates, accidentally pricked one of his own fingers. After Bousfield fixed the slide and examined it under the microscope, he was horrified to see that slide was full of Leishman-Donovan bodies. Naturally alarmed, concerned, and dreading the worst, he took a scalpel and cut the area of his inoculated finger. Fortunately, to his great relief, he did not contract that lethal disease, but this prompted him to draw the conclusion that there must definitely be an intermediate host for the parasite (9). Bousfield wrote an elegant report on his 'Observation on Kala-Azar in Kassala Province', published in the Third Report of the Wellcome Tropical Research Laboratories in 1908 (10). In that report, he summarized the clinical, laboratory, and pathological findings and observations he had made. He provided detailed statistics of proven and suspected cases, discussed the presence of 'bed bugs' (which at that time was thought to be the transmitting vector of the disease!), and touched on the historical background of Kala-azar in Sudan since the earliest observation made by Dr. Sheffield Neave. He tabulated the proven and suspected cases, elaborating fully on the clinical observations he had made of these cases, and then he wrote an account of the detailed laboratory findings. He went on ascertaining the outcome of various tests, including splenic punctures, blood and urine specimens, and finally autopsy details of two cases that perished during the work of the Commission. One could argue that this report, as well as the accompanying one in the same issue of Third Wellcome Report written by Captain Stevenson Lyle Cummins (11), was unique and probably second to none amongst the published papers covering Kala-azar at that time.

The work of the Kala Azar Commission was continued after Bousfield and Lyle Cummins by Captain Thomson and Captain Marshall, who published their findings in the Fourth Wellcome Report, in 1911 (12, 13). From 1911 onwards, the disease continued to show a paucity of cases and erratic distribution with some minor epidemic outbreaks from time to time. In 1923, Dr. Robert G. Archibald (by then, Director of WTRL) reported cases from the Kurmuk and Beni Shangol posts on the Abyssinian border. Dr. Robert Kirk thereafter reported some cases from Wad Arud in 1939, and in 1940 Dr. R. W. Stephenson reported several cases among the Dinka population of Melut (14).

The vector of the disease was not discovered till 1925, when Drs Knowles, Napier, and Smith at Calcutta, India, suggested that the sandfly, genus phlebotomus, was the culprit in the transmission of the parasite to man. It was Dr. Robert Kirk and David Lewis who suggested that other species of the genus phlebotomines are capable of transmitting the disease in the Sudan. Indeed, they later confirmed these species to be *P. orientalis, P. clydei,* and *P. martini* (15). In 1940, Kirk and Satti established the method of gland puncture as a reliable method for diagnosis during epidemics and outbreaks, as it does not require any preparation. It was Dr. Mohamed Hamad Satti's work that showed good results with the use of dimidine antimony, and as early as 1947 Kirk and Satti were obtaining good results by using pentostam to treat visceral leishmaniasis. According to Archibald and Haseeb, the disease in Sudan never occurred in an epidemic form, as it did in India, and continued to exhibit 'a smoldering fire of infection' (16). It was the prolific Robert Kirk who conducted the majority of research into Kala-azar in Sudan between 1930 and the early 1950s. Kirk first divided the clinical manifestations of visceral leishmaniasis into primary, secondary, and tertiary, according to the evolving immunity. Details are beyond the scope of this book.

B. Sleeping Sickness Commission

At the time of the great 'Scramble for Africa' and during the political turmoil in the Turco-Egyptian Sudan that culminated in the rise and rise of the Mahdi, the Equatorial Province of the Nile Basin, which was governed by Emin Pasha (Dr. Edward Schnietzer) on behalf of the Egyptian Khedive, remained one of the few territories not conquered by the Khalifa's troops. By 1888, Emin Pasha was besieged by Emir Fadallah Arabi, the leader of the Mahdist troops in southern Sudan. A relief expedition was dispatched by the British to rescue Emin Pasha, which went down in history as the 'Emin Pasha Relief Expedition'. That expedition was led by Henry Morton Stanley. The introduction of sleeping sickness into central Africa from east Africa was blamed on this expedition. We refer here to the fight between Dr. Patrick Manson and Henry Morton Stanley during the farewell dinner party organized by Henry Wellcome at the Piccadilly in London in honour of Dr. Balfour (see chapter V). After the relief of Emin by Stanley at Wadelai, many Sudanese soldiers who served under Emin, together with their women and slaves, settled in northern Uganda. Later, reports would blame the introduction of sleeping sickness into Uganda (from the western part of Albert N'yanza Congo) on the movement of soldiers and animals during that relief expedition (17). Trypanosomes in chronic forms were observed by Castellani and Bruce in these immigrant Sudanese soldiers (18, 19). Sleeping sickness was known to exist in West Africa for nearly a hundred years. Indeed, the parasite was named after Gambia, where it was first discovered. A Sleeping Sickness Commission was set up by the British Government in 1902 to investigate the exact culprit of such an epidemic, which was thought to have claimed the lives of half a million people in the Congo between 1896 and 1906. Further, two thirds of the population of Uganda between 1898 and 1908 were said to have succumbed to the disease (20). Through the efforts of Dr. Aldo Castellani, who was later joined by Colonel (later Sir) David Bruce (a descendant of James Bruce, the Scottish explorer), the vector (*Glossina palpalis*) and the parasite and its life cycle were mapped out and the species was named the east African trypanosome, or *trypanosome brucell* (after Colonel David Bruce). Captain Creig, a member of that Commission, was instructed to meet with Dr. Sheffield Neave, the 'traveling pathologist', at Gondokoro in 1904, as part of the investigation into whether sleeping sickness had spread into the Sudan or not. Since then, the disease was known to be endemic in the Belgian Congo, French Sudan, and Uganda (21).

Sheffield Neave was the first to discover the presence of the trypanosome in animals in the Sudan, in 1904 (22). Stemming from this important information, the Sudan Government established its own Sleeping Sickness Commission in 1905. It was led by Colonel G. D. Hunter, the Principal Medical Officer of the EA, with Dr. Andrew Balfour as a member. There was some concern about the spread of sleeping sickness into some parts of Equatoria and Bahr el-Ghazal. Those areas represented the first field work of the SSC. Indeed, the work of this Commission went on for several decades. The field work members were exclusively military British and Syrian doctors. First members of the Commission who conducted field work were Captain Ensor and Major Dansey of the RAMC. The report by Dr. Ensor in 1905 stated that, on surveying the border of the south along the frontiers of Bahr el-Ghazal, they were able to find that the tse-tse flies of genera *G. palpalis* and *G. moristans,* were both present but they could not determine any cases in the area. The maps prepared during these preliminary surveys proved to be quite accurate (23, 24, 25). Captain Ensor in his 1907-1908 SSC Report stated: 'we may be, and probably shall be, unable to prevent sleeping sickness from crossing the frontier into the Sudan, but with care we ought to be able to limit its spread' (26). Till 1910 not a single case of sleeping sickness was confirmed in the Sudan. The first one was reported from Raga on the north-western frontiers of Bahr el-Ghazal, close to the border of the French Sudan (now Central African Republic). That case was confirmed in an immigrant from there. Worth mentioning is that, since 1908, cases of sleeping sickness were known to exist in the Lado Enclave. The Enclave was the part of Southern Sudan that comprised the current area represented by the triangle of Yei/Juba and Kajo-Kaji, which was under the Belgian Congo Administration from 1898 till 1910, when it was handed back to the Anglo-Egyptian Government. From 1910, the disease was diagnosed in and around Yei. On June 8, 1910, Captain Colin MacKenzie and Dr. Yusef Derwish of the EAMC found 15 cases in Yei, and by 1911 there were 268 cases under treatment in that region (27). Until 1914 the disease was confined to the areas adjoining French Sudan/

Belgian Congo, and Anglo-Egyptian Sudan inter-borders (28). That primarily included the areas of Raga, Tembura, Meriedi, and Yei. It was only in 1914 that the first outbreak at the Sudan-Ugandan border at Kajo-Kaji, across the east bank of the Nile, occurred. This one was traced to cases imported from Uganda in the same way that cases around Yei were due to cases imported from Belgian Congo. The cases reported at Raga and Tembura were related to cases coming from the French Sudan (29). In other words, cases of sleeping sickness were primarily imported from the neighbouring countries prior to the disease becoming established in the Sudan. In 1916 and during the campaign to help the French in the French Sudan curb a native uprising, Sudanese troops were dispatched there to aid the French. Following the return of these troops to the Sudan by 1917, a major outbreak occurred in Raga, and this later extended to Tembura (30). By 1918, a major outbreak occurred in the regions of Tembura-Meridi, the homeland of the Azande. The efforts of the Syrian medical Officer, Yuzbashi Nessib Effendi Baz, and later Colonel Basil H. B. Spence of the RAMC, greatly helped to contain that outbreak, mapped out the extent of the geography of the epidemic, and set up camps where infected cases were segregated for treatment and isolation in order to curb the spread of the disease. These formed the bases of 'settlements' that were established at various locations in Azande Land. The famous ones were the Yubu and Yei settlements. This later innovation proved very effective in confining the disease to these areas and prevent its spread to other areas in Southern Sudan till 1922, when the disease started to appear further north and east of the originally affected areas. By 1924, the sleeping sickness epidemic was considered to be over (31). However, due to the perseverance of the SSC members, the number of cases declined thereafter, and by the 1930s only a few cases were seen sporadically in Tembora and Yei areas. By the 1940s, the trend of fewer cases continued and it remained so, well into the early 1950s (32).

The mainstay of the work of the SSC comprised public health work, namely mass examination of people's neck glands, and control of the disease via separating man and fly. This later included clearing the vegetation and trees close to rivers up to 200 yards wide (the flying range of the tsetse fly). A 'block' method was adopted.

According to this system, the river was divided into sections, termed 'blocks', between each of which a large clearing, 800 yards long and 200 yards wide on each side of the river was cleared of trees and vegetation. These blocks formed the basis of depriving the tsetse fly of its habitat. This method was combined with 'fly catching', in which many local boys were employed, supervised by Sudanese public health workers. That greatly helped reduce the number of flies. These approaches greatly helped to reduce the burden of the disease. During the 1930s, a different approach was adopted to curb the disease among the Azande, where attempts were made to establish villages in which the tribe could settle and get beyond the reach of the tsetse fly. That was started initially by moving the Azande to settle along roads that were erected in their districts. Later, agricultural and industrial establishments in Yambio and the new town of Nzara proved detrimental to the efforts to control sleeping sickness. One aspect of the social impact the work that the SSC had on the inhabitants of that part of Southern Sudan was the actual transformation of their lives. This was exemplified in a statement of Dr. K. G. K. Maurice, a member of the RAMC and SSC: 'In the course of the campaign against the sleeping sickness the habits of the natives were transformed….the task of extirpating disease had profoundly affected the life of a people' (33).

The SSC throughout the regime of the British Administration in the Sudan proved to be a success. In the period between 1950 and 1954, just prior to the Independence, the number of new cases per annum ranged between 60 and 100 cases (34). The task of the SSC was begun by the military doctors, and several notable ones were credited with outstanding efforts. Dr. Basil Spence was knighted in recognition of his role in the SSC, and Dr. Yusuf Effendi Derwish (a Syrian doctor) was made an MBE for his work with the SSC. However, following the expansion of civilian medical services into southern Sudan by the late 1920s, the civilian doctors began to take a more proactive role. British doctors like Alexander Cruickshank, John Bloss, and Peter Abbott had made their mark on these public health ventures.

Epidemics

I. Smallpox

The first medical dispatches of the Egyptian Army regularly contained statements about smallpox, which was known to have been 'endemic in the Soudan' for centuries. There were several reports of epidemics, firstly during the eighteenth and the early nineteenth centuries. Those were witnessed or reported by several European travelers, including James Bruce, William George Browne, and John Lewis Burckhardt. Several epidemics continued to ravage the Sudan throughout the era of the Turco-Egyptian Sudan and the Mahdiyya. Bayoumi (1970) stated that during the Mahdiyya five major outbreaks of smallpox occurred in the Sudan (35). In the Military Intelligence Reports for the year 1903, Colonel Penton, PMO of the EAMC, wrote that during the Mahdiyya, in Omdurman alone, not less than 25,000 had died of smallpox during the outbreak of 1895 (36). Following the Reconquest, there were active measures by the Anglo-Egyptian government to vaccinate the troops and the 'natives'. In the 1901 MIR, Colonel Major Penton writes: 'the absence of smallpox {is attributed} to the care taken in vaccinating the inhabitants of towns and villages near stations occupied by the troops' (37). In the 1902 MIR there was mention of the smallpox epidemic that broke out among soldiers of the 'Sudd Cutting Expedition' (as well as their 'Mahdists prisoners' and their families) soon after that expedition reached the Upper Nile. A field hospital was established near Tong, where cases were managed and vaccinations were given (38). That military dispatch was accompanied by a medical unit (which was later joined by Dr. Crispin during his early days in Sudan). This, and the major epidemic that occurred in 1899, probably represent one of the first official encounters of the new regime with the menace of smallpox in the Sudan.

During early 1903 a minor outbreak occurred in Omdurman, where Dr. J. B. Christopherson, the MO in charge of Omdurman, managed to contain it with good skilful measures of public health and clever clinical sense (39). In the MIR for that year, Dr. Penton asserted: 'A recent outbreak which also threatened to be serious, was averted by the skill and energy of the British Medical Officer, Dr.

Christopherson, on whom the brunt of the work fell, has written an interesting report on the subject. He commences by saying: 'it is not an exaggeration to say that a properly vaccinated person cannot contract smallpox'. He goes on to state that:

> I do not think the decrease of smallpox in the Sudan during the last few years was to be attributed to vaccination. It was attributed to the possible protection conveyed by previous outbreaks, the last of which in 1899 was severe. (40)

The subsequent Military Intelligence Reports, which contained extracts on health, continued to mention the occasional outbreaks of minor epidemics and sporadic cases of smallpox. In the 1904 Report, a mention was made of isolated cases of smallpox that were diagnosed in Khartoum, Suakin, and Wad Medani (41). In that year Captain Dansey-Brown of the RAMC conducted a vaccination campaign amongst children in Dongola, where 1,200 were vaccinated in two months, while Dr. Crispin was said to have left Khartoum with a large consignment of 'lymph vaccine' destined for the Blue Nile Province. From 1905 through 1919, only sporadic cases were reported from various parts of the country. In 1920, a severe outbreak occurred in several districts in Southern Sudan, involving Upper Nile, Mongalla, and Bahr el-Ghazal, and then extending to the nearby Nuba Mountains with high mortality. Following this, extensive vaccination was carried out in the South (42). In the same year, a smaller outbreak occurred at Berber and the source was traced to a man from Omdurman. During that year the total number of those vaccinated was 156,378. In 1922 a minor outbreak with a total number of 179 cases (with 13 fatalities) occurred in Khartoum among recent immigrants from Kordofan. The epidemic spread south along the Blue Nile up to the town of Rosiers, as well as north and east into Atbara, Sinkat, and Port Sudan. Extensive vaccinations were carried out, with the number vaccinated that year totaling 191,577 cases (43). Probably in the wake of this epidemic, from December 1922 till May 1923, an outbreak in Tokar and the surrounding district, in the Red Sea Province, affected 63 cases, following which extensive vaccination was carried out. It was mentioned in that year's report that the Red Sea Province was the only area in Northern Sudan where there had been no mass vaccination.

2. Cerebrospinal Meningitis

In Sudan, CSM is nicknamed 'Abu Farrar' (Arabic: the one with an axe). The first reported case from Sudan in the medical literature was a paper by Dr. H. Ensor of the RAMC, published in the *Journal of the Royal Army Medical Corps* in 1904 (44). The first epidemic on record following the Reconquest was in 1898 at Omdurman, with a mortality rate of 70% to 80%. In the pre-antibiotic era, treatment was mainly symptomatic and those who survived were liable to end up with permanent neurological damage. Public health measures—isolation and containment of suspected cases—were the mainstay of intervention during that era. In those days, lumbar puncture was one means of relieving the pressure and it used to be called 'spinal drainage'. The availability of sulphonamides (such as 'Prontosil')[1] in the late 1930s and early 1940s, was a major breakthrough in medical management. It was an irony that Dr. Pat Somers, the last Registrar of KSM, was the first one to use intrathecal injections of sulphonamides in Southern Sudan in the late 1930s (45). In 1898, the epidemic of CSM in Omdurman and Khartoum continued to linger on till early 1900. Squires quoted an extract from the Annual Report of 1900 by Colonel Penton, the Principal of the EAMC, which stated that the epidemic eventually subsided (46). The second epidemic did not occur until 1915, when it spread northward from Uganda, sweeping the southern provinces and moving to the Northern Sudan where it took its toll in the towns of el-Dueim and al-Kawa, on the White Nile south of Khartoum. Dr. Paul Squires was posted on board the barge attached to the 'Floating Laboratory' of the Wellcome TRL in Khartoum, to those areas in the White Nile, in futile attempts to curb the spread of the epidemic. That mission took several months, during which the epidemic spread across the Gezira District into Wad Medani and then further south into Singa and other reaches of the Upper Blue Nile. Dr. Squires attempted quarantines and isolation measures. Along the White Nile, the epidemic reached as far north as the town of Al-Getiena, and Khartoum and Omdurman had only a few cases (47).

Several other CSM epidemics were to follow. In 1936 an epidemic broke out that affected a total of 13,440 patients. In 1937-1938, another major outbreak took place in central and western Sudan, and by 1939 the epidemic became overwhelming in the south, especially in Bahr el-Ghazal Province. Dr. Bryant, Chief Medical Inspector, made a solution of crushed sulphonamide tablets and used it for injection (48). Several members of the SMS were commended for doing superb work to curb the menace of these epidemics. Dr. Bryant and Dr. Fairman and later Dr. Somers, who was credited with being the first one to use the intrathecal route for injecting sulphonamides to treat those cases, paralleled the more favourable contemporary European practice. The technique of the above three doctors was much applauded in the literature. Another clever attempt was that of Dr. N. L. Corkhill, who tried vaccination utilizing serum, but with little or no success. Dr. Corkhill, who had a special interest in nutrition, attempted using vitamin A during epidemics (49). The number of cases in the period of 1932-1941 totaled 30,802, with a mortality rate of 78.5%. Another major epidemic occurred in 1950, with 57,575 cases, and in the decade preceding that epidemic several small outbreaks had occurred. The total number of cases between 1942 and 1951 was 88,623, with a mortality rate of only 13.6%, reflecting the advances in medical management brought about in the post-antibiotic era.

Omdurman Midwifery Training School

'The work of this school, and the influence that spreads from it, I feel, is more appealing than anything else I know in medicine'

Sir Eardley Holland,

President of the Royal College of Obstetricians & Gynecologists, 1946

Early Beginnings

It was an irony that the training of midwives in the Anglo-Egyptian Sudan superseded the training of nurses. Several factors played a major role in this venture. According to the papers of the first Matron of the Midwifery Training School (MTS), Miss Mabel Elsie Wolff, a British nurse/midwife, who was born and brought up in Egypt, the idea of establishing the school came from Mrs Molly Crowfoot, wife of Mr John Crowfoot, who was Director of Education in Sudan during the period of the First World War. Mrs Crowfoot, who happened to have attended a birth at Omdurman when she began to formulate this idea, had already been 'horrified' at the practice of female genital mutilation. Having seen its consequences vis-a-vis the delivery process, she went on to persuade Dr. Crispin, the then director of SMD, to start training midwives in the Sudan. She went further and recommended Miss Mabel Wolff as the 'best person for the job' (50). Doubtless, this was not the major reason. Other needs, including the need to provide subordinate medical staff to meet the expanding service following the availability of more funds after the First World War, was probably another major factor. Further, development in other fields in the country, especially the building of 'Makkwar Dam' and the establishment of the Gezira Irrigation Scheme mandated improvement in maternal and child health, to meet the long-term supply of Sudanese labourers (51). The annual reports of the SMD over the preceding years had kept mentioning the fact that 'Sudan is very much under-populated following the wars, famines and epidemics that characterized the Mahdist's State' (52, 53). On January 1, 1921, the MTS at Omdurman was inaugurated, as the second major training scheme for allied healthcare professionals sponsored by SMD. It was preceded only by the training of medical assistants in 1918. The early successes of this school were due to the first two matrons, the 'Wolff Sisters', Mabel and her elder sister Gertrude Wolff. Both were born and brought up in Egypt, where their father was working as a clerk in a British company in Port Twefig, on the Suez Canal. Both were fluent in Arabic, and they had been prepared for such a difficult task by their earlier training as nurse/midwives in Britain. Also, they had already had experience with the training of midwives in Egypt.

Miss Mabel Elsie Wolff arrived in Sudan in November of 1920. At the time, Sudanese women had little or no passion at all to be trained in the nursing profession, and the profession was regarded as a low-class occupation. Even in Britain in those days, at the beginning of the twentieth century, nursing and midwifery were also considered low-class professions. The prime aim of the MTS in its beginning was to train the traditional Sudanese midwives, known as '*Dayas*' (plural [singular, *daya*]; Sudanese slang; meaning midwives) and then to create a class of 'modern midwives' out of and in rivalry to the existing ones (55). However, it wasn't to be an easy task. Recruitment of the first few batches of students proved to be very difficult. Some of the logistic difficulties that faced Miss Wolff in the beginning were the cultural barriers of the profile of the midwife herself in Sudanese society. Of the prerequisite criteria for a midwife in the Sudanese culture were: being married/or having been married; having already witnessed the experience of childbirth; and being relatively old. Miss Wolff herself didn't fit these criteria! She had stepped into an alien country. She was in her thirties and was unmarried. To 'accept training' from this 'Frankish uncircumcised White Woman' was repulsive to many of those traditional *Dayas*. The task of recruiting the first students for the school proved to be 'mission impossible'. Only two students joined the first batch. It was only intriguing that the first was a lady who was hitting 70 and the second was a 60-year-old widow with no experience! The elder of them poked Miss Wolff in the cheek and said, 'I was practicing midwifery before your mother was born!' (56). The first of these two was Nura bint Omar, of the Omdurman suburb of Farieg al-Suk; and the second was the wife of the *bawab* (gatekeeper), a young woman with no experience of midwifery. According to Janice Boddy and the SMD Report of 1922, Miss Wolff started her first class with 4 students (57, 58), the other two started only at the end of the first few months. The first of these was Aziza Bercy, an old midwife, 68 years of age, from beyond 'Abu Rouf' (an Omdurman suburb); and the second was Mastura Khidir, a youngish woman with previous midwifery experience. Mastura Khidir later became the first Sudanese midwife to receive a Medal from His Majesty King George V in 1945, as a tribute to be the only surviving pioneer midwife from the first batch that started their training in Omdurman (59, 60).

The major difficulty that faced Mabel Wolff was the fact that almost all her students were totally illiterate. Girls' education had just begun over a decade before (pioneered by Babiker Bedri, a Sudanese notable who had opened the first modern school to teach girls in Rufaa in 1907). The MTS mandate was to 'overcome, combat and improve harmful rites and customs'. The task would involve the teaching and mentoring of a new breed of '*Dayas*'—those of the 'Hakoma (Arabic for "The Government")—to counter-balance the conventional *Dayas*, the '*dayat Alhabil'* (Arabic; 'midwives of the ropes'). So, the primary aim of the MTS at the beginning was to improve the skills of the practicing 'traditional midwives', stressing the new concepts of cleanliness, hygiene, and safety. Later, sheer science was to follow. The criteria of age and literacy were not adhered to in the selection of the first candidates; indeed, the first wave of those who received this training were both old and illiterate. The average age of the first few groups of trainees was sixty (61, 62). The second batch consisted of six women from Omdurman, the youngest of whom was the widowed daughter of Aziza Bercy, a trainee from the first term. She was a bright, handsome, intelligent woman called Gindiya Salah, who later became the first Sudanese staff midwife at the school. Another, a woman from Omdurman called Umm Taiman Sharif Al-Hindi, was discovered by Miss Wolff delivering her first school case in a state of 'stark nudity', the reason given being that she did not want to soil the government uniform, which at the time was merely a surgeon's white overall! (63). Recruitment remained difficult in the first couple of years, however, as the length of the designed study course was initially only three months. By 1924, Miss Wolff had succeeded in training most of the traditional *Dayas* in Omdurman, Khartoum, and Khartoum North. The course of study evolved gradually, increasing to six months by 1924. Individual tutoring and coaching was the mainstay of the teaching style. The students had to attend 20 lectures and deliver a minimum of 20 cases. (During the author's training in the prefinal year of the Khartoum Medical School at Khartoum University, medical students were required to have delivered at least 20 cases.). Another 20 cases had to be observed with a co-pupil midwife. Practical and oral exams were conducted at the end of the study course by British Medical Officers from the SMD. On passing, the students were given a certificate to enable them to practice in the Sudan. The new principles taught to the students emphasized hygiene, cleanliness, and safety. Mabel Wolff stressed these principles when she wrote the following in the first elementary lessons she prepared for the students: '*The first lesson a midwife must learn, is the importance of good manners, morals and cleanliness*'. These principles had to be adopted by the student herself—her nails and hands, her family, her children, her husband, her own home, and her place of work (64). Miss Wolff's teaching style relied heavily on simple means and examples from local Sudanese homes, an art that she had mastered well. The heart of the instruction to the midwives was a cluster of basic concepts: hygiene, discipline, teamwork, orderly manner, and a personal and familial zest for cleanliness. The icon of these new principles was a photograph of a midwife displaying her 'Midwife box & kettle' The box would have all the items needed by the midwife to conduct a 'perfect hygienic job', and all the items had to be recognized by 'feel, taste and smell'. There was a special emphasis on being rational, and doses of various medicines had to be known by heart (65, 66).

The School persevered against the odds and the difficult enterprise triumphed against major stumbles at the beginning. The report of the SMD in 1922 stated that a total of 15 midwives had been trained at the MTS (67). The 1923 Report fetures the following extract:

> Progress made by the School is very gratifying. It has raised the 'local standard' of midwifery and it has also now begun to receive women from the provinces for training. It is thus hoped that the influence of the school will permeate gradually throughout the country and will result in the appreciable decline of in the maternal and infantile death rate of childbirth and consequently healthy increase in the population. Up to the present time 42 women have been trained of whom 25 are practicing at Omdurman and 8 in the provinces. (68)

By 1924 all traditional midwives in Khartoum, Omdurman, and Khartoum North had been trained, so Miss Wolff began her next phase: recruiting midwives from various provinces. She, like any other British staff in those days, would spend only nine months in the country each year, and of these she would spend six month at the School and three months touring the districts and provinces of the Sudan, advocating for the School and selecting her prospective candidates (photo, SMJ paper, courtesy of SAD). Thus, in 1925, she made a tour of the provinces, starting at Berber Province and then on to Dongola, meeting notable women to lobby them, and again her perseverance and dedication paid a dividend. That year she secured a total of 11 women to be trained (69). The provincial tours became a constant annual task Mabel would conduct, and that continued till the next stage of midwifery training was initiated with the opening of a series of satellite training schools in the provinces in the 1940s and beyond (70).

When the School was established, the premises were very limited. The funds allocated were little, so it could not finance a decent building that would include a lodging for the first Matron, who had to be housed in a two-room mud-brick building with a bathroom, but no bath. In one corner of the compound were a tiny kitchen and a servant's room. The School proper had two mud-brick buildings of two rooms each, one used as a dormitory for students, an office, a lecture theatre, and patient's examination room. In the corner of the building there was a little storeroom that was later converted into a 'labour room'. The furniture was very sparse, and lighting was by means of candles or paraffin lamp (71). Water was daily brought by gangs of prisoners while a well was being labouriously dug in the *'hosh'* (Arabic; courtyard). The only means of transportation for Miss Wolff was by a hired donkey or on her own feet.

In 1931 new premises were built for the School, and with the advent of expansion in the service with the creation of the SMS, the MTS was to enter a new era, with more funds, with the opening of the Women Hospital in 1925, and with the subsequent start of the nurses' training, which set a new milestones for the MTS role and vision. These milestones and new frontiers are covered in the section on SMS in Volume 2 (forthcoming).

Section V:
Hospitals

According to S. I. Khalil, the first modern hospital in the Sudan following the Turco-Egyptian conquest of 1821 was built around 1826 (72). At the time of the Mahdiyya uprising and during the fading years of Turco-Egyptian rule, there was a military hospital in each province of the Sudan. Following the Reconquest, there were only four hospitals in the country; however, the only surviving doctor was Dr. Hassan Effendi Zaki, an Egyptian doctor. By 1900 several small hospitals were built in Khartoum, Wadi Halfa, el-Obeid, Wad Medani, Atbara, and Suakin (see Section on SMD). All these hospitals began as military hospitals in the first few years of the Anglo-Egyptian Condominium. Later, civil hospitals began to be established in various major cities and towns in the Sudan. The main hospitals at the zenith of the SMD were at Khartoum, Omdurman, Atbara, and Port Sudan. The other hospitals in Wadi Halfa, Merwoe, Suakin, and Dueim remained small before the expansion years after 1924 (year of the establishment of the SMS). In this section we will focus on some of these hospitals, for which there is a dearth of records and what records there were difficult to trace.

I. Khartoum Civil Hospital

Built in 1909, the Khartoum Civil Hospital (KCH) was the first purposely built civil hospital in the whole of the Sudan. The building of this hospital lagged behind for a significant number of years after the establishment of the SMD. In Khartoum, the 'Military Hospital' during the Turco-Egyptian era was destroyed at the time of the fall of the city in 1885. Research is awaited to unravel the details of that hospital, its building, staffing, equipment, and various other descriptions. Following the Reconquest of 1898, the hospital that preceded KCH, and where medical care was delivered, was in a rented house owned by a Greek merchant named Mr. Ortalani, on Victoria Street (present-day Palace Street). We do not have details of that hospital, e.g., how many rooms/wards it had. In the 'Diary' of Dr. J. B. Christopherson, the first British Medical Officer of the Hospital, written in 1903, the 'Khartoum Civil Hospital' is described as a 'very primitive thirty-bed mud-brick building'. From these 'Diaries', more fragmented information has filtered out (e.g., 'I have 37 patients, 5 Wards, office, Kitchen, etc.') (73, 74).

The new hospital was designed by Mr Gorringe, of the Royal Engineers, the same architect who designed several other buildings in Khartoum and Wad Medani, including Gordon Memorial College and the Governor General's Palace (75). The hospital hosted the first British civilian nurse to work in Sudan, in 1907, Miss Maria Pye Moore (photo; see Illustration List). She was later joined by Miss Jones (later Mrs J. W. Sagar), who went on to be the first Matron of Khartoum Hospital. It was in KCH that Dr. J. B. Christopherson treated the first three Kala-azar patients (also co-infected with schistosomiasis) with sodium antimony tartarate. Dr. Christopherson was the first director of the hospital, and his term lasted from 1909 to1917. He was succeeded by Dr. Vincent Hodson (till 1922) and then by Dr. Paul Squires (till 1930). Following the establishment of the Kitchener School of Medicine in 1924, and the creation of the posts of senior physician and senior surgeon, the custom was for the senior physician of the SMS to be the director of KCH. The first to combine that title was Dr. Paul Squires. Following Dr. Squires, three more British doctors were in that post before the first Sudanese physician to hold it, did so in 1953. Those three British doctors were Dr. Roy Mervyn Humphreys (1930-1944), Alexander Cruickshank (1944-1948), and Dr. R. N. M. Buchanan (1948-1953). Dr. Halim was the first Sudanese physician to hold the post, which he did starting in 1953. From the tenure of Dr. Paul Squires when the Kitchener School of Medicine was inaugurated in 1924, it became a tradition from 1926 onward that the Director of KCH would also assume the position of Lecturer of Medicine at KSM as well as the post of senior physician for the SMS. This tradition would continue till the Independence of Sudan and beyond. The first Matron of KCH was Miss Maria Pye Moore, who held the post since it was created till 1930 (76). She was succeeded by Miss Elaine Hillis-Young, who also assumed the post of Lecturer of Nursing at KSM from 1935 onward. In 1937, Miss A. V. Butcher served in the position from 1942, when the post was taken over by Miss Gilchrist, an Australian. The last British Matron was Miss Noakes, who filled the post from 1947 till it was Sudanized in 1955.

2. The River Hospital

The other hospital in Khartoum was the Egyptian Army Military Hospital. This hospital survived the dismantling of Khartoum's buildings that took place following the fall of the city in the wake of the decisive Mahdist victory on January 25, 1885. The hospital had been established during the Turco-Egyptian era, possibly around 1826, as the first ever modern hospital in the Sudan (77). The hospital was then deserted following the demise of the regime by the Mahdists in 1885. During the Turco-Egyptian rule, the hospital didn't provide open service to the Sudanese natives and its services were primarily meant for the Turco-Egyptian rulers and for the army personnel and their families. Following the Reconquest, the hospital was rebuilt for the Egyptian Army as its main hospital serving its troops from 1901. It was known as the Egyptian Army Military Hospital, Khartoum. The hospital remained under the Egyptian Army Medical Corps and it provided service to the military as well as to the native Sudanese citizens. It was staffed by British doctors who were recruited to the Egyptian Army Medical Corps and seconded to the services of the Sudan Government. One of the earlier military doctors to have worked there was Dr. Steven Lyle Cummins, an Irish Bimbashi, who was the senior medical officer in the hospital during the early years of the Anglo-Egyptian Reconquest. During the 1924 mutiny and revolution by the Sudanese military corps, the incidents began when the Egyptian Army personnel were expelled from the Sudan following the assassination of Sir Lee Stack in Cairo. In direct response, a full-scale mutiny took place and some Sudanese military cadets took up arms in support of their Egyptian 'brethren'. During that uprising, the hospital sustained significant damage (78). Following that incident, the hospital was renovated and rebuilt and it was then incorporated into the SMS and became known as the 'The River Hospital'. The hospital subsequently hosted the earliest ophthalmology and respiratory services, especially for cases of tuberculosis, which was quite common in the country at the time.

3. Wad Medani & Other Gezira Hospitals

Wad Medani Hospital was built in 1904. After the establishment of the Gezira Scheme, the peasant populations were served mainly by two small hospitals built at Hag Abdalla and at Kilo 114 on the main canal. The hospital at Abu Usher was built in 1929 and it gained a special position during the construction of the Gezira Irrigation Scheme. It was usually manned by a British senior medical inspector.

4. Atbara Hospital

Atbara Hospital was the largest hospital north of Khartoum. The town sprawled when the headquarters of the Sudan Government Railways was made there in the early years following the Reconquest. Indeed, the hospital itself was designed and built by the British staff, and early patients were primarily employees of that service (79). It was the first hospital in the Anglo-Egyptian Sudan that had the amenities of electric lights and ceiling fans (80). One of the staff of the medical service, an Australian, Dr. Charles Eric Glasson Beveridge, who arrived in 1925 to take over as medical officer in charge of the hospital, described the hospital as being built of solid brick and being two storeys high, with 200 beds and 200 to 300 patients seen daily in the outpatient department, and it was staffed by two British and two Syrian doctors (81).

5. The 'Lady Baker'—the 'Ship Hospital'

With more expansion of medical services into rural areas, Dr. G. R. Footner, a British doctor who joined the SMD in 1911, was commissioned to work in Upper Nile Province from 1920, where he was based at Malakal, the capital. He was, in effect, the only civilian doctor in that region of southern Sudan. Much of his work was done on patrol, sometimes with the army patrols. The main method of transportation was via the river, especially during the seven months of the rainy season. The 1,500 miles of navigable waters in that province includes the White Nile, the Sobat and its tributaries, the Pibor and Akobo Rivers, the Zeraf, and Bahr el-Gebel. Dr. Footner proposed to Dr. Crispin, the then director of SMD, the idea of having a 'hospital ship'. Dr. Crispin approved of the idea and subsequently funds were secured (82). An old steamer ship, the *Atbara*, which belonged to the Sudan Development and Exploration Company, was converted into a hospital ship, which was ready to be used by 1922. The ship was named the 'Lady Baker', after the Hungarian wife of Sir Samuel Baker. Mrs (later, Lady) Baker was thought to have practiced simple means of nursing while in the Sudan between 1861 and 1865. Crispin happened to be a distant relative by marriage of Sir Samuel Baker, and the governor of Kassala, Mr R. Bailey, was also a relative of Sir Samuel. The approval of the name was subsequently granted by the Governor General, Sir Lee Stack. The ship had a dispensary and examination rooms on its lower deck, with an operating theatre and eight beds to accommodate patients, plus an accommodation for the medical staff, with a towing barge for overflow patients (83).

In the first year, when the Lady Baker was commissioned to join SMD on March 6, 1922, the ship made six tours to visit places where 'the natives' had had no previous opportunity to receive medical treatment (84). During those trips, a total of 1,040 injections of nova-arsenobenzol for yaws and syphilis were administered among a total of 1,094 patients who were seen. Dr. Footner was the physician in charge of the Lady Baker from 1922 till 1926, when he left the province to take the post of senior surgeon at Khartoum Civil Hospital and lecturer of surgery at KSM. Dr. E. A. H. Crouch replaced him in the Upper Nile and assumed responsibility of the hospital ship. The original ship was later replaced by a better and newer ship, which remained in service well into the years just prior to the independence of the Sudan (85). No more details could be traced about the hospital ship, especially how long it remained in service and what was its ultimate fate.

Quarantines

Wadi Halfa Quarantine:

Wadi Halfa Quarantine was established around 1902, following the Reconquest, with a mandate at the time to curb the spread of cholera from Egypt, where it once was endemic, to Sudan. The Quarantine was strengthened around 1919 when 'Sayiedi & Felaheen' labourers were recruited to help build the Sennar 'Makkwar' Dam. There was a well-perceived risk of 'importing' schistosomiasis and other helminthic infestations into the Gezira area through these Egyptian labourers, as those diseases were highly endemic in Egypt. The credit goes to Dr. William Byam and his moral stand over this vital issue.

Suakin Quarantine

This was established well before the era of the Anglo-Egyptian Sudan, during the Turco-Egyptian role to control cases of cholera and plague from entering Sudan. As Suakin was never taken by the Mahdists during their rule of the Sudan, the quarantine remained under Anglo-Egyptian control throughout the reign of the Mahdiyya. Following the Reconquest, it served as a filter point where the pilgrims coming from West Africa were also screened, especially for typhus and relapsing fever, among other conditions.

Endnote

1 https://en.wikipedia.org/wiki/Prontosil

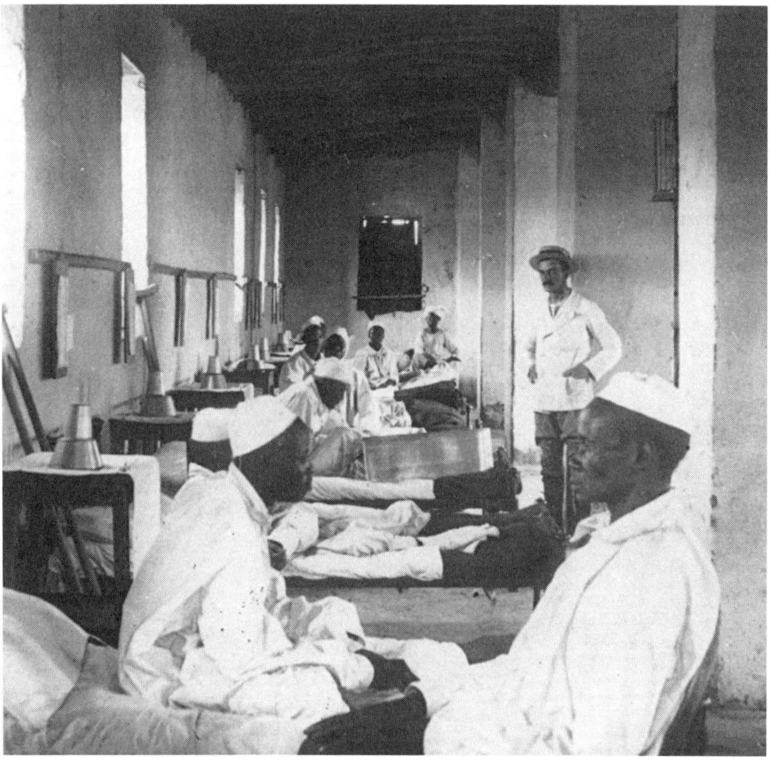

Dr. John Brian Christopherson in a male ward of Omdurman Civil Hospital, circa? 1904
(JB Christopherson collections, Sudan archive Durham, SAD, SD 02/02/11, Reproduced by permission of Durham University Library & Collections)

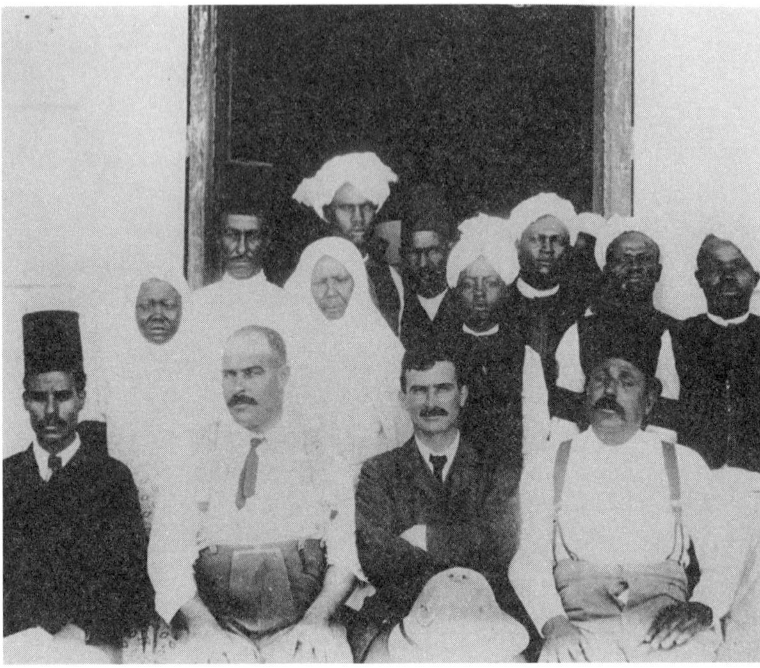

Group photograph, Khartoum Civil Hospital staff, Dr. John Brian Christopherson, Director of the hospital, (middle) Dr. Hassan Effendi Zaki {to his left with the fez)
(JB Christopherson collections, Sudan archive Durham, SAD, SD 02/02/12, Reproduced by permission of Durham University Library & Collections).

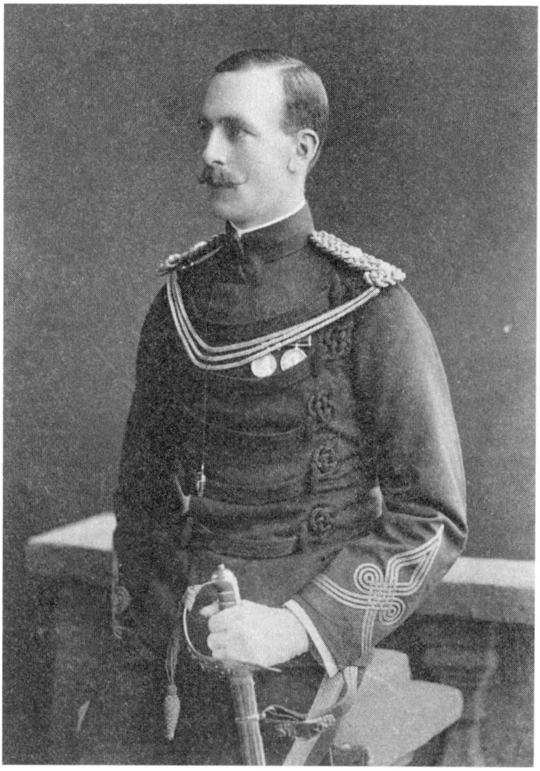

Dr. Edward Smyth Crispin
(Dr. ES Crispin collections, Sudan Archives Durham, 2/25/34, Reproduced by permission of Durham University Library & Collections)

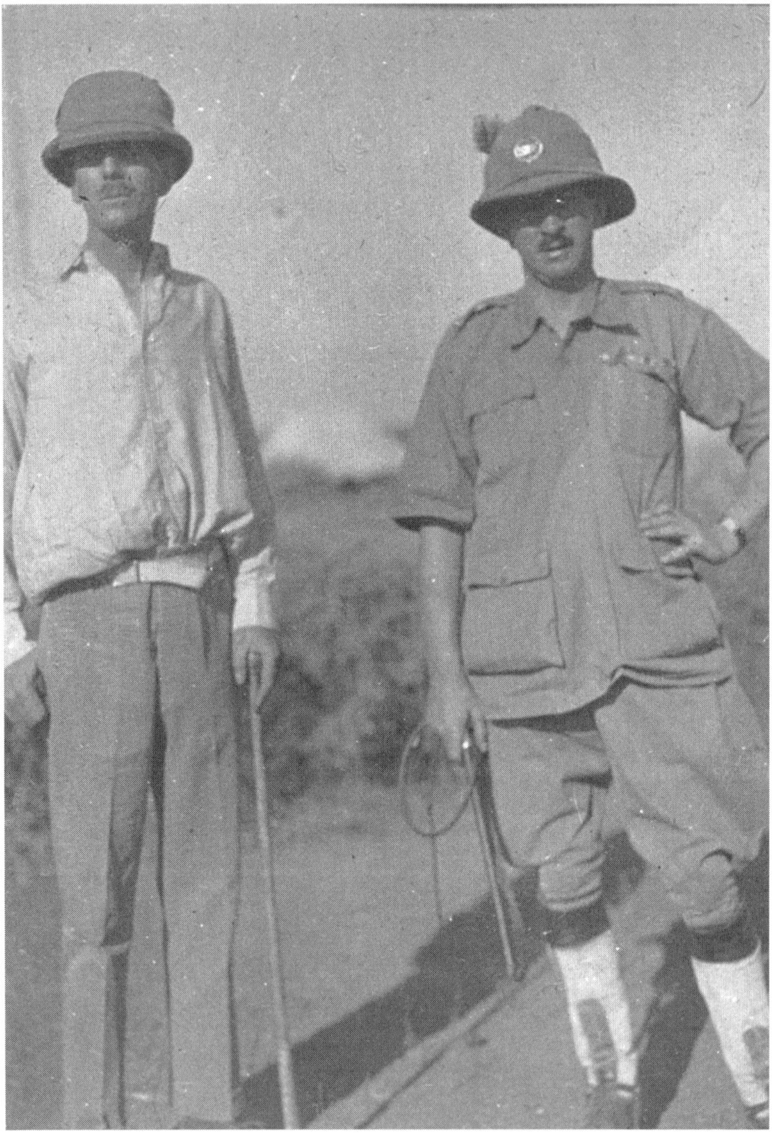

Dr. Oliver Francis Atkey
(Dr. OF Atkey collections, Durham SAD. 760/07/39, Reproduced by permission of Durham University Library & Collections).

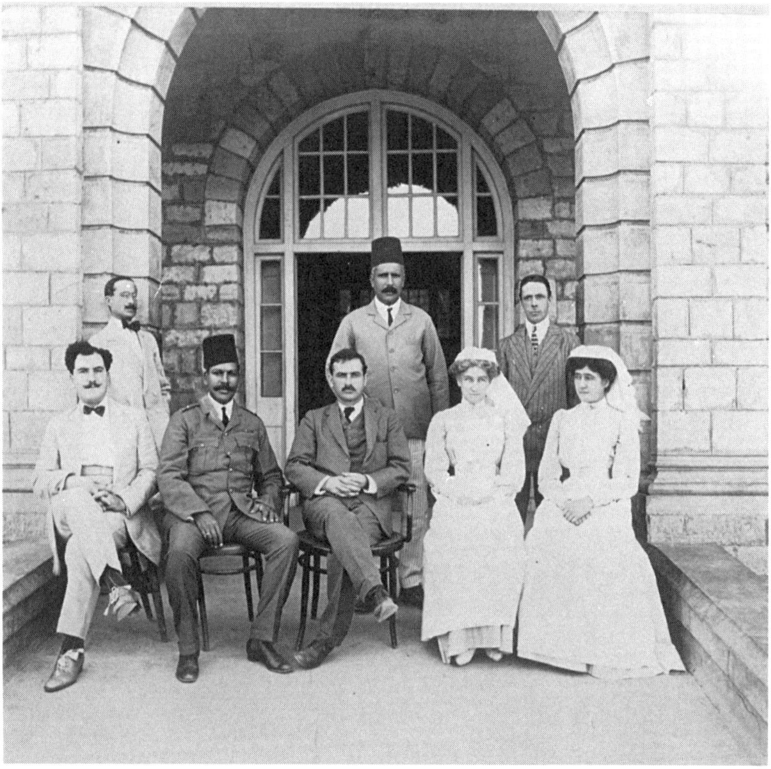

Dr. J B Christopherson with Staff of Khartoum Civil Hospital circa1912, sitting from left, Dr. Sassoun, (Senior Medical Officer), Dr. Muhammad Nikhlawi, a Bimbashi (Major), Egyptian Army, Dr. JB Christopherson, Director of the hospital, and the nurses, M Pye Moore (the first British nurse in the Sudan), and M. G. Jones (later Mrs J W Sagar). Standing from left Dr. Abd Latif, the dispenser, Hassan Labib and Mr. John R Newlove

(Dr. JB Christopherson collections, Sudan archive Durham, SAD 007/004/001, Reproduced by permission of Durham University Library & Collections)

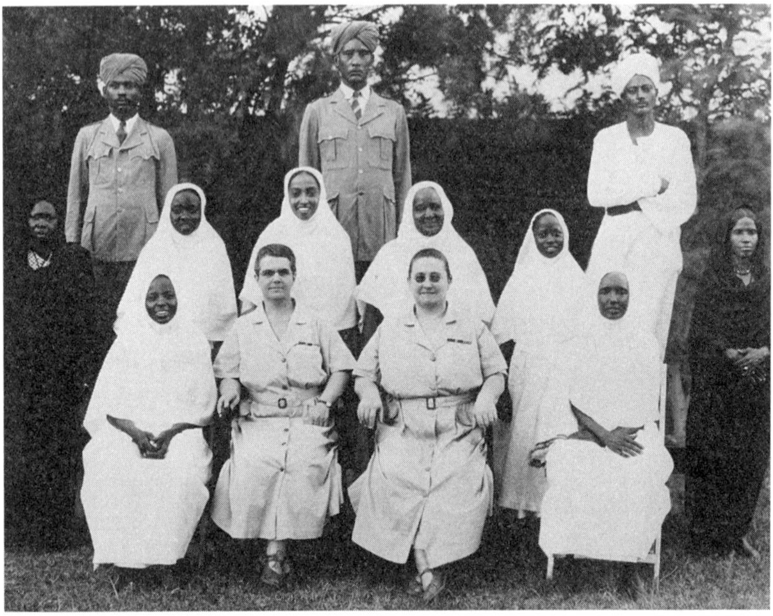

The Wolff's sisters, Mabel L. {to the right} & Gertrude Wolff with staff at Omdurman Midwifery Training School circa 1937. To the right of Mabel is Sitt Batul Mohammed Isa, a prominent Sudanese midwife on the staff of OMTS
(Sudan Archives at Durham, SAD, 583/05/02, Reproduced by permission of Durham University Library & Collections)

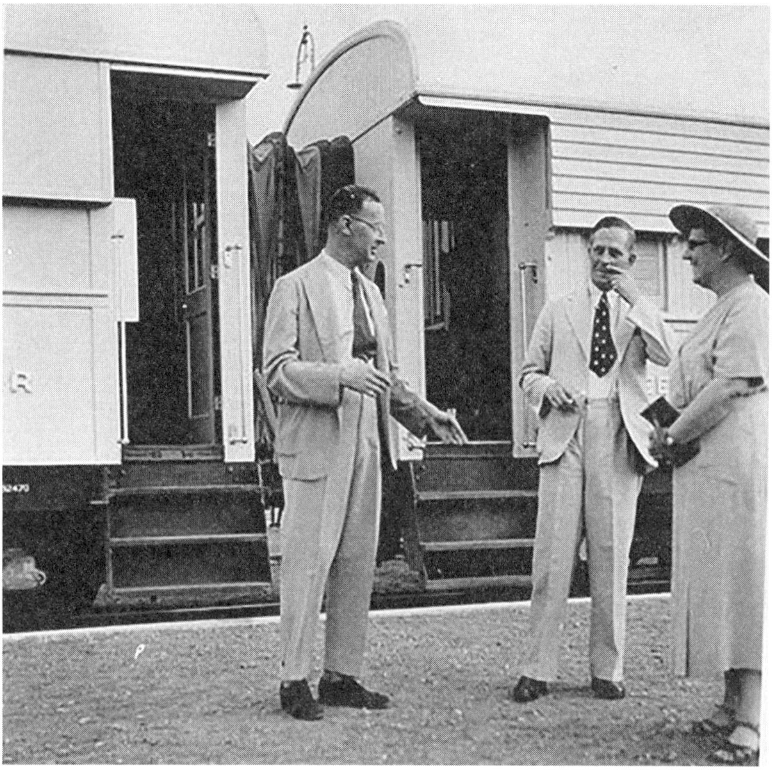

Mabel Wolff in tour of the provinces
(Image courtesy of Sudan Medical Journal).

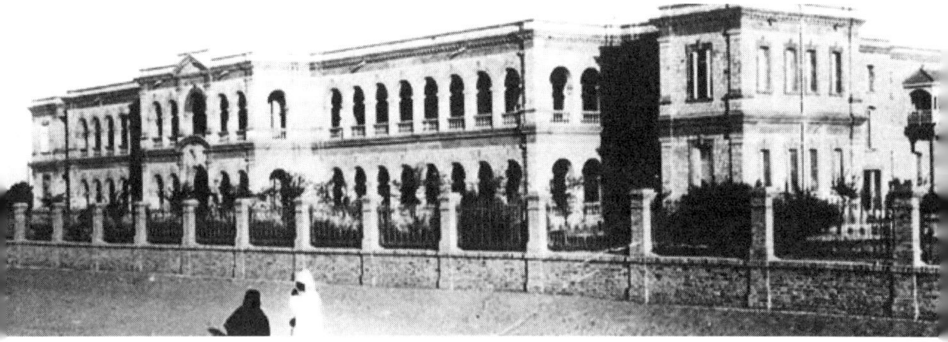

PART 4

THE WELLCOME TROPICAL RESEARCH LABORATORY AT KHARTOUM

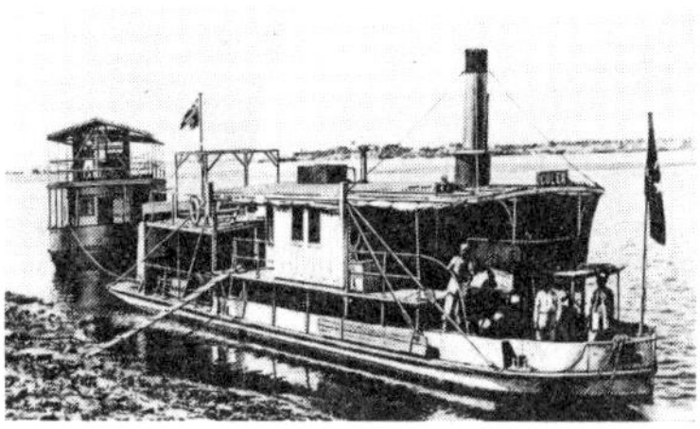

Chapter I

Wellcome & Balfour:
An Enterprise on the Nile

> It is from numberless diverse acts of courage and belief that human history is shaped. Each time a man stands for an ideal, or acts to improve the lots of others, or strikes out against injustice, he sends forth a tiny ripple of hope, and crossing each other from a million different centres of energy and daring, those ripples build a current that can sweep down the mightiest walls of oppression and resistance.
>
> –Robert F. Kennedy, US Attorney General, 1961-1964

Shortly after the Reconquest, the American industrialist, philanthropist, and pharmaceutical tycoon, Henry Solomon Wellcome, entered the scene. He was destined to play a decisive role in the history of modern medicine in the Sudan. The historical irony was that the relationship between Wellcome and this newly conquered British territory would prove to be both intriguing and curious. This relationship, which spanned over three decades in the life of one of the most iconic industrialists and philanthropists of the Victorian era, had also proven to be crucial to the history of research in tropical medicine. On the other hand, it was pivotal for the newly established, rudimentary Sudan health services and for the future of medical education in the Sudan, as it provided the foundation for first-class laboratory services that were second to none in the British colonial empire. Furthermore, apart from medicine, Wellcome's love of archaeology and his fondness for collecting antiquities led him in his later years to be involved in other spheres, such as social benevolence and philanthropy, as we shall see in subsequent sections. However, it was in the medical field that Wellcome's fingerprints were destined to survive. To understand such complex relations, one has to acquaint himself with the biography of Sir Henry Wellcome and the cascade of historical events in Victorian Britain and the British Empire in the last quarter of the nineteenth century.

Wellcome was born in 1853, on a farm in the American Midwest hinterlands of the State of Wisconsin, to a deeply religious family. When he was 16 years old, he moved to settle in Garden City, Minnesota, where he received a modern education and was first exposed to milestones of medicine and pharmacy. His uncle, George Wellcome, was a doctor. Young Henry was engaged to help him out in his surgery and in the small dispensary attached to the clinic. During his time with his uncle, the town was subjected to a fierce siege by the local Sioux Indians, an uprising that resulted in the massacre of several hundred of the white settlers. The subsequent reprisal by the authorities resulted in many Indians killed and their chiefs hanged. In the besieged city, Wellcome helped his uncle in looking after the dying and the wounded. The experience left a deep feeling and scars in young Henry's memory, such that he later became very sympathetic to the plight of the Red Indians and their cause. This very much sharpened his religious feeling and it proved decisive to his strong connection with Father Duncan and his missions among the Indians (1).

Following his studies at Philadelphia University, Wellcome graduated from the School of Pharmacy and elected to work as a pharmaceutical salesman. He was then invited by a fellow American, a university-mate and a friend, Silas Burroughs, to join him in London to establish a joint company, named Burroughs Wellcome & Co. In a short period, Wellcome became a prominent figure in business and in British public life. In London, he befriended another fellow American, the famous African explorer, Henry Morton Stanley.

Both Stanley and Wellcome were members of the May French-Sheldon salon of African explorers (2). Wellcome became deeply connected with the British colonial enterprises and the missionary activities destined for Africa. Further, he mastered the art of 'business publicity' and soon began to publicise his own *Tabloid Medicine Chest*. The first medicine chest he used accompanied Stanley in his adventures in the basin of the Congo River. According to his biographer, several factors drew Henry Wellcome's interest in the events in the Sudan. His imperial business dealings, the general public interest in the events at Khartoum following the death of Charles Gordon, his own religious upbringing, and his deep sense of humanity and egalitarianism—all formed a strong catalyst for him to seek to play a role in the Sudan. At Christmas of 1898, at the climax of the Kitchener-led campaigns, Wellcome bought and distributed to his friends and employees hundreds of copies of W. G. Steevens' book, *With Kitchener to Khartoum,* as well as *The Fire & Sword in the Soudan* by Rudolph von Slatin (3). In a written address to his employees, Wellcome said: 'The accompanying volumes; '*Fire & Sword in the Sudan*, and '*With Kitchener to Khartoum*'– contain a graphic description of the rise of Mahdism, the martyrdom of Gordon, and the reconquest of the Sudan by the Sirdar, Lord Kitchener of Khartoum. This struggle between civilization and barbarism forms one of the most remarkable and thrilling episodes in the history of the world. With best wishes for a Merry Christmas & A Happy New Year' (4).

Following the appeal of Lord Kitchener for the establishment of Gordon Memorial College in 1899, Wellcome wrote to him with a cheque of 100 gineas from Burroughs Wellcome & Co., 'offering to contribute as soon as the institution is ready for them, a complete medical equipment and stock for the dispensary in connection with the College' (5). Thereafter, Wellcome met Lord Kitchener (Kitchener having read Wellcome's book, *The Story of the Metalahktla*) (6). In that meeting, Kitchener provided Wellcome with personal letters to Lord Cromer, the British Agent in Egypt, and to Lieutenant Reginald Wingate, who succeeded Kitchener as the Sirdar of the Egyptian Army and Governor General of the Sudan. Wellcome was among the first Europeans to visit Sudan following the Reconquest.

In winter of 1899 he was in Egypt, where he met Lord Cromer, and proceeded up the Nile to Khartoum.

Henry Wellcome and His Tropical Research Laboratories in Khartoum

Gordon Memorial College was founded in 1900, and it hosted its first students on November 8, 1902. The buildings of GMC, a masterpiece of colonial architecture, were designed and executed by Sir George Gorringe, of the Royal Army Engineers. Gorringe later designed several other buildings in the Sudan, including the Governor General's Palace, made in a Venetian style, in addition to several other governmental buildings which are standing to this day (7). To Henry Wellcome, the visit to the Sudan was a moving experience. What he saw of the poor health and sanitation of this newly annexed country and its people is recorded in his diaries:

> It was my purpose to study the existing condition of the native people as well as observe their ethnographical characteristics. To aid me, the Sudan Government converted a native sailing craft into a Dahabeeyah to enable me to cruise on the Upper Nile and visit the native settlements. During my visit to one of the small islands of the Nile, just above the Shabaluka Cataract, there were perhaps thirty or forty inhabitant everyone lying helplessly prostrated, weak and emaciated suffering from malaria in an extremely virulent form. I am sure that no one could have seen those mere skeletons of men, women and children without being moved by deep emotions to do something to mitigate the pitiful conditions of these poor and surely distressed people…. (8)

Following the Reconquest, the health and sanitation of the country and its people were extremely poor and backward. However, the new masters were too busy with pacifying the people and establishing the basis of their new order. No plans were yet made to establish medical and public health services. The medical services conducted by the military medical personnel were primarily destined for the troops. In the build-up to the success of Kitchener's Reconquest campaigns, the country was ravaged by poverty, malnutrition, water-borne diseases, and malaria. There were successive series of famines in the aftermath of the waging wars of the Khalifa on several fronts. Epidemics of smallpox and cholera broke out in the absence of proper medical care and poor sanitation. Wellcome made suggestions to Wingate and ordered medicines and equipment for the dispensary he had donated to Gordon Memorial College, which kept his assistants in his Snow Hill London headquarters, Dawson and Powers, very busy dispatching those materials. Wellcome went further and made proposals to establish a tropical research laboratory, which he undertook to fully fund and equip. He unfolded his plans to Lord Cromer when he returned to Cairo, and his proposals were speedily accepted. In his remarkable letter to Colonel (later Sir) F. Reginald Wingate, Wellcome made his offer on September 28, 1901:

> Sir, I beg to offer for the acceptance of the Gordon Memorial College, Khartoum complete equipment for chemical and bacteriological laboratories for analytical and research work....'

Wellcome went on in this remarkable letter to set the objectives of his historic proposals:

> To promote technical education. To study bacteriologically and physiologically tropical disorder, especially the infective diseases of both man and beast, particular to the Sudan, and to render assistance to the officers of health and to the clinics of civil and military hospitals...It is anticipated that the work in the laboratories will prove beneficial to both the Europeans and the native populations....but the government of Sudan is to support it and maintain it by providing the salary of its director and staff. (9)

The offer was readily accepted by both Cromer and Wingate. It was a full donation, as said in Wellcome's letter to Wingate. The Wellcome grant, a generous donation and a unique philanthropist venture of its kind, later proved to be crucial not only for medical research, but for future public health and medical services in general in the Sudan. Further, it made Sudan a leader in research in tropical medicine, a vastly expanding discipline at the turn of the twentieth century.

Andrew Balfour: First Director of WTRL & First Medical Officer for Health, Khartoum, 1903-1912

On his return to London, Wellcome became preoccupied with his new tropical venture in the Sudan. His first task was to identify and choose a dedicated director for the laboratory. His friend, Dr. (later Sir) Patrick Manson suggested Dr. Andrew Balfour, a young and bright Scottish doctor from Edinburgh, whom Manson knew well. Andrew Balfour's father was a general practitioner in Edinburgh. Andrew was born in Edinburgh in 1873 and studied at George Watson College in Edinburgh, before qualifying from Edinburgh University with a Bachelor of Medicine in 1894. He then went on to obtain a Master of Surgery from Cambridge in 1897. Then he obtained an MD from Edinburgh University. Sir Patrick Manson came to know Balfour well, as Balfour later obtained a diploma in public health from London under Manson's guidance. Balfour served in the South African War as a surgeon. He was young, athletic, and played rugby for both Scotland and Cambridge. He had all the qualities Wellcome was looking for. Wellcome wrote to Mr James Currie, the Principal of Gordon Memorial College and Director of education in Sudan: 'Penton and I interviewed the candidates for the position of director and bacteriologist. The only two candidates, who are likely to be satisfactory, are both married men. Of these, Colonel Penton, Dr. Paton and I agree on favour of Dr. Andrew Balfour....' (10). Wellcome organized a farewell party for Balfour in a prestigious restaurant in Piccadilly, London, which was attended by a distinguished audience including several scientists who had a special interest in tropical medicine and the Sudan. Amongst them were Balfour's mentor, Dr. Manson, and the African explorer, Henry Morton Stanley. Balfour's mission in the Sudan would now begin.

Passing via Egypt, Balfour spent a few weeks in Cairo, where he had the opportunity to visit Qasr Al-Aini Hospital. There he had the chance to choose his laboratory assistant, Mr John Newlove, who would later prove to be a very useful aide in Balfour's ventures in public health and research in tropical medicine in the Sudan. Balfour was officially appointed as Medical Officer of Health of Khartoum on March 15, 1904, in addition to his capacity as Director of the Wellcome research laboratory (11). Balfour, a visionary and a perfectionist, set his priorities to improve the public health of Khartoum. His input into the health and sanitation of Khartoum in a relatively short period was both stunning and extraordinary. At its establishment, the Wellcome laboratory consisted of only five rooms on the second floor of the eastern wing of GMC. One was being used as the Director's office, trhe other as a museum. The staff were only the Director and Mr Newlove, who arrived from Cairo in April of 1902 to resume his duties, together with two Sudanese assistants, one of them a young boy (12).

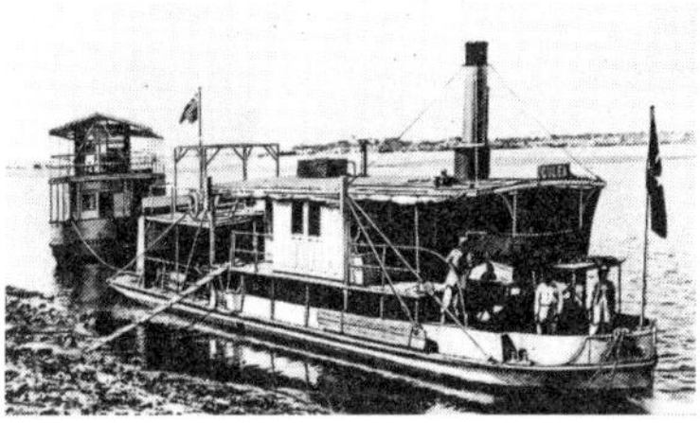

Chapter 2

The Foundation of Modern Public Health

Part A:

'Mission Not Impossible': Balfour & Byam and Mosquito Eradication & Malaria Control in Khartoum (1903-1913) & Kassala (1908)

Soon after he resumed office at Khartoum, Dr. Balfour began to set out his priorities. He identified four major areas that needed attention, in order to change the state of misery and squalor of Khartoum at the turn of the twentieth century, and to transform it into a decent and healthy city. He felt that his first task was to eradicate mosquitoes and control malaria, which was very devastating to the inhabitants (13). Earlier, Balfour, when he started his routine laboratory work, discovered that in the various blood slides he examined, the major forms of malaria were malignant tertian, quartan, and benign tertian. So, in his vision, the task to defeat malaria was to focus on finding its breeding sites, and then to tackle this via a group of 'sanitary workers', who were not available in the country at that time. The concept of the 'Mosquito Brigade' was well known in imperial medical circles. Here, a historical irony would point to the fact that Balfour's efforts coincided with efforts of other British personnel who were involved in improving the state of public health of the capital of the new Anglo-Egyptian dominion. Those were Colonel Talbot, of the Royal Engineers, and Colonel Lyle Cummins, Senior Medical Officer of Khartoum from the RAMC. The story of how the 'Mosquito Brigade' of Khartoum carried out this mission unfolds. Following some initiative from Colonel Talbot, some preliminary discussion was held with Colonel Lyle Cummins. Both were aware of Major Ronald Ross's work on mosquito control in India. In 1892, Ross, while working for the Indian Medical Service, had discovered the way the anopheline mosquito transmits malaria, a work that won him the Nobel Prize in 1902 (the year when Andrew Balfour was heading towards Khartoum). Ross designed an ingenious method of curbing mosquito transmission and controlling malaria, initially in India, and later in West Africa, Egypt, and Cyprus. This method proved to be effective wherever it was applied, and it became widely known in the British colonial circles. Colonel Talbot, who was by then the director of the Survey Department in Sudan, wrote to the Governor General, Sir Reginald Wingate:

> Do you think enough is being done to worry the mosquitoes? I think most persons are still blind or deaf to the beauties of the mosquito theory and I don't think the medical officers can do much unless cordially supported by laity'. He went on to assert 'how much does fever cost us every year and how much have we spent trying to prevent it?....this zeal on my part is due partly to the discovery that doctors don't hunt for mosquitoes as part of their regular work and secondly to my being a brand new convert to Ross' opinions from reading his books while up the White Nile. It is the hope that he may convert them in the same way as he has converted me, that makes me wish to see his pamphlets scattered broadcast in the Sudan. (14)

Following this, Balfour was asked to bring the matter to the fore. Balfour writes:

> Colonel Talbot being much interested in the matter, it was not long before one was asked to send to the SMO, Khartoum, a statement regarding the formation of a 'Mosquito Brigade', and one was subsequently requested to take complete charge of the work. I was

> very glad to do so, as it gives me an opportunity of studying the mosquito and their breeding places, of collecting specimens and of carrying some experiments.......two intelligent natives were from Colonel Stanton, the Mudir, and quickly trained to recognize mosquitoes, their eggs, larvae and pupae and to distinguish the culicidae from other insects. (15)

So, ironically, Balfour honestly asserted that the idea of the 'Mosquito Brigade' wasn't his. Secondly, he set out to do some research by investigating the breeding sites of the malaria vector, the mosquito. His first task proved to be a painstaking one. The first site that gave Balfour food for thoughts was the backyard of the Grand Hotel. There was a well that provided water to the hotel. In that well, Balfour realized, was one of the potential sites for mosquito breeding. Then, following thorough investigation, Balfour traced the source of the breeding sites to wells and waterways distributed in various parts of Khartoum. At that time, there were around 600 wells in Khartoum. In the essay on the subject he wrote for the Wellcome First Report in 1904, Balfour described the various types of common mosquitoes in Khartoum, including *culex fatigans* and several other species of the anopheline mosquito that transmit the parasites of several tropical scourges. These include the deadly malaria parasite, the microfilaria of elephantiasis, and the genus *stegomyia fasciata* that transmits Yellow Fever virus (16). The latter was traced to the bilges of the river steamers that traversed the Nile from Southern Sudan. Balfour adopted the concept of the 'Mosquito Brigade' pioneered first by Sir Ronald Ross in India. At first Balfour and Newlove made several innovations as well as modification of some ideas and techniques available at the time. The 'Balfour Brigade' consisted primarily of two Sudanese men who were obtained from Colonel Stanton's department. They were described by Balfour as intelligent. Balfour later wrote 'they were quickly trained to recognize mosquitoes, their eggs, larvae and pupae, and to distinguish the culicidae from other insects. Mr Newlove, the laboratory assistant...was placed in charge of these men' (17). Those first pioneering men were not mentioned by name and were referred to only anonymously. The necessary equipment was provided by Captain Rivers of the RAMC, acting SMO of Khartoum at the time. The initial plan of the 'Mosquito Brigade', at first, was to attack the mosquitoes at the larval stage. The breeding places, after initial research, were found to be the wells, Sakia pits (*Sakia*=Arabic, simple irrigation tool), garden tanks (primarily at the riverfront), bath waste pits, *zeers* (*Zeer*=Arabic. an earthenware vessel used by the natives to store and filter water for drinking and domestic use, made of special soil usually taken from the banks of the rivers in Sudan), permanent garden pools, and pools left in the banks by the falling Nile. The 'Mosquito Brigade' was to go around in the morning and again in the afternoon, inspecting wells, taking samples of water and examining them for egg boats, larvae, and pupae (18). Those wells found infested were sprayed with a mixture of petroleum distillate that Balfour found to be safe for both humans and animals, non-volatile, and effective. Besides, the crude mixture of oil was available in abundance and lasted a long time. The 'Brigade' would revisit all water sources, including *zeers* in the households. During his surveys, Balfour found that *zeers* were important reservoirs for mosquito breeding.

The work of the 'Mosquito Brigade' had to be codified in laws that would ensure that the cycle of mosquito-breeding control not be broken. A fine was to be imposed on those households that breached the regulation of keeping their *zeers* free from evidence of mosquito or its larvae breeding. This entailed regular inspection of all household water sources. That law was made very strict, with no exemption for any delinquents. Interestingly, the Inspector General of the Sudan Government, Sir Rudolph von Slatin Pasha, was fined for breaking this rule when on inspection of his house, the *zeer* was found to be a rife breeding site for mosquitoes. The Austrian became very furious, and his rage abated only after Balfour himself ten days later was caught red handed, when the *zeer* in his office was also found to have mosquito larvae. This tells the tale of how efficient and fair the regulations were during that era. No wonder that with the steady fall in the number of breeding sites, the incidence of malaria continued to fall accordingly, year after year (19). The wells in Khartoum were owned by individuals and not by the government. Without the cooperation of those owners, the mission of Andrew Balfour would not have been possible. He also used other, supplementary measures to hone his method to perfection. Wells were to be provided with covers, pumps were used to draw water, and 'Blue Nile fish' were used. This fish was famous for feeding on larvae, but even so, it was not successful, as the fish did not last long in those wells (20). The task of the 'Mosquito Brigade' was not an easy one. To accomplish such wide inspection of water sources, the men had to enter and inspect each household water source. The cultural barriers were not easy to overcome in those days, as the custom of the Sudanese people did not allow their families to be in contact with strangers. A notice both in Arabic and English had to appear regularly in the local newspaper, the *Sudan Gazette*, instructing the people about these important public health measures and how they could be implemented (21).

Another challenge that Balfour faced was to deal with the water vessels that accompanied the Nile steamers. Those were a dreaded source of 'imported malaria'. At the time, many of these steamers were traveling up and down the country, and those that traversed the southern frontiers were the most notorious for bringing in the deadly mosquito. The risk did not involve transmission only of malaria, but also Yellow Fever. These vessels also included the military gunboat, Zafir, and the geological research boat SS Nubia (22). Balfour, Newlove, and their 'Mosquito Brigade' tried several measures, including crude petroleum distillate and fumigation with sulphur squibs. Other measures included educating the crew staff and engineers of these vessels to deal with adult insects. Such measures were somewhat successful in keeping the mosquito at bay. By 1906, Balfour wrote in the Second Wellcome Report: 'I have not seen a living wild adult Anopheline in Khartoum for more than a year and a half and I am always on the outlook for these insects' (23) On the eve of the start of the campaign against the mosquito in the summer of 1903, around 50% of the wells in Khartoum were found to be infected. That was reduced to only 9.5% after six months of hard work and dramatically to 3.6% after one year (24). Such success had to be maintained by tackling other confounding elements that feed into the pipeline of the mosquito life cycle. Balfour had to deal with the issue of water drainage following the summer rainy seasons. Khartoum was initially built on a ground level below that of its two natural boundaries, the Blue and the White Nile. Following rain spells in summer, water pools tended to collect, and these formed an excellent environment for mosquito breeding. Those proved to be difficult to deal with. Balfour went on to suggest to the authorities the most effective ways of draining such waste water. He was also visionary in suggesting the creation of a 'dry zone' at least one mile wide in the area south of Khartoum and in the area north of Khartoum North. He made another suggestion: growing sunflower plants, especially in the southern swamps of the White Nile. He argued that those plants would be excellent for draining the marsh via their water absorbing capacity, so they would help in breaking the mosquito-breeding cycle, in addition to the economic value of their seeds (for oil) and fibre. Balfour went even further and advocated a comprehensive system of a new water supply to the town by establishing a pipeline system that would use the water from the Blue Nile rather than from wells (25).

Over the years, Balfour and his 'Mosquito Brigade' pressed on with their efforts to control malaria and eradicate the mosquito despite the odds of having a small work force and scant financial resources. Their perseverance was not to be without reward. The mosquito was eradicated, and the incidence of malaria dropped to its lowest levels in under one year (26). Lt-Colonel Penton, Principal MO of the EA, commented in his 1903 Report:

> Dr. Balfour, the Director of the Research Laboratory at GMC, has waged a vigorous campaign against mosquitoes at Khartoum. His Report is special is especially interesting showing what is possible in a populous town in the direction of carrying out Major Ross' System. I have already in my Egyptian Report, dwelt on the remarkable results attained in the fever-striken (sic) town of Ismailia by the adoption of that System. (27).

By 1906, Khartoum was a clean, healthy city second to none in the whole of Africa. This fascinating public health achievement was not confined to the capital, as Balfour was asked by the SMO to make suggestions and recommendations for this work to be emulated by other RAMC members who were in charge of the various provinces. Colonel Bray (who later became the Director of SMD in 1912), conducted some work in Kassala, in eastern Sudan, aiming to reduce the mosquito breeding and curb the menace of malaria (28). A few years later, in 1908, Captain William Byam elegantly executed a similar work to that of Balfour, by waging a war against malaria in Kassala. In his autobiography (ironically, written nearly fifty years later!), Byam stated that his first task was to devise a plan to curb the menace of the mosquito and the dreaded malaria in Kassala. Those efforts helped to reduce the number of malaria cases amongst the troops under his command from twelve hundred cases to only twenty (29). He made a thorough observation and investigational research of the roots of the problem. He discovered that the town's fortified wall (built during the time when the city was established during the Turco-Egyptian rule) had numerous pits adjacent to it and so too did those that encircled the troop's barracks. These and the moat around the fort tended to retain water during and soon after the rainy season. This enabled vegetation to grow, producing gardens, and served as an excellent breeding site for mosquito. Byam then created his own mini- 'Mosquito Brigade', headed by his subordinate, the Syrian medical officer, Dr. Asad Malouf (30). Byam's quest to eradicate mosquitoes and control malaria was a 'Balfourian experiment in miniature'. It wasn't clear from his writing about this venture whether he was influenced by his fellow Briton. Interestingly, later in 1911, Byam, who had moved to Khartoum as senior medical officer, befriended Balfour and his deputy, Dr. Robert Archibald, and lived with them in the same compound. Byam's encounter with Balfour's earlier mentor, Patrick Manson, at St George's Hospital in London, and later with William Leishman prior to his work in the Sudan, might have provided him with the knowledge needed for such an accomplishment.

Part B:

Balfour & Newlove: Sanitation & Refuse Disposition of Modern Khartoum

Balfour's second task was to handle the issue of sewage collection and its disposal. Careful and thoughtful research again characterized Balfour work in this area. He abolished the use of the *Crowly cart* and replaced it with 'latrine buckets' (31). Disposal of these buckets was carried out in trenches outside the southern part of Khartoum. Secured measures were taken to ensure their safe and effective transport to the disposal sites. Such safe disposal kept enteric diseases like dysentery and enteric fever to the minimum, and the breeding of flies was also kept down. It is intriguing that this system of sewage disposal adopted by Balfour continued to be in use in Khartoum (and many other Sudanese cities and towns) till the 1960s and early 1970s, when it was finally abolished.

Balfour and Newlove went even further to handle their third priority: refuse collection and its disposal. Balfour proposed the creation of large pits to collect the wastewater, and those large pits were cemented over and provided with hoses and pumps and later drained and disposed of outside the town. That proved to be an excellent solution. Other public health endeavours conducted by Balfour were to ensure a safe water supply and clean and healthy meat and milk provision (32). Again, novel measures were made and brilliantly executed and supervised. To ensure proper implementation of those measures, legislation was strictly imposed. The research facilities of WTRL were used to their best effect, ensuring that those ventures were backed up by scientific means. As communicable diseases were so rampant at that time, the best remedy was to prevent them. In those days, modern drugs and treatments were not yet available. The outcome was a clean healthy town, which remained a prototype in the African British colonial mosaic.

The public health work of Andrew Balfour is recorded in detail in the series of four reports published by the Wellcome Laboratory in Khartoum. These volumes are available at the Wellcome Archives, and an excellent summary is provided in the historical narrative by Patrick D'Arcy (1999) (33).

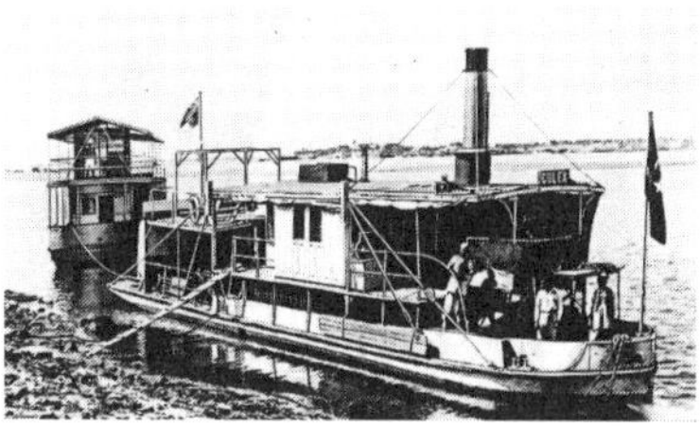

Chapter 3

Balfour & the Early Foundation of Medical Research in the Sudan

Part I:

Neave &Wenyon; The Traveling Pathologists, the Floating Laboratory& New Frontiers of Tropical Medicine

Wellcome's involvement with 'his laboratory' in Khartoum did not cease with his 'full donation'. He was to remain on the scene and behind the curtains. A continuous flow of correspondence between him and Balfour was maintained throughout Balfour's tenure at Khartoum. Knowing Wellcome's generosity and his willingness to provide on-going support, Balfour maximized his access to the networking group in London, who were very interested in research in tropical medicine and in the Sudan. Many of them had gathered at his farewell party in Piccadilly before Christmas 1903. In 1904, just under two years since Balfour's arrival at Khartoum, he furnished yet another, new pioneering venture to explore more frontiers of tropical medicine beyond his base at Khartoum. Early research focused primarily on sleeping sickness (trypanosomiasis), a menace that the new rulers were anxious about, as it was spreading to the southern Sudan from neighbouring Uganda and the Belgian Congo. That involved a visiting pathologist, Dr. Sheffield Neave, from the London Institute of Tropical Medicine. It is likely that Balfour proposed the idea of a visiting pathologist to the Sudan Government and possibly also to Wellcome. It is not clear how the idea was executed. Henry Wellcome naturally supported his protégé's proposals. An able pathologist, Dr. Sheffield Neave, was selected to go to Khartoum, with a specific mandate to travel up the White Nile in the capacity of a 'traveling pathologist'. He was seconded from the London Institute of Tropical Medicine for six months in 1904-1905. Dr. Neave was the son of the Governor of the Bank of England, who was known to have a lifelong interest in natural history and had an excellent reputation as a collector. Sheffield Neave, Jr, who ironically embarked upon his studies in medicine well into his forties, qualified from St Bartholomew's Hospital in 1900, and immediately obtained the MRCP in 1902 (34). He was a prolific character with excellent personal qualities. His assignment was planned to be for one year. Part of his mission was to participate in the investigation by the Royal Society's Sleeping Sickness Commission sent by the British Government. That commission was stationed in Uganda and began the investigation that led to the discovery of the cause and extent of trypanosomiasis in Central Africa. An Italian pathologist, Dr. Aldo Castellani, went there first, and was followed by Dr. (later, Sir) David Bruce. Their joint efforts culminated in the discovery of the parasite and its vector, which was named after David Bruce, in 1902-1903, as *trypanosome bruceii*. (35). Dr. Bruce was a descendant of the Scottish explorer James Bruce.

Dr. Neave began his journey from England in November of 1903 and arrived in Khartoum in the same year. While in Khartoum in 1904, he made the diagnosis of the first case of visceral leishmaniasis in Sudan, in a boy from Omdurman. Neave performed a splenic puncture and observed the Leishman Donovan bodies in the pathological smear he examined (36). Neave then left Khartoum on board a 'Gayyasa' (a boat), on December 16, 1904, heading towards Gondokoro, a spot close to the present-day city of Juba in Southern Sudan. The plan was for Dr. Neave to meet with Captain Creig (of the RAMC), who was part of the Sleeping Sickness Commission in Uganda at Gondokoro, investigating the possible presence and distribution of the tse-tse fly in southern Sudan (37). Both failed to confirm the finding of the fly south of Gondokoro. Later Neave was informed by a Dr. Hodges (Probably a missionary doctor) that the fly *was* present at Gondokoro, just further inland. After he met with Captain Creig, Neave travelled down the White Nile tributaries towards Bahr el-Ghazal. In all, he spent 127 days away from Khartoum, collecting mosquitoes and other insects, examining the blood of various birds, reptiles, fish, and other animals for parasites. He prepared a total of 800 blood slides and mounted many dissected insects and stored specimens that were later taken as museum specimens (38). While in Bahr el-Ghazal, Neave received orders to map out the tse-tse fly belt. He was the first to report the presence of the tse-tse fly species, *G. moristans*, in Bahr el-Ghazal. It appears that most of his work was geared towards finding trypanosomes of various genera. Dr. Neave had also done extensive work in entomology, especially dipetra mosquitoes, and here he found two new culex, one of which was named after Dr. Neave, as *culex naevei* (*vide infra*), by Mr Theobold, an eminent entomologist in London. Neave also collected significant numbers of medicinal plants used by the Bari tribe of Southern Sudan. He described many cases of syphilis, leprosy, hydrocoele, and actinomycosis. He also reported that the tubercle bacilli were rife in the South. He went further, making interesting remarks on the anthropology of the some of the southern Nilotic Sudanese people he met. He stated that their legs are longer in proportion to their trunk and that they also exhibit a narrow pelvis (39). He also stated that Sudanese children up to 16 years of age, especially females, tend to have marked lordosis, more so than the white races, suggesting that they attain an erect attitude later in life. His report published in the second Wellcome Report in 1906 represents a treatise of the earliest data on tropical medicine and anthropology in the Sudan. It was likely that his anthropological remarks tempted Balfour to support the hiring of Dr. Alexander MacTier Pirrie of Edinburgh, to conduct the first medical anthropology work in the following years. Further, his remarks in this area were used by later professional anthropologists, like Dr. Seligman and Evans Pritchard, to formally study the Nilotic tribes (*vide infra*). During his journeys in the Upper Nile, Neave was accompanied by a Ugandan boy who was brought by Captain Creig to catch flies. The boy later on proved to be infected by the trypanososmes protozoa and Neave had to start treating him with atoxyl (the only treatment on trial at the time for trypanosomiasis). In addition to setting the scene for early scientific research on trypansomiasis, Neave also made excellent clinical observations on several other diseases in southern Sudan, including leprosy. His joint work with Captain Craig, of the Royal Society's Sleeping Sickness Commission in Uganda, helped the colonial administration of both Uganda and the Sudan to map out the extent of sleeping sickness in the two neighbouring countries.

Wellcome's benevolent enterprises in connection with his laboratory took yet another major step when he was approached by the great Egyptologist, Dr. (later Sir) Ernst Alfred Wallis Budge, of the Egyptian and Assyrian Antiquities at the British Museum. Budge, who had visited Sudan and met Balfour, suggested to Wellcome to explore the possibility of providing a 'Floating Laboratory', to be attached to the parent laboratory in Khartoum! In his letter he wrote to Wellcome:

> I went and saw Dr. Andrew Balfour. The work that he has done is in my opinion amazing and you ought to feel very proud that this work has only been possible through your munificence.... Now there is another question which I would like to put before you. As you know well, they are doing wonderful work up the White Nile in respect of the cattle disease, but the distance of the field work from Khartoum kills some of the results. What is really wanted is a laboratory in a boat, which could move about from place to place.... It is hopeless to look at the government for such a thing. Only scientifically minded people like yourself will help in such a case. (40)

Andrew Balfour wrote about the idea in the introductory section of the Second Report of WTRL. He pointed out that the addition of a 'floating laboratory' would add much benefit to the scientific work they were trying to do. He stressed that the difficulty in obtaining pathological specimens in a viable and intact state would be very much alleviated. 'Material occasionally reaches us in Khartoum from these distant regions but it is too often in a damaged state.

Blood slides are dirty and spoiled, insects broken, notes incomplete. If the condition would be studied in a proper manner, I am certain that much of value would be generated. I tried doing blood work and microscopic work in a native hut, and it is disheartening. Dr. Neave had similar experiences. A laboratory either on a barge towed by a launch, or on a small steamer would be an excellent way of meeting the problem…'.

In a footnote, seemingly added on the proof of the Report, he confirmed that 'It gives me much pleasure to state that this request has also been favourably considered and that ere long a laboratory will be at our disposal'.(41), and it was to be. Naturally, the idea was quite appealing to Mr Wellcome, as he previously had had similar experience by fitting a hospital ship during the South African War. The floating laboratory became a reality early in 1907. The Sudan Government built the barge at Khartoum shipyard, and Henry Wellcome provided the fittings and equipment at his own expense. Further, 'the old boys' network' went into action. The Khartoum Laboratory and the London School of Tropical Medicine jointly staffed the floating laboratory and planned the medical research (42).

The first voyage of the Floating Laboratory was undertaken by Dr. Charles Morley Wenyon, a distinguished pathologist of his era. Like Andrew Balfour, Wenyon was another protégé of Sir Patrick Manson. In that first journey, he traversed the White Nile and its tributaries up and down the southern and central Sudan. He built on the work done by Sheffield Neave, especially his research into sleeping sickness. Wenyon had the advantage of laboratory equipment at hand to further explore this deadly disease, and to expand research into other diseases, especially leishmaniasis (Kala-azar). The latter disease proved to be a significant endemic disease in most parts of the Sudan, especially the east, the west, and the north. Wenyon also conducted research on other tropical parasitic diseases. One of his distinguished accomplishments was his confirmation of the earlier work of Fritz Schaudinn, a German bacteriologist, on the life cycle of entamoeba histolytica, the parasite of amoebic dysentery. Furthermore, Wenyon conducted some of the earliest research into malaria in southern Sudan, and he also described cases of leprosy and mycetoma (43). In the same report, he asserted that syphilis was common in southern Sudanese, even in children as young as ten years of age. However, it was his research into trypanosomiasis that gained him fame in the field of pathology. That made the basis of his later famous treatise, 'Wenyon Protozoology', which was published in two volumes in 1926 (44). Wenyon went on to have a lasting relationship with Wellcome Laboratories till his death in 1948. The subsequent many scientific voyages of the 'Floating Laboratory' were to last for decades. The subject was well researched by D'Arcy in his excellent book on the Wellcome laboratory at Khartoum (45).

Part 2:
Research on Entomology

Andrew Balfour's protean interests included a special focus on entomology. His novel research into entomology was greatly assisted by other members of the RAMC who were in the habit of conducting various military and medical missions in various branches and tributaries of the Nile. Among those was captain Lyle Cummins, Captain Ensor, and even non-medical personnel like Captain Stanton (the designer of the Sudan Camel stamps). The task of finding and mapping out the locations of different types of mosquitoes was indeed one of the first public health tasks for Balfour. It was the backbone of his work to eradicate mosquitoes, curb malaria, and prevent the potential spread of other mosquito-borne diseases like Yellow Fever, Dengue Fever, and filariasis. Being pre-occupied with this pressing task, Balfour made his first entomological research to help him in his practical enterprise. The various types of mosquitoes he identified to be rampant in Khartoum were the nuisant *Culex fatigans*, which he first discovered in the wells of the Grand Hotel in Khartoum. Next, he discovered the major anopheline genus, *Pyrotophruscos-talis,* which was also highly prevalent in Khartoum and is a known vector for malaria. He also discovered *Stegomyia fasciata*, a vector of Yellow Fever (46). The quest to map the presence of various types of mosquitoes took place along the banks of the Nile from Dongola down to the Pibor, Rosiers, the Lado Enclave, and the hinterlands of Bahr el-Ghazal. The four Reports of the Wellcome Laboratories, which were published between 1904 and 1911, included various articles on entomology written by various authors. Early entomological work was published in the First Report in 1904. Balfour in that Report wrote an article on 'Biting and Noxious Insects Other than Mosquitoes' (47). He followed this with a second article bearing the same title in the Second Report (48). In the first article, Bal four pointed to a discovery that 'has to be chronicled', verbatim. He meant to point out the important discovery by Lt-Colonel Griffith, who, after beeing provided with a small entomological outfit prior to a trip up the White Nile; brought from the area around the Pongo River in Bahr-el-Ghazal, to the laboratory, specimens of several insects, among them was *G. moristans* (49). That discovery of the tse-tse fly was a landmark one, which alerted the government to the potential presence or spread of the deadly sleeping sickness across the southern frontier. That proved to be the case a few years later (see Part III, Section on the Medical Health Commissions). Balfour didn't stop there; he even went into researching the insects and other vegetable parasites that were primarily harmful to crops, published in the First Report of the Laboratories (50). This work was done well ahead of getting a dedicated staff. It was a piece of an ingenious work. Balfour would use his networking connection to secure that his efforts—and those of others—to collect various types of insects when going out trekking on the Blue and White Nile, would not be in vain. In a very concise and detailed report written by Mr Ernest E. Austen, of the Zoological Department of the British Museum (Natural History), various blood-sucking flies (*Diptera*) found in Sudan were described (51). In that report, two new, hitherto undescribed Diptera species were mentioned. Dr. Fred V. Theobald, one of the most eminent British entomologists of his time, wrote a comprehensive article about the mosquitoes of the Sudan (52). Theobald was then the president of the Association of Economic Biologists of Britain and was a foreign member of the Economic Entomologists of Washington, D.C., USA. Dr. Theobald had earlier examined in detail the various mosquitoes that had been collected by Balfour and his colleagues, and he made description of some new species that were discovered by Balfour and others. Among these new species was a culex that resembles *Culex fatigans* (a known vector of yellow Fever), which he named *C. pallidocephala*, and a second one discovered by captain Lyle Cummins and named after him as *C. cumminsii*. Several new anopheline mosquitoes were discovered by Dr. Balfour. One was named after Mr Wellcome as *A. wellcomei*, and another new member of the genus Uranotaenia which was named after Balfour himself as *U. balfouri*. This latter one was discovered along the Pibor branch of the Sobat River (53). Some work on entomology was also part of the task assigned to the travelling pathologists, Dr. Sheffield Neave and Dr. Charles Morley Wenyon. Dr. Theobald wrote the second part of his scholarly review of the various mosquito work of the Laboratory staff in the Second Report of the WTRL (54).

The above is only part of the extensive work Andrew Balfour masterminded in the field of entomology during the impressive ten years he spent in the Sudan. His contribution to other fields of parasitology was truly unprecedented. It is worth noting that he had discovered some new species in this field. One day he made a discovery of a new blood parasite, which he stumbled upon while examining blood specimens of the 'Jerboa of the desert rat (*J. gordoni*)'. Balfour one day observed that there were peculiar intra-corpuscular parasites in the red blood cells of this animal, while conducting some work on trypanosomiasis. Balfour wrote in the Second Report of WTRL:

> ...while carrying out work in connection with trypanosmiasis, I have had to make occasions of numerous examination of the blood of the jerboa or desert rat...in the first blood examined I was surprised to see that a large proportion of red blood corpuscles harboured an unpigmented and non-motile parasite.... In the stained specimens it was at once apparent that we are dealing with some kind of trophozoite. (55)

He sent a specimen to Professor Charles Laveran (the French Nobel Laureate and discoverer of the plasmodium of malaria and the trypanosome of sleeping sickness). Balfour went on to confirm that 'Professor Laveran at once declared the parasite to be a haemogregarine and has kindly informed me that the discovery is one of much interest'. Professor Laveran named the parasite after Balfour as *H. Balfouri* (56). In a similar encounter, and stemming out from his earlier finding, Balfour went on to see whether that parasite could be seen in other rats. He studied blood specimens of Norway rat. He was only intrigued to observe a yet different parasite. However, Balfour felt that the parasite is closely allied to, if not identical with, the parasite that had recently been discovered by Patton in one of the Indian palm squirrels. He requested Dr. Patton to send him a blood film containing the parasite. Balfour felt that his parasite was different, and he proposed to give the name of *Leucocyto zooamuris* to the rat parasite (57).

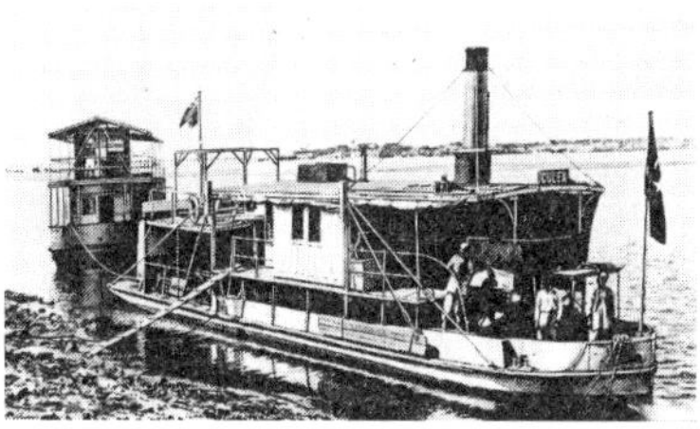

Chapter 4

Balfour & the Earlier Research in Anthropology in the Sudan

In a different sphere, Balfour used his earlier connections with Edinburgh to secure a Carnegie Research Fellowship for Alexander MacTier Pirrie, a well-qualified medical anthropologist, to conduct research in anthropology. Balfour probably realised that this important field, which has its interface with medical sciences, had not been studied formally in Sudan. Apart from some crude description by several European and British explorers who traversed the Sudanese hinterland, the field needed a more specialist input. Those travellers, which included John Speke, Charles Grant, Samuel Baker, John Petherick, and the German Schweinfurth, made useful descriptions on physical characteristics of the different tribes they saw. Dr. MacTier Pirrie was trained at the anatomical department of Edinburgh University, where he obtained degrees in both medicine and anthropology. This enabled him, under Balfour's guidance, to conduct one of the earliest anthropological studies on the tribes of Sudan. Dr. Pirrie and his companion set foot in Sudan in autumn of 1906, travelling via Cairo. He soon began to implement a plan for what would be a landmark enterprise in the history of anthropology in the Sudan. MacTiere Pirrie began his work initially at Khartoum by taking anthropometric measurements of some students from the GMC, some native soldiers, and some natives from the prison. That sample represented several Sudanese tribes. He then set off on a journey to study the tribes that dwell in the triangle lying between the Blue Nile, Sobat River, and White Nile. The work of Pirrie, which was done in a scholarly fashion, covered the Nilotic tribes—the Dinka, the Shilluk, and the Nuer. He also studied a small tribe, hitherto unknown, called the Burun, which occupy the strip of land west of the Abyssinian border, north of Sobat River, and east of Melot, on the White Nile. His accounts on this tribe represented a major part of his anthropological work. He also took the opportunity to examine some members of several other tribes that he encountered during his trip south of Khartoum, which included the Nuba, Furs, and Fertit, to mention but a few.

The work of Dr. Alexander MacTier Pirrie was cut short after he, and his assistant, O. E. Inglis were infected by the deadly visceral leishmaniasis parasite, to which Pirrie succumbed months later in Chalmers Hospital in Edinburgh. Later Inglis died in England. The research and work of MacTiere Pirrie was later collected and written up by Dr. David Waterston, one of his colleagues in the department of anatomy at Edinburgh. This was published posthumously in Balfour's Third Report of the WTRL (58). In this section we will give a short account and the salient features of the report prepared by Dr. Waterston, who obviously faced a difficult task of piecing together the various hand-written notes of Dr. Pirrie. Dr. Waterston examined a great many photos taken by MacTier Pirrie of the many tribes he studied in his short but very fruitful enterprise that proved to be to the death of him. Dr. Waterston asserted that:

> Dr. Pirrie unfortunately did not survive to work up the extensive material which he had in this way obtained, and the loss which was entailed by his sad death is a severe one and in many ways irreparable. The cards on which the records of the various measurements had been made had been handed to me in order to find out whether they could be made to yield any results of value. I have also seen large number of photographs.... As a result I have not been able to take up all the threads of his work and to weave them into a complete memoir on the indigenous tribes of this portion of the Sudan, nor could this work have been done by any person except Dr. Pirrie himself. (59).

However, from the excellent report Dr. Waterston did, it is clear that Dr. Pirrie had managed to do an excellent job. Herein, we shall try to give a short account of that report, concentrating primarily on its salient features. Even though some of the notes Dr. Pirrie had jotted down on language and customs were fragmentary and incomplete, Dr. Waterston did find that the cards that had records of anthropometric measurements were generally complete. He then gave a comprehensive account of hitherto undescribed anthropological features of the tribes examined by the deceased scholar. On the Burun tribe, a previously unknown populace, Dr. Pirrie located the exact boundaries of their country. He also gave details about their customs. He stated that, apart from those living on the northern boundaries of their country (those adjacent to the Fung and the Hameg), they are '*shiekhless*', i.e., without leaders. This was likely related to the influence of the Fung and Hameg, who were the rulers of the first Islamic Sultanate, the Fung Kingdom of Sennar, which lasted for over 300 years. Pirrie realized that the 'Burun country' didn't have any cattle, and that their sheep and goats were the poorest (compared to those of other tribes). He also stated that:

> …they have few women, they are overrun with syphilis, and they offer poor resistance to disease…and that they are addicted to merrisa…with a system of merrissa meetings in neighbouring village by which man attend about three in a week. Fighting is common at these orgies, the poisoned arrow being the usual implement employed. I consider that the lack of women has largely to do with their addiction to drink, facilitated by the superabundance of their grain. (60)

The report also highlighted the dialects of the Burun, stating that it is more closely related to the Nuer, and pointed out that both the Fung and the Hamg speak the tongue of the Buruns. Pirrie also studied other tribes, including the Nuer, the Shilluk, the Bongo, and the Nyam Nyam (the Azande). On the Bongos, Pirrie commented that:

> …they appear to be devoted almost exclusively to agriculture, and were of a docile and yielding disposition, unlike the Dinkas, and a large number of them had been reduced to slavery by the invading Khartoumers (sic). By the Dinka they are known as the Dohr. In complexion, they are much less dark, or black, than the Dinkas,

> and in colour they are similar to the red-brown soil upon which they reside. (61)

He went further to assert:

> ...the jet-black Shilluks, Nuers, and Dinkas natives of the dark alluvial flats, stand out in marked distinction to the dwellers upon the iron-red rocks, who notwithstanding their diversity in dialect, in habitor in mode of life, present the characteristics of a connected whole. (61)

The customs, beliefs, and superstitions of several tribes were elaborated. The way these tribes salute and greet each other was discussed. There was significant variation between them. For the Buruns, the author stated that the concept of 'snake magic' held by the three Nilotic groups, the Dinka, the Nuer, and the Shilluks, was discussed in detail as Dr. Pirrie understood it. He also stated that other animal magic was used for practising magic. He went on to write about the mythology of those tribes, pointing out that the Nilotic tribes believe in a 'rain god' who, among the Dinka and Nuer, bears the name of 'Deng-Dit', and by the Shilluk is called 'Nekang' (62). Dr. Pirrie also took the opportunity of writing about some customs of other tribes that he did not study as closely as he did the Fung and Hameg.

An important part of Dr. Pirrie's work, as reported by Dr. Waterston, had been his anthropometric measurement of the physical characteristics of the tribes that occupy the aforementioned area. This also included measurements of members of other tribes who Dr. Pirrie encountered during his trek in the south, including Furs, Nubas, and another group he called 'Furwais', which is clearly a confusion with the Fur. (The word 'Furawi' is the adjective of the eponym 'Fur' in Arabic.) Another point of confusion was between the Nuba and the Gebellawi. The author and Dr. Pirrie put them down as separate entities. There is no such tribe in Sudan as 'Gebelawi' and the word is just another Arabic corruption of the term 'Nuba'. It is the adjective of Gebel, which in Arabic means 'hill' or 'mountain'. The description included the appearance and colour of the hair, the shape of the skull and nose, different colour of skin, and the degree of prognathism (which is considered an important discriminatory feature to distinguish between races) (63). On the Shilluks, the report states:

> Their physiognomy hardly offers that decided negro type which their swarthy complexion would lead one to expect, but, judged by the shape of the skull, this people belong to a less degraded race of Central Africa... The stature of the Shilluks is very moderate, and, as a general rule, is short compared with that of the lank and long-legged Dinka inhabitants. (64)

Measurements were made into tables.

In a supplementary report to that of Dr. Waterston, D. J. Vallance, Curator of the Royal Scottish Museum at Edinburgh, wrote 'Notes on the Ethnographical Specimens Collected by Dr. A MacTier Pirrie' (65). This primarily added a valuable dimension to Dr. Waterston's report. Mr Vallance, who appears to have been an expert in the field, examined the specimens that Dr. Pirrie had collected from various tribes, primarily the Dinka, the Nuer, and the Buruns. Only few specimens wre germane to to the Nuer (66). The specimens included weapons, tobacco pipes, dress, musical instruments, some domestic utensils, and surgical and medical appliances. In his short but detailed description, Mr Vallance was able to draw some very useful assumptions, remarks, and conclusions. Mr Vallance compared the throwing stick of the Buruns to the boomerang of the Australian aborigines. He could draw an analogy between the dress of the Burun women to that of the Massai and the Kaffir in Kenya. He commented that it was believed that the latter tribe had moved to its current land from a more northerly position. After examining the pipe of the Buruns, he commented that it was probably copied from the neighbouring Arabs or the Abyssinians (67). The most interesting part of Mr Vallance's report was his remarks on the Dinka method of 'cupping' after examining the surgical tools used for this. He included the written account of a witness to the procedure (68) that reads as follows:

> The skin was wetted and the end of five cow horns with holes bored in their ends were applied. The doctor then sucked the ends and plugged the holes with some cotton which he had in his mouth. Then after a short while, when the pores has been opened,

> the horns were removed and incisions were made with a small knife. The horns were then sucked on and sucked as before. After a little they were taken off and found to contain a lot of thick blood that had been drawn from the skin. The last operation was to rub the incision with butter.

Mr Vallance further commented that:

> ...the use of the horn for this purpose is widely spread in Africa, and it is interesting to note that it has been applied in the same way in Scotland. A specimen identical with that just referred to but coming from Shetland is in the collection of the Royal Scottish Museum. (69)

The earlier work by Alexander MacTier Pirrie on anthropology in the Anglo-Egyptian Sudan set the scene for later anthropological work led by Charles Gabriel Seligman and his wife Brenda Zalaman Seligman. It was no surprise that Sir James Currie, the then Director of Education, induced the Sudan Government to secure some funds for ethnographical research. Currie was advised by D. G. Hogarth, the famous British archaeologist. Currie invited Seligman and his wife to come and undertake research among various tribes of the Sudan (70). Seligman; who had started his career as a physician and pathologist after qualifying from St Thomas' in London, became one of the most celebrated pioneers of anthropology. Seligman and his wife began their anthropological research among the Nilotic tribes of the south as early as 1909. They made their trips with the help of the 'Floating Laboratory' up and down the White Nile (71). They undertook two trips, the first during 1909 and 1910, when they traversed the White Nile from north to south. The second trip was undertaken in 1911 and 1912, covering the country from west to east. In the second trip they studied the tribes of the Kababish in the west and the Beja in the east. However, it was mostly their work among the pagan tribes of the south that received great publicity. Later on, his pupil, E. E. Evans-Pritchard, conducted much work among the southern Sudanese tribes, especially the Zande and the Nuer (see Volume 2).

Wellcome Laboratories was ravaged by a fire in June of 1908 that destroyed much valuable work and equipment. Henry Wellcome cabled Balfour, who had written to him earlier following the tragic incident:

> I had neither the heart nor the time to write to you by the first mail leaving after our sad calamity and indeed even now there is much to do if we are to rise like a phoenix from the ashes…. (72)

In a second letter to Wellcome, in the same month as the tragedy, Balfour went on to emphasize to Wellcome their efforts to salvage what could be salvaged, stressing that their morale was still high and that their spirit had not been broken, using the Scottish phrase 'stout heart to a stay brae' and asking for help and support from his sponsor. Wellcome's munificence was always there for Sudan and its cause. He aided Balfour by sending replacements of various items and equipment that was damaged by the fire. He also offered his moral support to Balfour and his colleagues:

> With all my heart I sympathise with you in all the misfortunes with which you are beset. This fire has been a serious set-back, but with men like yourself these misfortunes are only incidents in the great chapter of life.... I beg you will not fail to let me know anything that I can do to assist you in your difficulties…. (73)

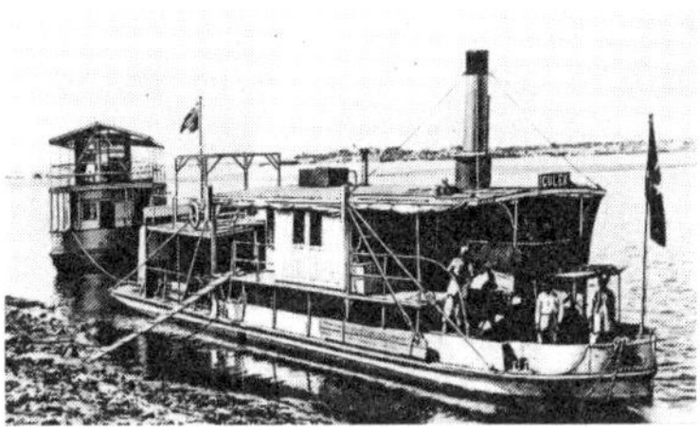

Chapter 5

Milestones of Development of the Laboratory:
Scope, Facilities, and Staff

The time Andrew Balfour spent in Sudan, spanning ten years (1903-1913), was full of scientific innovations and ventures and witnessed extensive research into tropical medicine, public health, anthropology, and native and traditional medicine, to name but a few. Here, we would like to shed some light on the milestones of development of the Wellcome laboratory at Khartoum during the Balfour era. As mentioned earlier, WTRL at Khartoum began with only two members, Balfour and his laboratory assistant, Mr John Newlove, together with two Sudanese staff, one of them a young boy tasked with preparing the bottles and cleaning them (74). It was a shame that the name of the Sudanese staff remained anonymous. The laboratories comprised only five rooms, with one of them used as a kitchen, another as an office for the director, and a third as museum. Routine work began energetically with the arrival of Mr Newlove from Cairo in April of 1903. By the end of the first year, the laboratory became a hub of activities, including routine laboratory work for Khartoum, and the museum by then contained scores of mounted specimens illustrative of human pathology and tropical diseases. There were specimens of mycetoma, small collection of skulls, and what promised to be a very fine and complete set of photographs illustrative of 'native' diseases of the Sudan, taken by Mr Turstig for Dr. Christopherson, who donated it to the museum (75). Several members of the RAMC and EA were flocking to the laboratory to help with routine work and to use the facilities of the library. Dr. Balfour began an energetic process of networking with London and Liverpool Schools of Tropical Medicine as well as the US Department of Agriculture to help with journals and periodicals and to receive pathology specimens (76)

By 1906, significant progress in the laboratory work had been attained. That included both routine work and research. Addition of more staff, which was always the ambition of Dr. Balfour, led to expansion. Support from Mr Wellcome and the Governor General, Sir Reginald Wingate, helped to employ an economic entomologist, Dr. Harold King, who joined in January of 1906 (77). By the end of 1904, Mr Newlove had left the laboratory to take up the post of Sanitary Officer for Khartoum, and Mr H. R. Friedrich replaced him. A second laboratory assistant, Mr J. A. Goodson, and a Sudanese graduate of the GMC, Mr Mohamed Effendi Khalil, were appointed. Earlier, in October of 1904, Mr William Beam was appointed as a chemist. His inclusion enabled much routine and research work to be conducted on river water, grains, and salts. His research on gum arabic was a pioneering work that helped in later years to place the commodity confidently on the world market. During the same year, the premises of the lab were extended by two rooms. One was used as a library and the other as a water analysis room by Dr. Beam. The laboratory, after receiving a grant of £E320, managed to secure a purchase of several equipments for the chemical and bacteriological sections, as well as ordering some journals and periodicals for the library. The laboratory continued to grow in content. The museum had a marked increase in its pathological materials from various doctors working in various districts. These included insects, ticks, native drugs, and other pathological materials that included interesting photographs, which were added to the earlier collection by Dr. Christopherson. Further, a veterinary component was included for the first time, by Colonel Griffith (possibly the first veterinary surgeon in the Sudan). Sir Rudolph von Slatin presented a goat with some malformation (78). Further, the laboratories also received a fine Zeiss microscope adapted for photographic work by a Mr MacMillan, who was probably a British businessman/photographer. Various doctors from the RAMC and EA Medical Services continued to make themselves available for work and study in the laboratory. Dr. Balfour, with the help of Mr James Currie, the Principal of GMC, managed to obtain recognition from the Carnegie Research Fund, University of Edinburgh, to recognize the Wellcome Laboratory for training purposes of its Fellows (*vide supra*).

The staff of the laboratory didn't increase further till early in 1908, when Captain Robert Archibald joined as assistant pathologist and bacteriologist. Before coming to Sudan, Dr. Archibald had a distinguished career. It appears that it was the networking and the excellent connection of Andrew Balfour with Sir David Bruce and Colonel Leishman (under whose guidance Dr. Archibald had had some earlier training), that secured the hiring of Dr. Archibald to the post in the Sudan. Dr. Archibald would later become the third and last director of the laboratory (*vide infra*). Following the appointment of Dr. Archibald, Mr Vitale (probably a Greek), joined as a clerk who was also assisted by a Sudanese junior clerk, Mr Ibrahim Effendi Hafiz. By this time, the staff also included two Sudanese attendants, one of them referred to as 'chief laboratory attendant' by Dr. Balfour, who commended his abilities 'to make excellent blood films and attend to the sterilization of bacteriological media' (79). Dr. Balfour commented that both of the attendants were among the fighting 'Dervish troops' during the Reconquest. In September of 1908, Mr H. E. Friedrichs, the laboratory assistant, left the laboratory, and his replacement, Mr E. Inglis, joined in January of 1909. During the winter of 1907, a Carnegie Research Fellow, Mr E. S. Edie, joined the laboratory as a chemical research fellow. His main task was to conduct research into the chemistry and bacteriology of gum arabic. The earlier pioneering work of Dr. William Beam into the subject demonstrated that the scientific knowledge of gum arabic was scarce, hence the tasks were assigned to Mr Edie (80). On other frontiers, the Chemical Section, now flourishing under the guidance of Dr. Beam and his assistant, Mr Goodson, was very busy conducting extensive investigation and research into various areas that affected sanitary, public health, medico-legal issues, and agriculture. On the other hand, Dr. Harold King, the 'economic entomologist', conducted extensive research on various insects of the Sudan. Dr. Balfour commented that his work had earned for him the name of 'Father of Flies', and 'it is interesting to see the Sudan fieldworkers crowding around him and listening eagerly to his explanations and instructions' (81). Dr. King's research into mosquitoes paved the way for future workers in the field. During 1908, Dr. Balfour, with the help of Dr. Archibald, furnished an excellent supplement to the Third Report of the Laboratory. That supplement included an overview of the latest developments in Tropical and Veterinary Medicine. In the Third Report of the Wellcome Laboratory, Dr. Balfour asserted:

> I am aware that it is very difficult for medical and veterinary officers stationed in the Sudan to keep in close touch with current literature…it is quite impossible for those working in out-stations or travelling about. Hence it occurred to me that these officials, to many of whom the laboratories are indebted for notes and specimens, might appreciate a paper of this kind. (82)

The laboratory remained an important hub for medical and veterinary doctors stationed in Khartoum or nearby, who avail themselves of its facilities for work or study. A further grant of £E150 received from the Government towards periodicals and journals helped greatly in that direction (83). By 1908, other amenities and facilities of the laboratory had been added. The museum expanded further in its contents with addition of more pathological and entomological materials in addition to exhibits of 'Solaro' tropical clothing and tablets for water sterilization. Colonel Hunter presented some native drugs from the Kassala regions, and similar materials from Kordofan were provided by some other British officials (84). The laboratory continued to support the civilian medical service by performing routine pathological and bacteriological work that also covered cases of suspected cancer, and medico-legal specimens (85).

Before Dr. Balfour left in early 1913, the laboratory continued to grow both in the number of staff and in the scope of work. By 1911, the senior staff included a senior assistant chemist, Dr. J. Thompson, and Captain W. B. Fry, who was appointed as a protozoologist and assistant pathologist. Mr Inglis, unfortunately, died before the end of 1909, after having been in the country for only six months. He was replaced by a senior laboratory assistant, Mr George Buchanan, who had trained earlier in the pathology department of Edinburgh University. Later on, Mr Marshall was also appointed as a junior laboratory assistant. A new junior clerk, Mr Nicholas Effendi Hakim, was appointed to help Mr Vitale, the laboratory clerk who had been in the post since 1908. Hence, the volume of the work of the laboratory was so immense that the Fourth Report of the laboratory, which came out in 1911, had to be split into two volumes, medical and scientific. In the foreword section of the medical volume of the Fourth Report, Dr. Balfour stated that the routine work continued to grow, with over 1,800 examinations having been conducted in the Bacteriology Section alone, which included pathological specimens sent from various hospitals, Wasserman tests, bacterial vaccines, and reporting on veterinary materials (86). A major undertaking of the laboratory was the work employed to test for the new water supply of Khartoum, from a chemical and bacteriological point of view. That work proved to be of vital help in conducting that enterprise (87). The Wellcome Laboratories, which by then had acquired the additional title of 'Tropical' upon the request of its major sponsor and benefactor, Mr Wellcome, began to accumulate fame and reputation as a centre of excellence in the emerging field of tropical medicine. No wonder that it soon began to attract freelance researchers, who came at their own expense, requesting to conduct research in various fields. Among these were Dr. A. C. Stevenson, of the University College, London, and Dr. W. M. Ader, who both came in winter 1908-1909 and spent a good spell at Khartoum. Dr. Stevenson, who appeared to be a very renowned researcher in pathology, discovered a coccidosis in the Sudanese goats. That discovery helped the Sudanese veterinary officers stamp out the disease in the affected herds (88). He also made other contributions to research in veterinary medicine. He wrote papers for the 1911 Report. The fame attained by the Khartoum Laboratories attracted other 'freelancers'. Dr. Balfour subsequently received applications from a medical missionary in Iran, an American Professor, and an Italian scientist, to come and station themselves at Khartoum to conduct research. He had to turn them down and welcomed only Professor E. F. McCampbell, of Ohio State University, to join research ventures at Khartoum and on board the 'floating laboratory' (89). The Wellcome Laboratory had earlier hosted Sir David Bruce and his wife on their way from Uganda back to Britain. Sir David Bruce took the opportunity to discuss the issue of trypanosomiasis in animals with Dr. Balfour. Lady Bruce helped by making an extensive series of measurements of the trypanosomes held in the laboratory and made some careful drawings from them (90). Other visitors during the last few years of Dr. Balfour's tenure were Monsieur Solvay, a Belgian, who gave a generous donation to the laboratories, used for buying some microscopes and journals. It is noteworthy that Lord Kitchener made a visit to the laboratory in his last trip to the Sudan in 1911.

The scope of the research of both the chemical and bacteriological sections of the laboratory continued to grow and expand. Dr. Harold King made further immense contributions to the knowledge of insects and mosquitoes. His chemical counterpart, Dr. Beam, conducted extensive research into the soil of the Gezira. The plans to set a mammoth irrigation project was reaching a critical stage and sound knowledge of the nature of the area was of paramount importance to the success of the project, which was afoot since the early days of the Reconquest. The ambition to exploit the immense agricultural facilities of the Anglo-Egyptian Sudan was by no means restricted to the Gezira region. Dr. Beam's soil research included the region of Dongola on the main Nile basin in the north and other districts (91). With the addition of more staff to the Chemical Section of the Laboratory, with Dr. Thompson and the Carnegie Research fellow, Mr Edie, the scale and scope of research was extended into other, wider frontiers, including water, poisons, commercial products, and pharmacology of local plants. Mr Edie's research on gum arabic added more insight to that gained earlier through the research of Dr. Beam. An impressive feat was the discovery by Dr. Beam of a colour test for detection of 'hashish', a finding that was later confirmed by Professor Schmidt and Dr. Lucas in Cairo (92). The field work of the laboratory remained a strong component of research, which was enhanced by the availability of the steamer, S. W. 'Culex, to tow the 'Floating Laboratory'. By 1911, the museum was moved into a new and wider room granted by Mr Currie. The library continued to grow steadily despite limited funds (93).

Dr. Balfour's ten years of extraordinary efforts and energies which he selflessly put into his work was not to be without a hefty price. He suffered bad health in his last years. This forced him eventually to resign his post and to return to the UK early in 1913. His legacy at Khartoum was destined to stay, however, despite the eventual demise of his laboratory at Khartoum, as it was inscribed into the stones of the modern Sudanese history. Balfour was of a breed of extraordinary doctors. Beyond doubt, he was a genius, and his protean and diverse interests place him undoubtedly as a polymath of science. His many feats were difficult to enumerate and also hard to emulate. His accomplishments spanned several frontiers of medical sciences that included public health, pathology, pharmacology, entomology, biology, sociology, and anthropology, to name but a few. His ambitions crossed many boundaries and his vision was far-reaching. His extraordinary abilities of networking would pay dividends in orchestrating the complex and multi-disciplinary work he performed. Connection with world-renowned scientists during his heyday, beyond doubt, gave his work in Sudan a first-class quality scarcely seen elsewhere in the British Empire in the early twentieth century. The program he established had laid a strong foundation for an exemplary health service and medical and scientific research center that flourished for many decades.

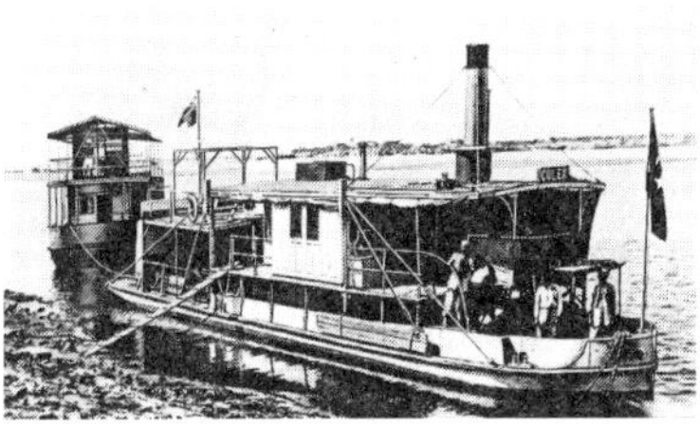

Chapter 6

The Wellcome Reports & Supplements: CME for Doctors in the Sudan

The various feats of Dr. Balfour continued to extend into new frontiers in accord with his ingenious mind and his polymath character. In 1908, soon after the Third Report of his laboratory at Khartoum was ready to go to print, he went to yet another new frontier. This time, it was to publish a supplement to the Third Report. In what he called a 'Prefatory Note', Balfour asserted that:

> It is a difficult matter for medical and veterinary officers stationed in the Sudan...to keep in touch with the current literature. This review is intended to help them in some measure, to serve as a guide to new books, papers, and to present in a small compass the most recent discoveries on the subject indicated. (94)

Balfour wanted to provide for all doctors of the Sudan a means of keeping them 'up-to-date' and equipping them with a quick reference to all new developments in tropical medicine, a vastly expanding speciality at the time. In that prefatory note, Balfour outlined what the exercise was all about. He stated that:

> ...while in the main intended for the medical and veterinary officers, who have rendered the laboratories with vast assistance, it is hoped that workers in other tropical countries, where conditions

are similar to those obtaining in the Sudan may find the Review of service.

He also affirmed that the work would be of value to students of tropical medicine, emphasising its academic credentials. Two volumes came out. A second one would follow with the Fourth (and last) Wellcome Report from Khartoum in 1911. The first volume, which spanned 260 pages, was the outcome of painstaking work carried out by Balfour, helped by the new recruit to the Laboratory, the prolific 'Archie', Dr. Robert Archibald, who had joined the Laboratory less than a year before. Subjects were discussed in alphabetical order. A more or less similar format, as appropriate, was followed. The treatise encompassed all subjects related to tropical medicine. A theme would be chosen, covered in depth in terms of latest published articles. Papers were discussed in depth, difference in opinions would be pointed out. The author (A. B. or RGA) would state his opinion(s) and points of critique on each paper. At the end of each section, the authors would point out any specific and relevant data relative to the Sudan, including any published work. Subjects included were very diverse, from infections, to infestations, to aspects of bacteriology and parasitology, to public health aspects of water, milk, filters, ice, beverages, and clothing. A section related to cancer in the tropics was included. A few interesting points in this regard are worth further elaboration. Dr. Balfour commented in the 'Cancer' section that he had records of only 10 cases of cancer over a period of 5 years (1903-1908). Although he acknowledged the limitations of his position, not being a clinician in the country, he assumed that cancer in general must be very rare 'amongst the natives of the Sudan'. From the time of inauguration of the Laboratories at Khartoum early in 1903, all cases for pathological examination from both the military and the civil hospitals in Khartoum were sent there. The observation at the time was of special interest to Balfour, who asked the help of Colonel Hunter, the PMO of the EA in the Sudan. The latter wrote to his medical officers scattered in various provinces. Four medical officers responded and their statements were identical. They all confirmed the rarity of cases of cancer. Some of those officers had worked in more than one province, and one had spent 21 months at Bahr-El-Ghazal. A few cases described by a couple of them were breast and skin cancer, referred to as scirrhus breast tumour and epithelioma of the foot (95). Before accepting the above statement, one has to understand that the medical services at the time were very rudimentary, and that most patients would seek treatment at their native doctors, and cases of cancer would most likely perish before they could come to the attention of those British doctors. Captain Thompson, in his response to his chief, Colonel Hunter, commented that of the two cases of suspected cancer he saw at Wad Medani, one of them never turned up for treatment (96).

The second part of 'Recent Advances in Tropical Medicine & Hygiene' came out also as a supplement to the Fourth and last WTRL Report, published in 1911 (97). It was vastly bigger than the first supplement, amounting to 458 pages. The format was more or less similar to the first supplement. Subjects were again organised in alphabetical order. There were four authors this time, including Dr. Balfour and Dr. Archibald; Captain W. B. Fry, who was also an employee of the WTRL seconded from the EA; and Captain W. R. O'Farrell, of the EA. The latter was a volunteer. Subjects were divided between various authors, and the initials of each of them was inserted against the appropriate topic in the contents list. Dr. Balfour, in his 'Prefatory Note' would assert:

> ...a good many letters have been received testifying to the usefulness of the First Review Supplement', and expressing the hope that a Second might be forthcoming. After some hesitation it was decided to accede to these requests and, at the same time, slightly to widen the scope of the second Review, so that it might deal in a more general manner with Tropical Medicine as a whole, and not only with diseases only represented in the Anglo-Egyptian Sudan. In this way it was felt that it would appeal to a wide public and become a better book of reference. (98)

Obviously, following the first Review, Dr. Balfour had received several letters from various readers, possibly from inside and outside the Sudan, making suggestions for the next volume. Balfour did not disappoint. He indeed came up with a more comprehensive and more detailed Review. The Second Review thus was bigger, more detailed, and wider in scope. It had been three years since the First Review appeared, so more advances had been made in tropical medicine and many more papers dealing with various subjects. Balfour addressed this fact, and even though the volume of the Second Review was almost double that of the First Review, he commented that 'we have only space to deal briefly with other papers' (99).

Subjects were covered in a very elaborate and detailed way. The literature on each theme was covered in depth, not only reviewing the latest papers and pointing out differences in opinions and findings of different authors, but also the latest advances in understanding of pathophysiology, advances in diagnostic and laboratory methods, and the latest breakthroughs in treatment modalities. Further, subjects were dealt with in a scholarly way: general accounts were given first, referring to past knowledge and disease concepts; then the latest findings and discoveries regarding aetiology, diagnosis, and laboratory results; and, where appropriate, pathological diagnostic methods would be thoroughly covered and discussed. Various papers then would be referred to, and full bibliographical references would be provided. Areas of uncertainty would be pointed out. A regular feature in this volume was the inclusion of 'Additional Notes' (likely written by Dr. Balfour himself in proof). These usually highlighted areas of interest or controversy, as well as raising points relevant to the Sudan. Here we give an example. Writing in the 'Additional Notes' on the Section on Anthrax, A. B. would state that 'The Strasburg method of diagnosis was mentioned in our First Review. This has now been perfected by Muller and Engler, who searched for some porous substances on which the suspected blood might be sent with the bacilli under favourable condition….' (100).

The subjects were again diverse, ranging from infection to infestations, from viruses to climate, from flies to filters, from heat stroke to hydrophobia (the old name for Rabies), from faeces to fevers, from diarrhoea to disinfection, and from vaccination to veterinary medicine. One could count 94 different headings, with Dr. Balfour authoring 54 of them.

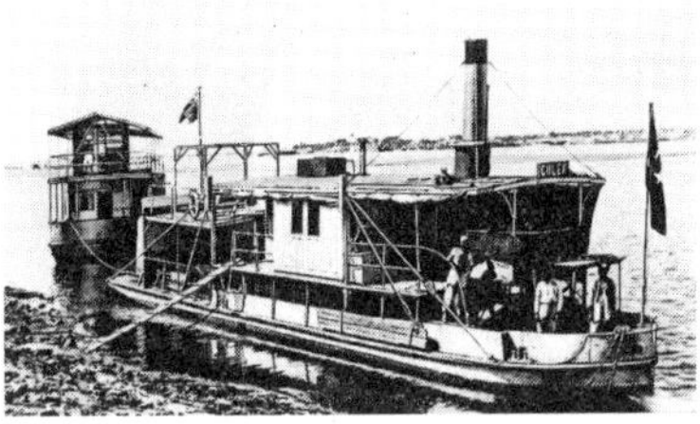

Chapter 7

The Post- Balfour Era

The Chalmers' Years: 'The Second Leap'

Following the resignation of Andrew Balfour in 1913, the Wellcome Laboratories entered a new stage under the leadership of Dr. Albert Chalmers. Chalmers, a shrewd researcher, built on the strong foundation that Balfour had set, and he explored other frontiers (101). Research into schistosomiasis (bilharziasis) led Chalmers himself to confirm Leiper's discovery of the schistosomiaisis snails. Further research in this area led to the first use of the chemical compound, potassium antimony tartrate, by Dr. John Bryan Christopherson. Christopherson treated around 70 Sudanese (and some Egyptian soldier) patients with this agent in 1915 in Ward 7G in Khartoum Civil Hospital (102). Chalmers took research started by Balfour into a second stage. Research in other tropical diseases was to be more systematic and the contribution of Albert Chalmers to the field of tropical medicine led to his recognition by the Royal Society of Tropical Medicine & Hygiene. Chalmer's Medal, awarded by the Society, was a prestigious distinction to researchers in the field. Sadly, Chalmers succumbed to acute viral hepatitis when he was touring India with his wife in 1920.

The Archibald Years: The Second Leap and the Fading Horizons

Dr. (later Sir) Robert Archibald had long connections with Wellcome Laboratories in Khartoum. A pathologist and assistant bacteriologist, Archibald joined WTRL in 1908 from the RAMC following a spell with the SSC in Uganda, where he worked with Dr. (later Sir) David Bruce and Aldo Castellani. Archibald trained with the distinguished pathologist, Colonel Leishman, the co-discoverer of Leishman-Donovan bodies, the pathological hallmark of the visceral leishmaniasis. Archibald took over the directorship of WTRL following the untimely death of Albert Chalmers early in 1920 (103). He steered the laboratories into further frontiers of research, and his directorship witnessed the tumultuous years of 1927 through 1935, when the WTRL ceased to exist as a leader and independent stakeholder of medical research in the Sudan. Several newly qualified Sudanese doctors worked under his guidance, including Dr. Mansour Ali Haseeb, the first Sudanese bacteriologist and the first Sudanese dean of medicine at Khartoum University (see section on Kitchener School of Medicine). Haseeb and Archibald further explored the scene of leishmaniasis in Sudan (104).

In the late 1920s, it transpired that further extension in the educational role of Gordon Memorial College would necessitate that the laboratory be relocated within the premises of the newly built Stack Laboratory, near the newly inaugurated Kitchener Medical School and Khartoum Civil Hospital. In 1927, WTRL was moved permanently from Gordon Memorial College to be housed in the Stack Laboratory complex. The latter was built in Khartoum in memory of Sir Lee Stack, who was assassinated in Cairo in 1924. Earlier, there were some signs of further extension of the Wellcome Laboratory's role by establishing some satellite branches of the laboratory. A branch was opened at Wad Medani in 1924, primarily to focus on conducting soil and agricultural research. Another branch was opened at Atbara in January 1925, primarily to assist with the chemical work of the Departments of Railways and Steamers of the Sudan Government. Research in this latter branch dealt primarily with the boiler water supplies and corrosion. This branch was closed in

1932 during the great recession (105). In that year, Wellcome made an offer to the Sudan Government to build a new, purposely built laboratory on the Nile. Wellcome offered to finance the whole enterprise, including buildings and equipment. The offer was considered by the Government of Sudan (or its representatives), but there was disagreement over the details of the project. Wellcome insisted on a first-class river-front site building, which unfortunately did not meet with approval from the government, so Wellcome, unfortunately, withdrew his offer. It was a sad personality clash, highlighted in the letter by N. R. Udal, the then Principal of GMC, to Wellcome:

> …I heard from Sir James Currie the other day and he is terribly upset at the discontinuance of your laboratories as I knew he would be, and it is a cruel and bitter blow to all of friends of the Sudan and it is incredible that such a thing should happen.I only pray that Syme {Sir Stewart Syme} may realize the folly of his action and try to repair the mischief he has allowed his advisors to do. (106)

By 1935 the dismantling of WTRL had taken place. The original Chemical Laboratories was divided into two sections. The Chemical and Entomological Section was joined to the Geological Surveys of the Public Works Department and was placed under the Department of Agriculture to form the Agricultural Research Institute. To this, the Soil Research Section at Wad Medani was added. The second part of the Chemical Laboratory became the Chemical Analytical Section, which remained at Khartoum, retaining the name of 'Wellcome Research Laboratory'. In July 1939, further re-organization took place. This time, the Wellcome Research Laboratory was transferred to the Sudan Medical Services as part of the research service of SMS and the name was modified again to 'Wellcome Chemical Laboratories'. In September 1940, the laboratories were evacuated as 'per war necessities' and placed in Shambat, a suburb of Khartoum North. This transfer was made in a very short time, with little notice, and the new premises that hosted the Laboratories were only half the size of its original space. Those premises were not prepared as laboratory, so it was during this move that much of the equipment of the Laboratories was either lost or damaged. After the Second World War, it took until 1948 for the decision to be made to move the Laboratories back to Khartoum. This time, not to its original premises at the GMC, but instead to the first floor of the River Hospital (which later became the first Eye & Chest Hospital in Khartoum), not far away from GMC. The Laboratory moved into a single floor, which was to undergo some alterations so that it could accommodate the WTRL. This took place in May / June 1949, when the move was completed. The new area was finally equal to the original area of the Laboratories at the GMC. That new area comprised seven laboratories, dark rooms, small laboratories for distillation, milling operations and repairs, storage, four offices, and a library (107). As D'Arcy put it, 'popular or not, justifiable or not, necessary or not, the discontinuation of Wellcome Tropical Research Laboratories marked the end of an era of medical research in the Sudan' (108).

The Tragic Death of Andrew Balfour

Following his resignation from his post at Khartoum, Andrew Balfour moved to London to take up the post of Director of the Wellcome Bureau of Research. He then went on to be the first director of the London School of Tropical Medicine and Hygiene when it was founded and oversaw the building of the new school. He was knighted in 1929. However, from 1927 onward, he was noted to be suffering from depression, which eventually led to his demise in 1931.

> It became known yesterday that the death of Sir Andrew Balfour, Director of the London School of Tropical Medicine, whose funeral took place at Edinburgh on Thursday, was the subject of an inquest on Monday last.... Dr. Thomas Arthur Rose, Medical Director of the hospital, said that he received Sir Andrew on 5th January. Sir Andrew was sent to him by Professor Bramwell of Edinburgh, with a report that he had been suffering from insomnia and was greatly worried at the possibility of having to resign his position.... The Coroner expressed his sympathy with the relatives and said that Sir Andrew was a man bearing a distinguished name and who had performed splendid work. He felt very distressed that his end should come in this way.

This posting appeared in the *Times* Feb 7, 1931, under the headline 'Late Sir Andrew Balfour, Tragedy of Nervous Breakdown' (109). Dr. Balfour had earlier been admitted to Cassel Hospital, Penshurst, a psychiatric Hospital in Kent, a few weeks prior to strangling himself in one of many bouts of severe depression. His wife, Lady Balfour (*nee* Grace Nutter), passed away in April 1951. She had been married to Balfour since 1902. It is interesting to note that his son, Elliot Archibald, who was born in 1909 when his father was in Sudan, went on to join the Sudan Political Service in 1932 (the year following the tragic death of his father). He worked in several posts in Khartoum and in Blue Nile and Darfur Provinces and he remained in Sudan till Independence, serving lastly as Deputy Governor of the Northern Province. In April of 1952, he married Ivy Potter (*vide infra*), who was Supervisor of Health Visitors at the Midwives Training School, Omdurman. He made many friends in the Sudan and enjoyed his long service there, and he used to say: 'We are the end of a rare breed. They don't make them any more'. He died at Kent (same county in which his father had died) in July 1995, at 86 years of age.

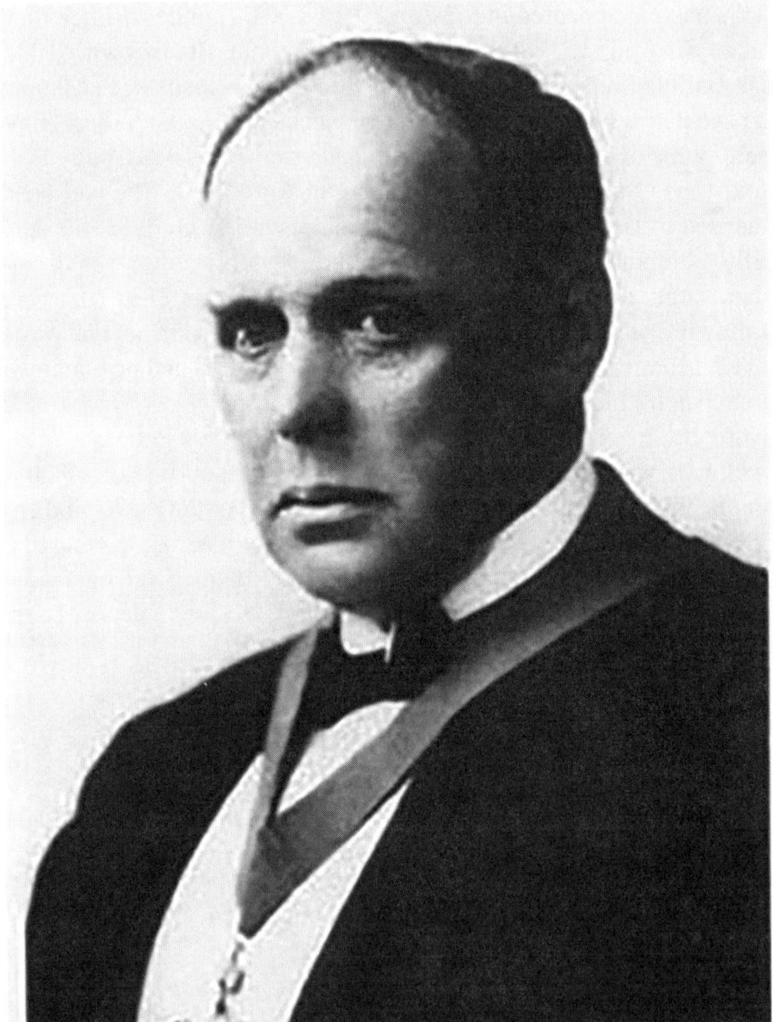

Sir Andrew Balfour
(Images courtesy of Wellcome Foundation for history of Medicine)

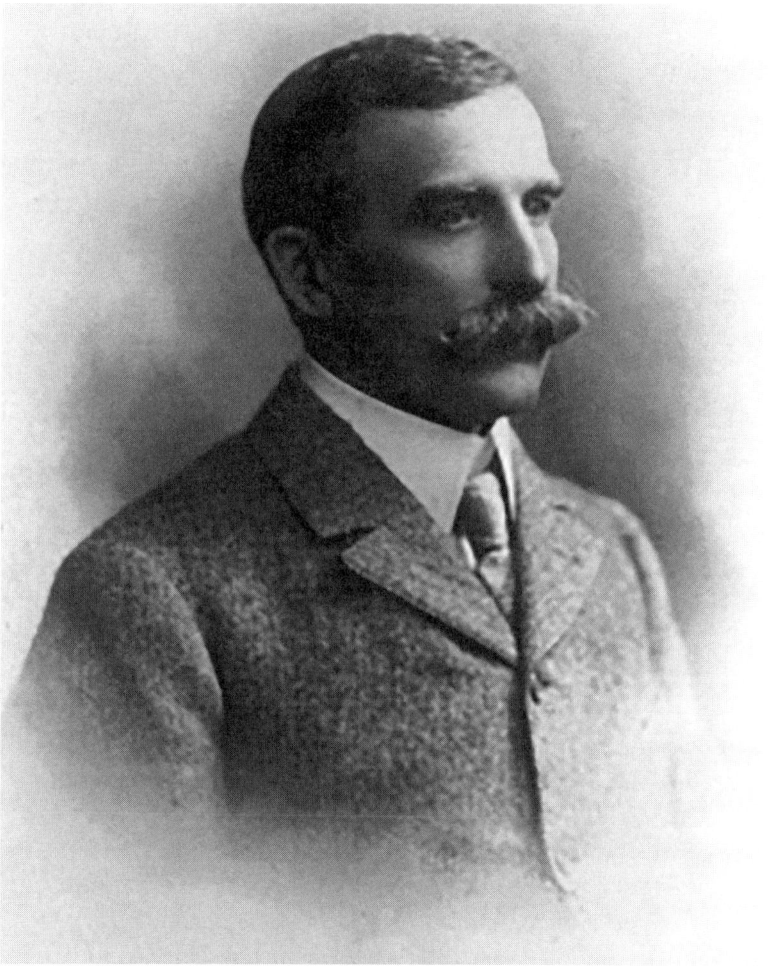

Sir Henry Solomon Wellcome
(Images courtesy of Wellcome Foundation for history of Medicine)

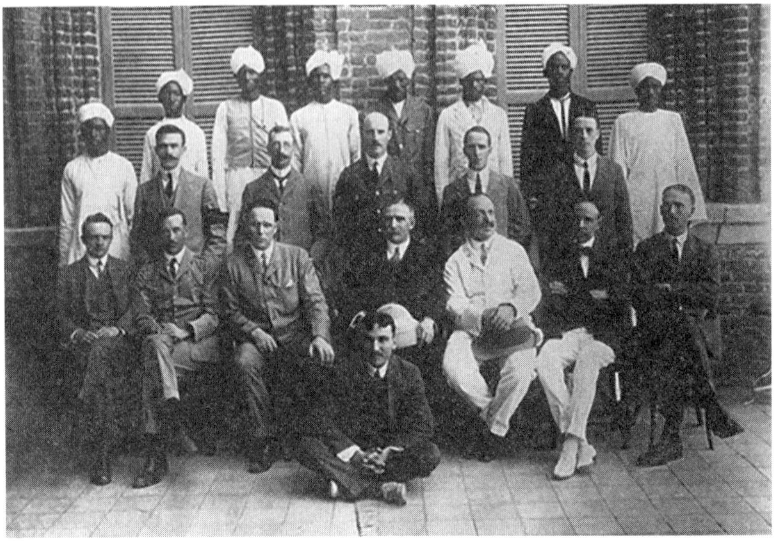

Wellcome with staff of the Wellcome Tropical Research Laboratory: circa, 1910.

FRONT ROW (from left to right): Dr. J Thompson (Senior Assistant Chemist)- Captain Fry RAMC (Protozoologist)-Andew Balfour (Director of Laboratories)-Mr Henry Wellcome – Mr James Currie (Director of Education Department, Sudan Government) William Beam (Research Chemist)- Mr Harold King (Entomologist).

MIDDLE ROW: Mr JJ Vitale (Senior Clerk)-Mr J Goodson (Assistant Chemist) – Captain Dr. Archibald RAMC (Pathologist)- Mr George Buchanan (Senior Laboratory Assistant)- Mr Alexander Marshall (Senior Laboratory Assistant).

BACK ROW: Laboratory Attendants: Mohamed Ibrahim, Abdullahi Nurin, Omar Kuwais, Bashari Mohamed, Mahdi Sharaf El-Din, Said Yunis, Adam Farah El-Dar, Ali Nimir FRONT: Nicola Effendi Hakim, (Senior Clerk)

(Images courtesy of Wellcome Foundation for history of Medicine)

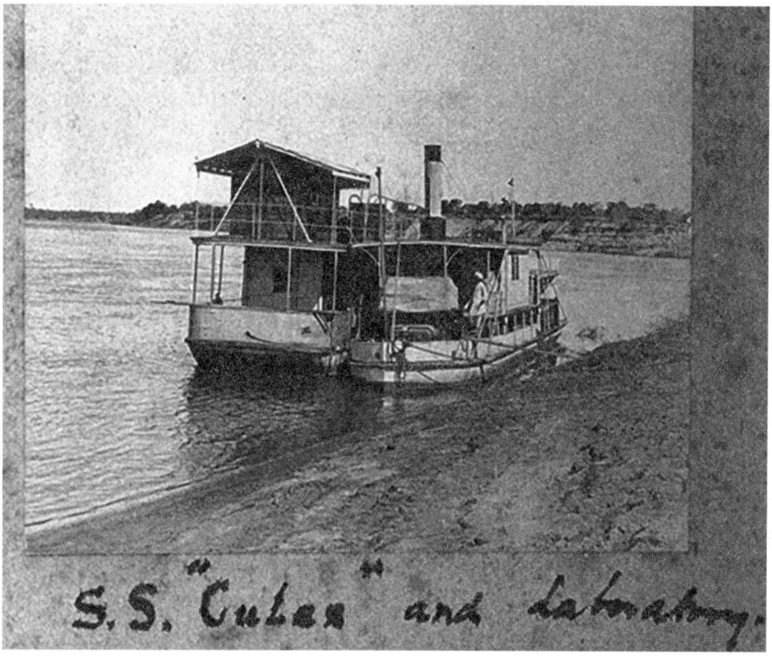

The Floating Laboratory, 'Culex'
(Images courtesy of Wellcome Foundation for history of Medicine)

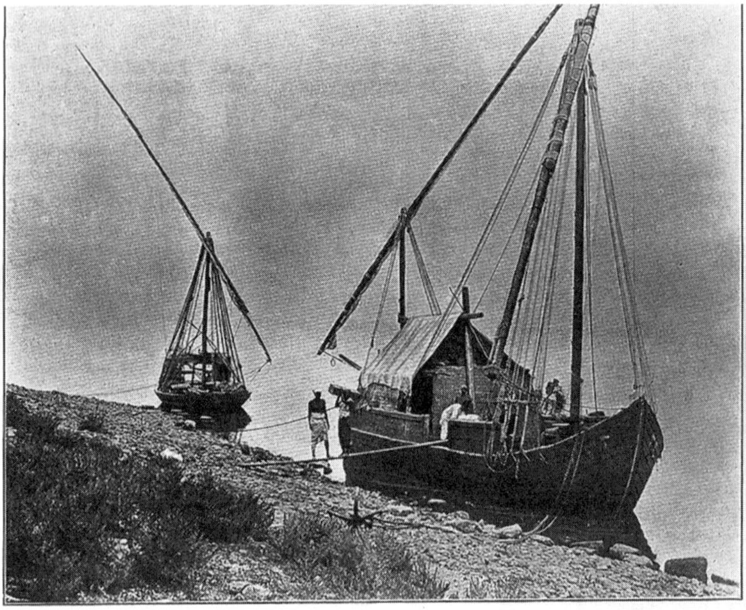

Gyassa used by Dr. Sheffield Neave, circa. 1904-1905
(Images courtesy of Wellcome Foundation for history of Medicine)

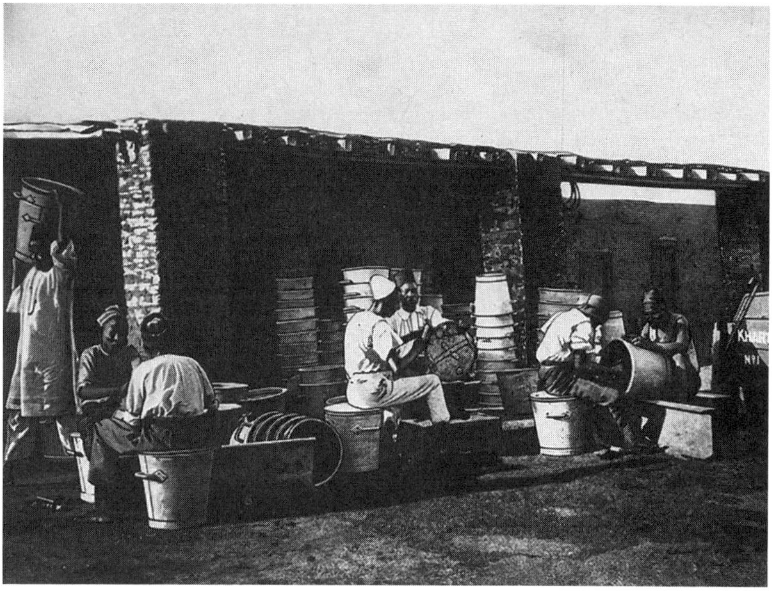

Khartoum Sanitary Service, Sudanese men repairing buckets, circa.1911
(Images courtesy of Wellcome Foundation for history of Medicine))

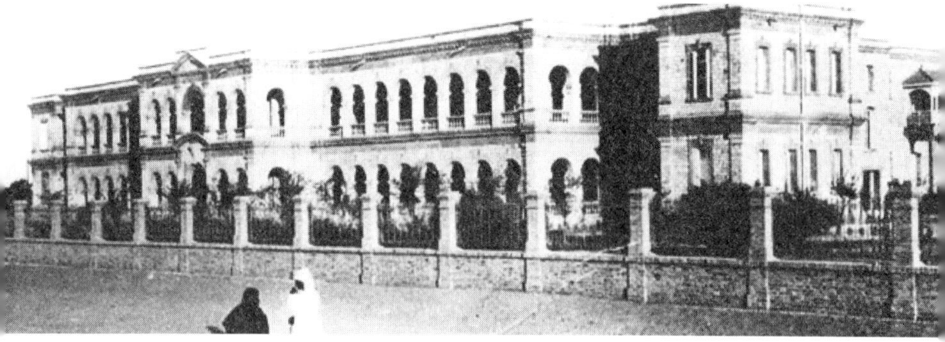

APPENDICES

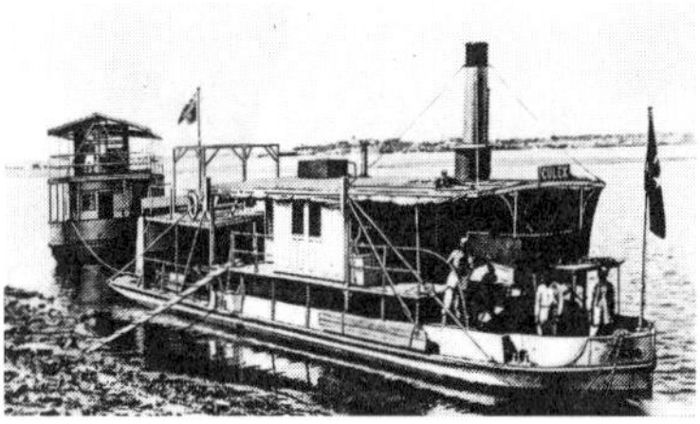

Appendix I

Jack Christopherson, Forefather of Modern Sudanese Medicine & Bilharzia Cure Discovery at Khartoum Civil Hospital

When Earth's last picture is painted and the tubes are twisted and dried,
When the oldest colours have faded, and the youngest critic has died,
We shall rest, and, faith, we shall need it—lie down for an aeon or two
Till the master of All Good Workmen shall put us to work anew
And only The Master shall praise us and only The Master shall blame
And no one shall work for money and no one shall work for fame
But each for the joy of the working, and each, in the separate star,
Shall draw the Thing as he sees It for the God of Things as They are!

–Rudyard Kipling

A landmark feature of the SMD was the historical contribution of its first director and one of the first few civil doctors to work in Sudan. To Dr. Jack Christopherson goes the credit for researching and then masterminding the discovery of the first cure for bilharziasis. Bilharzia, at the turn of the twentieth century, was a major scourge and an ominous medical condition with no cure. The full story and the biography of Jack Christopherson was published some time ago by his great niece, who spent long and painstaking years researching the footsteps of her great uncle and placed him back on the map of medical history. I have devoted a full chapter to this fascinating saga in Sudan's medical history. The core of this chapter was written well in advance of publication of the aforementioned biography of Jack Christopherson, and the opinion of the biographer, Ann Crichton Harris, to whom I am greatly indebted, has been sought as to the content of the original section, early in 2009, before the publication of her book. Some additional information was added to the original text after her book was published in the summer of 2009.

To understand this period better, one has to know more than what was earlier known about John Brian Christopherson. He could well be the 'Forefather of modern medicine in the Sudan'. Much has surfaced about Dr. Christopherson in recent years, e.g.: reappraisal of his role in the establishment of modern medical services in the Sudan; his pioneering discovery of a cure to a dreaded ailment, bilharziasis; and his great contribution to tropical medicine in general. Christopherson, a brilliant physician and a very fine surgeon, did not receive his rightful place in medical history, nor the recognition, acclaim, and fame he deserved, except very lately. His obituary in the *British Medical Journal*, in the July 30, 1955 issue, read as follows:

> Dr. J B Christopherson, who died at his home at Lyden-on-Severn in July 21st, made some important contribution to the knowledge of tropical diseases.... (1)

He was described in another tribute, by Sir Russell Brain in the Presidential Address of the Royal College of Physicians of London, as 'a versatile man who turned his mind into many branches of medicine and served with distinction in tropical medicine' (2). It was intriguing that Christopherson was regarded otherwise by many of his fellow Britons who were his contemporaries in the Sudan. His early few years were indeed happy and blissful, but despite all his qualities, he was not a 'man of politics' but rather, as described by

Ann Crichton-Harris, 'a man who would rashly speak out his mind' (3). Hence, he was to suffer greatly. He was labelled by his administrative British seniors, Sir Reginald Wingate and Sir P.R. Phipps, after an initial 'honeymoon period', as a 'trouble-maker' (4).

John Brian Christopherson was born in Batley, West Yorkshire, in 1868, the son of Cannon Brian Christopherson, Rector of Falmouth. He was educated at Newcastle-upon-Tyne Grammar School, Clifton College, and Gonville & Caius College at Cambridge, before completing his medical training at St Bartholomew's Hospital in London. He graduated as MB ChB in 1893, and then held the post of house physician, house surgeon, and anatomy demonstrator at 'Barts' before obtaining his FRCS in 1897. Shortly thereafter, in 1898, he obtained both his MA and MD degrees from Cambridge. Between the years 1896 and 1902, he was on the surgical staff of Albert Dock and Evelina Hospitals in London, before joining the medical troops at the Imperial Yeomanry Base Hospital at Deelfontein during the Boer War in 1902. In the same year he went to the Sudan, initially as private physician to the 'ruling elite'. Here there is some confusion about to whom he was actually appointed. Some records say that he was 'Physician to the Governor General, Sir Reginald Wingate' (5), while other sources state that he came as private physician to Sir Rudolph Von Slatin Pasha, the Inspector General of Sudan. In this relationship, however, lies some of 'the boon and the bane' of Christopherson. Rudolph von Slatin Pasha, an Austrian, was in the service of the Turco-Egyptian Sudan Government before the Mahdist uprising as Governor of Darfur starting in 1878, and was later a captive of the Mahdi and a prisoner and confidante of his successor, Khalifa Abdullahi, from 1884 till 1896. Slatin played a decisive role in the Reconquest of the Sudan following his successful escape to Cairo and was among the invading troops led by Lord Kitchener. Following the defeat of his old foes, the Mahdists, Slatin was appointed Inspector General of the Sudan Government. Christopherson was said to have become his physician, close friend, and confidante. On the other hand, Rudolph Slatin was to be Christopherson's saviour following his capture by the Austrians in Serbia during the First World War. The life and times of Christopherson in the Sudan were to be full of events, turmoil, personality clashes, and sound medical achievements. He was to be a foe and a friend to many of his fellow native Britons, both medical and non-medical. He was labelled as a 'troublemaker' by some senior officials, such as Sir P. R. Phipps, the private secretary to the Governor General and sometime Assistant Civil Secretary. Sir Reginald Wingate was also to write in a private letter to Phipps expressing his wish for 'this troublesome doctor to pack up and go home' (6).

Christopherson's Personality Clashes & Professional Feuds

The 'Appointment Blunder'[1] & the Crispin Affair

There is certainly a cloud surrounding the establishment of the Sudan Medical Department in 1904, and the ensuing conflict and dispute over the appointment of its first director. What filtered out, was conflicting stories of what is described by Crichton Harris as 'the appointment blunder' of the first director of the SMD (7). By 1904, Dr. Christopherson had been in the Sudan for over two years and his star was rising. Edward Smyth Crispin, who came to Sudan earlier than Christopherson, was approached by the Principal Medical Officer of the Egyptian Army (Dr. S. Lyle Cummins) to take up the post, totally unaware that Dr. Theodore Dyke Acland, the medical advisor to the Sirdar, had also approached Dr. Christopherson and offered him the post. Both accepted the offer. Later, it was felt that Christopherson was more suitable for the post, so Crispin protested and threatened to resign (8). Eventually, Crispin accepted an offer to take up the post of Medical Officer for Port Sudan, which was in the process of being built as the new harbour for the country. In the aftermath, relations between Crispin and Christopherson were never mended, and that cast a significant pall over their working relationship, which was to last many more years. Christopherson remained director from 1904/1905 till 1908, when he was dismissed, and replaced by Colonel Mathias, Principal Medical Officer of the Egyptian Army. What made things more complicated was that Crispin was appointed as his Assistant Director (9).

The Rift between Balfour & His Circle

As mentioned earlier, Andrew Balfour arrived in Sudan in January of 1903, a few months after Christopherson had joined the service of Sudan's Government. Balfour was to 'reign supreme' in his own 'Laboratory Kingdom', and although he was appointed as Medical Officer of Health of Khartoum, he was working completely independently, but not out of tandem with his other medical colleagues. Little is known about the professional and personal relationship between Balfour and Christopherson for the full decade that followed, but from the limited information available we can say that, during the first few years, probably till 1906, their encounters were more cordial (10). Balfour made several comments in praise of Christopherson's contribution to the flourishing laboratories, and these comments were made in the First Wellcome Report, published in 1904 (11), but not so in the Second Report, published in 1906 (12). However, the last two, issued in 1908 and 1911 respectively, made no mention of any contribution by Christopherson. As Ann Crichton-Harris argues, it was very much open to speculation that Christopherson was subject to the 'policy of exclusion' practiced by Balfour and his associates (13). On the other hand, Christopherson's medical papers at Durham do contain a substantive collection of articles on the subject of 'Sudanese Medicine & Tribal Customs'. It was obvious that Christopherson had made significant efforts to gather as much material relating to these topics as possible, using his network of subordinates scattered all over Sudan when he was director of the Medical Department. The responses Christopherson received from a list of many Syrian and Egyptian doctors were used to compile a paper he was writing on the subject (14). Possibly it was not sheer coincidence that the same subject was written about in detail in the Third Wellcome Report, published in 1908. In that Report, there were four articles, one by D. G. Anderson, another by Leonard Bousfield, the third by Dr. Hassan Zaki, and the last consisting of supplementary notes by Rudolph von Slatin Pasha[2]. It was not clear whether Balfour had commissioned Christopherson to deal with the subject and he then changed his mind, or whether it was just a coincidence. One can only speculate. Christopherson himself had written a not dissimilar report titled 'Description of Sudanese Native

Remedies in the Mahdi and Khalifa's Time in Omdurman', including an account by Khalifa Ahmad Sharfi (a maternal uncle of the Mahdi) (15), and none of these contributions were ever published!

As documented by Ann Crichton-Harris, there was an open rift between Christopherson and Balfour on 'naming a spirochete', or on reporting the 'first case of relapsing fever from the Sudan' (16). The actual conflict between the two men was to the subject of several stories, but it was so intense, as came out later, that Balfour was considering taking legal action against Christopherson (17). The rift between Balfour and Christopherson seems to have also involved, in a kind of a 'silent war', some of Balfour's friends and associates. Leonard Bousfield, who was close to Balfour and who succeeded him as Khartoum Medical Officer of Health in 1913, never mentioned Christopherson in his memoirs, *Sudan Doctor*, published in 1954 (a year before Christopherson's death) (18). Further, although it is not clear how close William Byam was to Andrew Balfour, but Byam in his personal memoirs; *The Road to Harley Street,* Byam made no mention of Christopherson. This is despite him being Senior Medical Officer of Khartoum District in 1911, when Christopherson was the director of both the Khartoum and the Omdurman Civil Hospitals. The number of British doctors and the size of the British community in Khartoum during that time were relatively small, and one would expect people of the same profession to know each other. Further, when Byam joined the headquarters of SMD in 1911, he lived in the same Doctors Mess with Andrew Balfour and his deputy, Robert Archibald (19). Colonel Byam, as was learned later from his autobiography, appears to have been on good terms with both Balfour and Crispin. He was also a known close friend of Robert Archibald with whom they co-wrote one of the prominent books on tropical medicine at the time, *The Practice of Medicine in the Tropics*, published in 1923. Furthermore, although Christopherson was one of the earlier staff of Albert Dock Hospital in London, following his return to London in 1919 he was not added to the staff of the London School of Tropical Medicine, despite his being an authority on tropical medicine. One may also only speculate that the 'bad blood' between him and Andrew Balfour may have played a role in this. Christopherson, on the other hand, seemed to have been on good terms with Andrew Balfour's successor, Albert Chalmers, with whom he co-authored some papers (20).

3. Bilharzia Drug Discovery & the 'McDonnagh Case'

During Christopherson's time in Sudan, bilharzia was rampant in both Egypt and the Sudan. Prior to the establishment of the Gezira Scheme, cases were rather sporadic, with a significant proportion of those cases actually occurring amongst the Egyptian troops. Indeed, most cases that were to be treated by the newly discovered drug were Egyptian soldiers. Sir Leonard Rogers in Calcutta in 1912 was the first to have started effective treatment of cases of leishmaniasis by sodium antimony tartarate. Christopherson would treat leishmaniasis cases, and while he was assessing the effectiveness of this treatment, he realized that those patients who were co-infected with 'bilharziosis' had some intriguing findings in their urine. He realized that the bilharzia ova were rendered sterile, with eggs no longer hatching, when submerged in fresh water, and some even had dead miracidia. He decided to try treatment with tartar emetic in cases of 'schistosomum haematobuim' (sic), a disease that was then totally incurable. In his famous *Lancet* paper published in 1918 titled 'The Successful Use of Antimony in Bilharziosis', Christopherson asserted that:

> …after trying and confirming the conclusion of previous workers on the use of intravenous injection of antimony tartarate (tartar emetic) in cases of Oriental sore, internal leishmanisis and naso-oral leishmanisis (Espundia) as found in the Sudan.
>
> In May 1917, I commenced at the Khartoum Civil Hospital to treat bilharziosis (both vesical and rectal) by the same drug…. The treatment of bilharzioisis up to the present has been altogether palliative and unsatisfactory. It has baffled all attempts to find a satisfactory remedy.

He would go on to state:

> There is no doubt that antimony given as intravenous injection of tartar emetic considerably interferes with bilharzias and suspend its activities, even when it does not actually kill. My own opinion, based on the cases treated during the last year, is that antimony (antimony tartarate) is a definite cure for bilharziosis, and that intravenous injection of tartar emetic kills the shistosomum haematobium and renders it harmless.... These observations are based on 13 cases of schistosomum haematobium, more than 13 however were treated by the method. (21)

Christopherson later compiled details of 70 cases he had treated at KCH. In that paper he acknowledged the efforts and help of his colleague, Dr. V. S. Hodson, Senior Medical Inspector at Atbara, who had treated several cases at KCH during his leave of absence in 1917, and also subsequently treated some cases successfully at Atbara Hospital. He also acknowledged the help of his subordinates, Dr. Mustafa Izzedin (possibly an Egyptian or perhaps a Syrian doctor) and Mr John Newlove. Such an achievement was not destined to garner immediate fame and recognition, and yet another 'cloud was to stand over the portrait'. After Christopherson published his famous *Lancet* paper, another British doctor, Dr. J. E. R. McDonagh, had claimed that he had cured three cases of urinary bilharziasis three years before Christopherson (22). A long feud then ensued that left its shadows on Christopherson's achievement. However, he was nominated for Noble Prize of Medicine, but it was never to be.

In Sudan, Christopherson was very popular among his non-British colleagues, patients, and subordinates. He was famously known as 'Christo'. Several records indicate that he was much beloved, even by some notable Sudanese public and religious figures. Documents kept at the Sudan Archives in Durham document that he had a long friendship with Syed Al-Shareef Yusuf Mohamed Al-Ameen al-Hindi, a notable religious leader (23). A letter sent to Christopherson by one of his longtime subordinates and confidantes, Dr. Hassan Effendi Zaki, paid tribute to 'Christo' for all his good contributions to the welfare of his Sudanese patients and friends (24).

Christopherson, following his return to Britain in 1919, worked as a consultant at London Chest Hospital, Victoria Park. Further, from his fame and authority in treating bilharziasis, he founded and ran a 'Bilharzia Clinic' at the Ministry of Pension, which dealt with many British service men who had contracted the disease overseas. He became a Fellow of the Royal College of Surgeons of England and of the Royal College of Physicians of London. For a while he was examiner at the London School of Tropical Medicine and Hygiene. He was awarded the C.B.E. in 1919. He also received the Order of The Nile (Third Class) from the Sultan of Egypt (25). Christopherson retired for the last twenty years of his life to a country home in Lydney-on-Severn in Gloucestershire, which he called 'Heaven's Gate'. He died at 87 years of age, on July 21, 1955. A close friend would write the following words of tribute following his death in 1955:

> Christo, a name by which he was known by his many friends in Khartoum, was most popular with the Sudanese who worked with him in his researches, but had little time for the social life in the British Community, by whom he was much admired. He was very humble and retiring never seeking any high honour which he richly deserved. He was well known for his many selfless kindness to his patients and would often ask me to visit some special patient in whom he was interested. (26)

Sir Philip Manson-Bahr[3] wrote, in Christopherson's obituary in the *British Medical Journal* (July 30, 1955), words of praise, appreciation, and tribute:

> Christo to his friends- has passed on at age of 87. His name is but a memory to the present generation, for he had been living in retirement in his country home appropriately named 'Heaven's Gate' for nearly twenty years, yet his fame is known to all students of tropical medicine. To Christopherson is undoubtedly due the modern treatment of schistosomiasis with antimony: he was the first to put this method on a proper basis. It is only fair to him that the facts should now be set forth, as they are apt to be forgotten..... I was fortunate to be able to visit him in April 1919, in Khartoum, where he most convincingly demonstrated his technique of injection and the results he had obtained.... It should be stated that this work of Christopherson was quite original, and it was only when the results had been published that he became aware that J E R McDonagh had claimed to have cured two cases of urinary schistosomiaisis by antimony three years previously.... From this time onwards, I was to see a great deal of Christo. He

was a kind, considerate soul, with a keen inquisitive look and an inquiring mind.... He played a great part in the medical history of the Sudan....we shall all mourn the passing of Christo for a man of great worth and great attainments, who became a guide, philosopher, and a friend to all who came into contact with him. (27)

Endnotes

1 The 'Appointment Blunder' is a descriptive term first used by Ann Crichton Harris, a great niece of Dr. Christopherson, who researched the records of her great uncle for eight years and eventually wrote his biography, published in 2009 by Brill, titled *Poison in Small Measures: Dr. Christopeherson and the Cure for Bilharzia.*

2 Rodulph Carl von Slatin, an Austrian of Jewish ancestry, was born in Vienna in 1857, and died in 1932. He came to Sudan in 1874 as an aide to the Austrian Consul and was thereafter appointed by Charles Gordon as Governor of Darfur, in 1878. He became a captive of the Mahdi and his successor, Khalifa Abdullahi, and managed to escape to Egypt in 1896. His escape as well as his book, *Fire & Sword in the Sudan*, was a major pretext for the Sudan Reconquest operation, and the support from the swinging of public opinion in London for the Nile Expedition proved decisive for the success of the operation. The book was translated from German by Reginald Wingate, who was in charge of the Intelligence Service of the Egyptian Army. Slatin was amongst the invading troops led by Kitchener. Following the Reconquest, in 1900, Slatin was appointed Inspector-General of the Sudan, a post that was purposely created for him, and which he held till 1914, when he was compelled to leave upon the eruption of the First World War, being an Austrian citizen. He became a Baron of the Austrian Empire in 1906, Knight and Commander of St Michael & St George in 1898, and Knight Commander of the Victorian Order in 1908. On the medical side, Slatin had a sound knowledge of Sudanese medical practices during the Turkkiya & the Mahdiyyia. His additional notes to the article written by Dr. Hassan Effendi Zaki, 'The Healing Art & Practices by the Dervishes in the Sudan During the Rule of the Mahdi and the Khalifa', was a sound reference work for medical practices during that era (see Part II, Chapter 3).

3 Sir Philip Manson-Bahr, was a zoologist and physician known for his contribution to tropical medicine. He was of German origin and he changed his name to Manson-Bahr after marrying Edith Margaret

Manson, daughter of the doyen of tropical medicine Sir Patrick Manson.

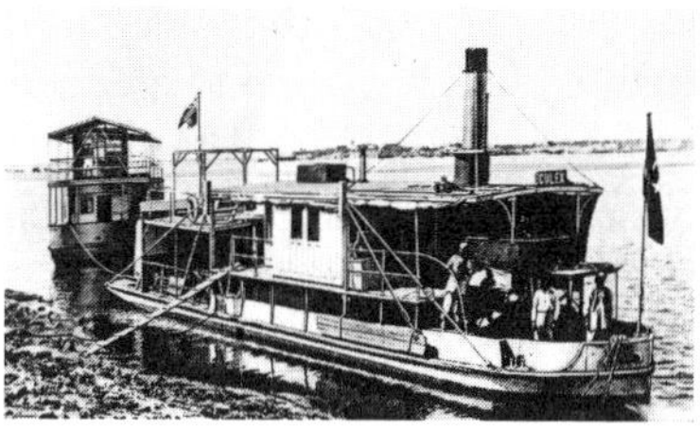

Appendix 2

Bimbashi Stanton & Sudan Camel Stamp

Philately is the art of collecting and studying stamps and related items, so it is a science in its own right. In this section we will give a short account of the story of the origin of the famous Sudanese Camel stamps (See Illustrations Section). It transpired that this story was narrated by Dr. William Byam, who worked in the Anglo-Egyptian Sudan from 1908 to 1912. Byam had a lifelong love and passion for the art/science of 'Philately'. While Byam was in Egypt in 1935, he co-founded the 'Egyptian Philatelic Society'. His Wikepedia page mentions that Byam took up philately in 1923 as a method of relaxation from his stressful medical practice in Harley Street (1). He joined the Royal Philately Society in 1924 and took up a special interest in the philately of Egypt, a country that very much had shaped his early career. Later he went on to found the 'Egypt Study Circle', in 1935 (2). That was a feat, the first of its kind, and, following a presentation to the Philatelic Congress of Great Britain in 1938, in a paper titled 'Organization of a Study Circle', he inspired others to establish similar study circles in the areas of their own interest (3). It is noteworthy that Byam had a house in Guernsey, which was occupied by the Germans during the Second World War, where he kept most of his philatelic collections.

Here, I reproduce an article from the *Canadian Philatelist Journal,* published posthumously in 1964 in his memory (4). The article was written by Byam as a chapter in his second autobiographical book, *Dr. Byam in Harley Street* (5). The chapter narrates the story of the Sudan 'Camel stamps', which was the hallmark of the Sudan postal services for many years beyond Independence. The article is an entertaining account of the origin of the 'Sudan Stamps' and, as it was quoted in the journal, it gives more personal details than had hitherto appeared in the philatelic press.

> Byam wrote: My first efforts at serious work was an attempt to build a picture of postal development in the Sudan. This collection began with the stamps used in the days of Gordon Pasha, when only Egyptian stamps were available in the Sudan. These are recognized as having been used in the Sudan by the town names in the postmarks on them.
>
> Then followed evidence of the posts organized for use by the Army during Kitchener campaign to re-conquer the Sudan from the Dervishes. To illustrate this phase I acquired letters sent by members of the fighting force after the various battles. Some of these letters were marked 'No stamps available'. Others provided evidence of railway development, being certified by postal officials as sent from rail-head. For a short time stamps of Egypt were in use overprinted SOUDAN, repeated in Arabic. The Sirdar (Kitchener) disapproved of this practice as he was determined to avoid anything of political significance. Egyptian stamps in any form, Kitchener considered, would suggest the Sudan was being conquered to become a part of Egypt. He therefore told Colonel Jimmy Watson, a member of his personal staff, to obtain designs for a special stamp and gave instructions that his own portrait was not to be included neither was the design to have any propaganda value. Watson approached one of the artists war correspondents with the force and obtained from him a sketch of the outside of Abu Simbul rock temple, showing the four colossal statues of Ramses II. The figure of value of the stamps was inserted in the entrance to the temple which is situated between the two central statues. Watson presented the work of art for the approval of the Sirdar. Under it the artist had written: 'My price for this sketch is 20 guineas'. Kitchener without looking at the sketch added, 'my price isn't'. Watson was then told to order Bimbashi Stanton* to prepare designs for a Sudan stamp which the Sirdar would inspect in four days. Stanton, a British officer serving with one of the Egyptian battalions, was acting correspondent to the *Illustrated London News*. All he had with him, as artists material; was a small supply of water colour paints and some sheets of very ordinary foolscap paper. This order from the Sirdar came as a most

unpleasant surprise. Stanton had no experience or knowledge of designing stamps. He knew if he failed to satisfy the Sirdar he would certainly be sent home to rejoin the British regiment.

In depressed mood and bemoaning his fate, he sat idly turning over the pages of the latest number of the *Illustrated London News* when his eye fell on an advertisement for Treloar's Carpets. It was full-page picture of a camel laden with original rugs, being ridden up Ludgate Hill. Stanton, with relief, seized the idea that here was the design for his stamp. He at once went out from his tent, camera in hand and persuaded a friendly Arab to allow photographs to be taken of him in his camel. The animal was made to trot, so that Stanton might record the proper movements of his legs. In the sketch that resulted, the camel was portrayed with an Arab postman on its back, trotting past a range of desert hills. By the sandy track lay the skeleton of a camel, one of the many which perished during the long trek to the South. Slung behind the rider were two spears. Treloar's rugs were replaced by saddle bags for carriage of mail. On these bags were names of Berber and Khartoum, two towns yet unconquered; flattery intended to appease Kitchener wrath if he rejected the design. This was conceived of the most famous of all time- the Sudan Camel Postman- a design which remained in use for longer than almost any in the history of the Post of the World.

Under the main drawing, Stanton sketched a series of the miniatures of the stamp in colours which differed for the various denominations he believed would be required. Kitchener approved the design without comment and equally without praise. Stanton was ordered to take it to England and be responsible for its correct reproduction by the world-famous stamp printers, Messer's De La Rue.

When Stanton returned to his place in the front line, up the Nile, he asked Jimmy Watson if he would approach the Sirdar with a request for a set of the new stamps certified as designed by him and bearing the signature of the Sirdar in confirmation of the statement. Watson agreed and made the request to which he received the reply, 'Yes, but see he pays for them'. Watson himself paid for a set the stamps. When mounted and certified as the work of Stanton, Kitchener designed to append his autograph but left Watson to make the actual presentation.

This story was told me when I visited Stanton in his West Country home. There I saw the set with Kitchener signature appended. Of the stamps themselves little could be seen, as the sheet on which they had been mounted had been framed and hung on the wall of Stanton bathroom where steam had dealt faithfully with De La Rue's fugitive printing ink.

Stanton wrote this story for my collection. He also gave me a number of envelops addressed to his parents carrying the letters he had written after the battles in which he fought as the victorious army advanced to Khartoum.

---

*Colonel E. A. Stanton, C.M.G., later became Governor of Khartoum.

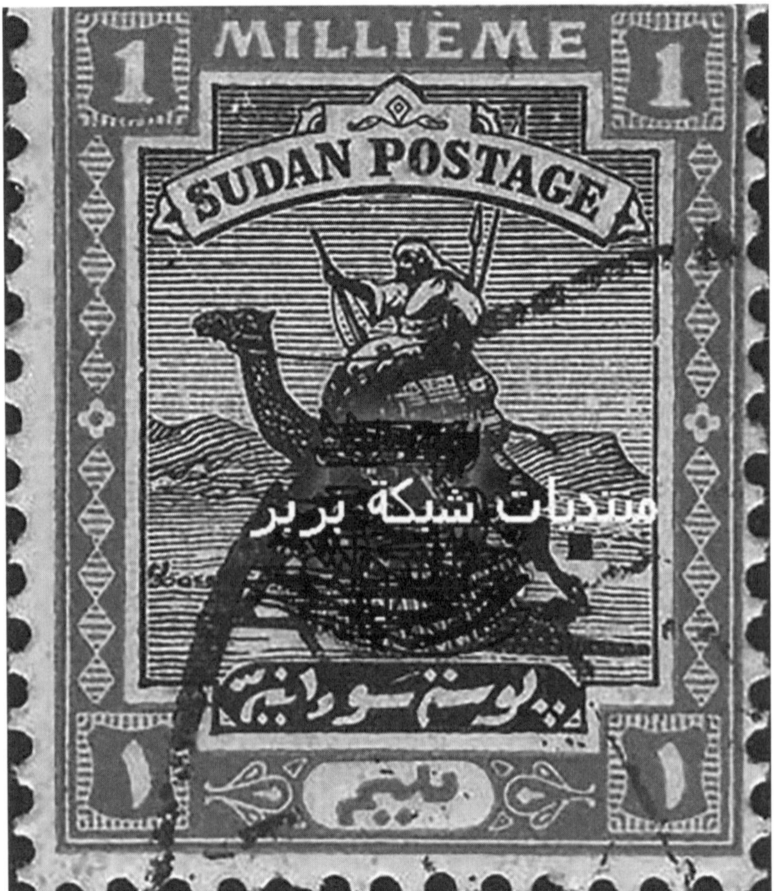

Sudan Camel Stamp

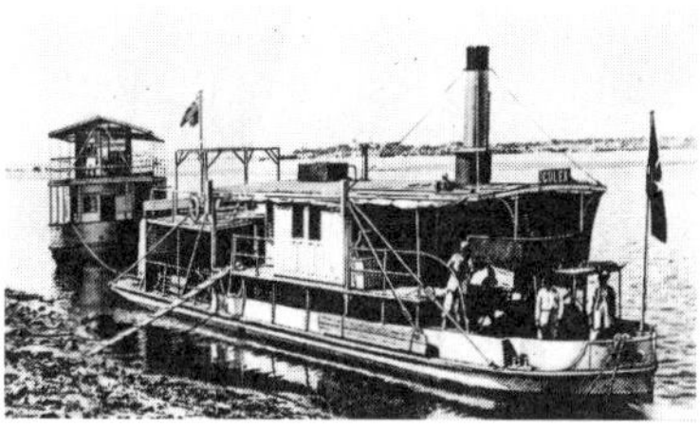

Appendix 3

Henry Wellcome in Gebel Moya, Sennar: Archeology Zeal or Social Benevolence?

Henry Wellcome had varied interests. A special one was his love and passion for archaeology and archaeological research. This indeed dated back to his childhood, when he first became fascinated by archaeology. When he was four years old, he found a Neolithic stone implement and his father explained to him that the perfecting of that tool had been more important to its markers than the electricity, telegraph, or the steam railway engine are to contemporary man (1). In 1911, Wellcome visited Sudan and, after having taken a trip on a gayyassa up the Blue Nile with one thing in mind: to pick a site where he may succeed in adding something to what was already known about Old World archaeology. The archaeological discoveries in Egypt and the common history and geography of the Nile Valley may have tempted him to try his luck in this part of the Sudan. Landing at Sennar, Wellcome chose the site near Gebel Moya, a hilly outpost to the south of Sennar, to start his excavation. Here, Wellcome stayed for the whole of the period from January to April 1911. Wellcome began his project, which would not only involve digging for ancient buried materials; but also involved transforming the landscape of the whole of the area of Gebel Moya. In his various projects, Wellcome employed as many as 4,000 people throughout the four seasons that his archaeological site excavation was going on, relentlessly. Not only were job opportunities created but also a dispensary would be established, a school would be built, and even the social habits and lifestyle of the local inhabitants would be changed. Wellcome discovered that the natives heavily indulged in consuming the local liquor, *'merissa',* which was behind many local troubles and crimes. He would write: 'They (the people of Gebel Moya) were unaccustomed to discipline and habituated to unbridled licence and acts of violence. The local beer, merissa, was the cause of "hideous all-night drunken orgies".' Wellcome would then launch a campaign aimed at curbing this bad habit of the natives, which was also behind some of their idleness, not only among those who were employed by him in the archaeological excavation, but also others. For those who would abstain from drinking 'merissa' for up to eight weeks, an incentive was given in the form of the 'Order of the Peacock' award, adorned with peacock feathers. And as peacocks are not readily available in the Sudan, Wellcome imported several from England and created a small local zoo where these birds were kept. He would even use verses from the *Quran* to support his quest for abstinence from the local beer. He went even further and imposed a compulsory alcohol ban on his British and other foreign workers. The mass employment, the supply of water from wells dug by Wellcome, and even sport days very much changed the way of life of the local inhabitants. A 'House of Boulders' was built on the top of Gebel Moya, the remains of which can still be seen today. The building was meant to be a private accommodation for Wellcome during his visits to the site. This house continued to be occupied by Major Julio Uribe, an Ecuadorian army officer employed by Wellcome to oversee the progress of the work in his absence. Pioneering ventures would be executed. Aerial photography to take pictures of the excavation sites was carried out using a camera with a shutter attached to a kite. Also, the equipment that needed to be transported to the plateau of Gebel Moya was carried on an aerial ropeway called the 'flying camel', which was erected on the plain below the hill. Even a motor car was brought to the site, only the second in the Sudan after the Governor General's! At some stage, the excavation site was like a military camp, with guards and unaccustomed discipline, amid houses built for the local labourers and the foreign archaeology staff alike (photo; see Illustrations section). Wellcome's archaeological venture was the best of the archaeological digs in the Sudan for many years. The outcome, although it did not fulfill the ambitions of the benefactor, was successful in unearthing material that proved that there was a community living in the area between 1,000 B.C. and 400 A.D. A late Neolithic combined cemetery and settlement locality was found, with nearly 3,000 graves excavated.

Despite the fact that the work at the site never resumed after it ceased with the onset of the First World War, Wellcome's zeal for the whole project never declined, and he would return to spend a few days in some winter seasons, or sending Major Uribe. This continued for many years. However, the onset of the First World War brought an end to the active archaeological zeal of Mr Wellcome in the Sudan. Major Uribe kept coming to the house till 1938, years after the death of Henry Wellcome in 1936 (2). Following this, the Trustees of the Wellcome Foundation made a decision that it would be pointless to resume any further work at the site (even though the licence was still valid). Many years later, in 1949, two monumental volumes covering the archaeological and anthropological aspects of the work were compiled and published by Frank Addison (3). In 1955, the anatomical report was published by Mukherjee, Rao, and Trevor. These helped to shed some light on the whole enterprise, and beyond doubt it made a significant contribution to the ancient history of the Sudan. In 2010, a new edition in a single volume covering both aspects was published by Cambridge University Press (4).

Recently, interest in the excavation at Gebel Moya has been revived, especially since the items discovered were dated to the period between the 5th and the 1st millennia B.C. (5, 6). Currently, some work is underway to utilise advances in science to understand more about these archaeological collections and unravel some of the mysteries of the earlier inhabitants of the Sudan.

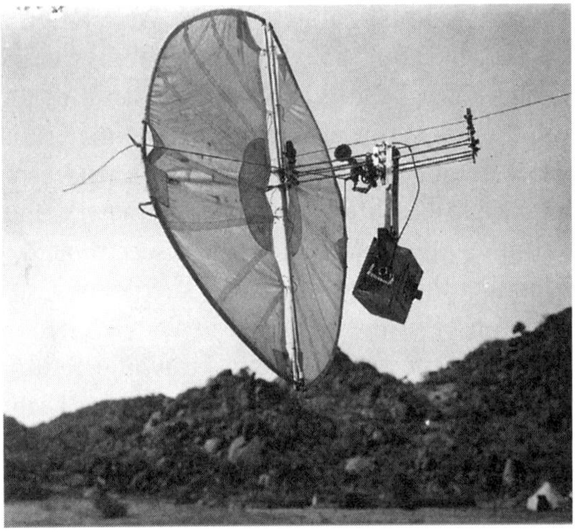

Aerial photography at Gebel Moya

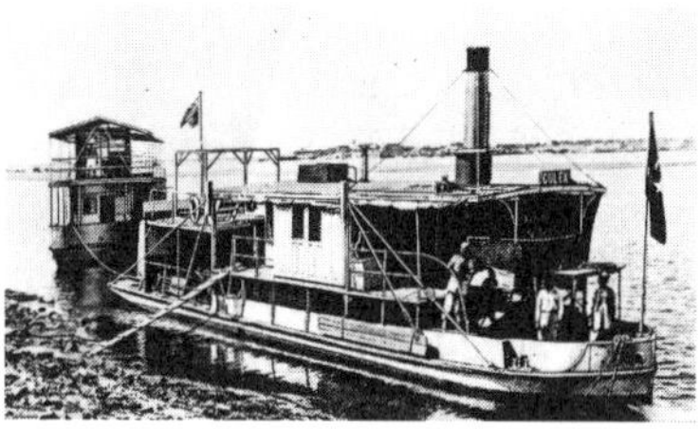

Appendix 4

Traditional Medical Practices & Superstitions

Traditional Sudanese Medicine in the Pre-Turco-Egyptian Era

Possibly the early evidence of traditional Sudanese medicine in the literature (in English) surfaced in the writings of several European travellers and explorers who trudged across the Nubian and other Sudanese hinterlands since the late medieval times. The first medical person who came to Nubia and Sennar was the Frenchman Charles Jaques Poncet, who was accompanied by the Jesuit Father Charles Francis Xavier de Brevedent, in 1699. Although Poncet was a reputable physician and apothecary who spent many years practicing amongst the European and Turkish elite at Alexandria before his trip to Abyssinia via Sennar, his writing didn't include much about what he may have encountered of the native Sudanese methods of traditional healing (1). A few years later, in 1701, another Jesuit priest, the German Theodoro Krump came to Sennar from Egypt. Prior to Krump, another Jesuit priest, Father Pasqual, seems to have lived and practiced medicine in Sennar and was taken as private physician to the Fung Sultan (Krump, 1708) (2). It was through the writings of Krump that we come to know some aspects of health and disease in the Fung Kingdom of Sennar. After another three-quarters of a century, the Scottish explorer James Bruce came to Sudan on his return journey from Ethiopia back to Europe. Bruce described the native methods of vaccination against smallpox, which the natives called 'buying the pox' (يردجال ريطشت). Here a rag would be wrapped around the arm of an infected person, and the person wanting to be 'vaccinated' would be standing by. Usually the old women of the tribe were the ones who carried out the procedure. A price had to be placed on the 'rag' and after haggling and bargaining on the price, when it was agreed, the rag would be taken away by the person wanting to be vaccinated. The rag would be tied on the arm and when the recipient contracted the disease, he would only have the number of pocks he had paid for! (3). Bruce commented on the expertise of the native healers in extracting the Guinea (Medina) worm from the body of those infected with it (4), and on their practice of treating patients with liver disease and epilepsy by herbal remedies (5).

The next European explorer who became enthralled by the stories of James Bruce and decided to follow in the footsteps of the Sudan was the Englishman William George Browne (6) (see Part II). Contemporary medical practices and various medicines used by the natives to treat various diseases were also documented by him, ranging from 'natrun' to 'tamarind' to phlebotomy and to the ancient practice of leeching and the use of some substances as aphrodisiacs. This last, he remarked, were in high demand, not surprisingly (7). He also described at length the practice of female circumcision, which he stated is less in Darfur. Following Browne was the prolific Anglo-Swiss John Lewis Burckhardt, who also described the method of inoculation, called *'dak-el-Jedri',* that was practiced in the Nile Valley and the medicine used by the natives to attempt to cure those infected, by stating 'the only cure for the smallpox was to rub the whole body with butter three or four times a day and to keep themselves closely shut up' (8).

During his one-month stay at Shendy, the most important trading post in Central Sudan during that time, Burckhardt wrote about various medicines used by the native medical practitioners, stating that 'grocers and druggists are the most frequented of any' (9) and would sell various herbs and native medicines imported from either India, Egypt, or other parts of the Sudan, such as Sennar, Kordofan, and Darfur. Those items included substances like Fenugreek (called *Helba*), antimony (local name: *Kohol*), *gerfa* (cinnamon shrub), Sembil, Mehalab, and a fruit called '*tamr el-Berr*', imported from Kordofan, which is used to treat flatulence, on which Burckhardt commented that 'it is believed here to be a remedy for flatulence, of which many people here complain' (ibid.) (10).

Native Sudanese Medical Practice during the Turco-Egyptian Era

The previous section highlighted the scope of the medical services available in the Turco-Egyptian Sudan. This section will deal with the native medicine and medical superstitions that were documented during the same era. These are primarily found in the writings of some European travellers who had mentioned their encounters with the native Sudanese medicine and medical practitioners. An earlier traveller to Kordofan was the Austrian Bohemian trader Ignatius Pallme, who was mentioned in preceding sections. Pallme referred to the native medical practices as 'domestic quack remedies and superstitions' (11). Here we extract from his description of treating the common malady, fever:

> Those attacked with fever after the amulets and other mystic charms have proved useless, drinks for three or four days a cup containing about a pound of melted butter daily, or a large quantity of milk, in which a sandal-wood has been steeped during twenty four hours. Both these remedies produce a powerful alternative effect, as I saw several persons cured of fever by them. (12)

He also described the treatment of other common problems, including dysentery and dropsy:

> For allaying dysentery, use of sour milk, in which tabaldia, the fruit of a tree, causing constipation, has been steeped overnight. The same fruit taken in small quantity acts as a gentle purgative, but those modes of treatment are adapted to the natives and always prove fatal to the Europeans. For dropsy they know of no

> remedy and persons attacked with this disease die, with but few exceptions' (ibid p. 195) (13). Pallme also described the ways the native people deal with the common parasitic infestation, jiggers (flea = Sarcoptylla penetrans'). He stated that the natives use red hot iron to burn the part inflamed. Smallpox sufferers had the habit of rubbing their whole body with earth or roll in the sand until the pustules were broken and the entire surface covered with incrustation. He also described the way tapeworms were extracted when 'the native seize the portion of the animal protruding through the opening, wind it carefully around a small piece of wood, and proceed in this manner until they have gradually extremed (sic) the whole.... (ibid., p.196) (14)

Dr. Arthur Todd Holroyd, an English physician, wrote a first-hand description of native medical practices, stemming from a personal experience when he was attacked with a severe febrile illness, likely malaria, while he was in Ambukol in northern Sudan in 1838. Here we reproduce his account of his vivid experience:

> After leaving old Dongola and on the 4th I was attacked with intermittent fever, which in spite of quinine and other remedies, assumed a continuous form, and when I arrived at Ambukol I was so exhausted with exertion.... My fever continued to increase, and I became delirious with occasional lucid intervals. Sheikh Mohamed and the Hajji held a consultation, the result of which was that the former persuaded the later to permit him to burn under my coverlet some amulets which he had written, and which he asserted were a certain remedy for my complaint. I was asked to submit to this plan of treatment, and being unconscious of what was going on, I was informed afterwards by Hajji that I acceded (sic) their request. Subsequently I learned that the Sheikh wrote some passages from the Quran on slips of paper, and having placed a small earthenware stone under my coverlet burnt each amulet separately, at the same time placing his right hand on my forehead and repeating prayers, until the papers were consumed, a remedy which almost roasted me alive and stifled me with carbonic acid gas produced.... During the night the delirium decreased, Towards the morning I began to doze, and at noon the formidable symptom disappeared. The Sheikh was extremely anxious to repeat the remedy, and I obstinately refused to submit though I had his assurance that I should suffer less every time the remedy

> was repeated seven successive evenings and convalescence would soon be established.... (15)

Another European traveller was Sir Samuel W. Baker, who first came to the Sudan in 1861. In his book, *Nile Tributaries of Abyssinia*, Baker wrote down his observations in the eastern part of the Sudan (16). Like most of his preceding fellow European travellers, Baker presented himself to the Sudanese as a 'physician':

> I was in full practice as physician and we congratulated ourselves upon the healthiness of our little isolated camp. (17)

> My success as a physician had gained me so many friends, as I studiously avoided the acceptance of any present in return for my services, which I wished them to receive as simple acts of kindness; thus I had placed Sheikh Hassan bel Kader under an obligation, by curing him of a fever.... (18)

His large 'Medicine Chest' gave him special status among those with whom he became acquainted in his journeys in those Sudanese hinterlands. Baker, in his thesis, described his medical observations, a first-hand account of the medical practice of that era:

> The plagues of Egypt were upon us; the common house flies were in billions, in addition to the cattle tormentor....the plagues of boils broke out and every one was attacked more or less severely.... this was species of itch, which affected all ages and both sexes equally. It attacked all parts of the body, but particularly the extremities. The irritation was beyond description; small vesicles rose above the skin, containing watery fluid, which, upon bursting, appeared to spread the disease. The Arabs had no control over this malady which they called 'coorash', and the whole country was scratching. The popular belief attributes the disease to the waters of the Atbara at this particular season; although a horrible plague, I do not believe it to have any connexion with the well known itch or scabies of Europe. (19)

Interestingly enough, Baker invented a remedy for this '*coorash*' by making a 'medical paste' from gunpowder mixed with sulphuric acid. Baker also made intelligent medical observations by the standards of today's modern medicine. He stated that nearly 50% of the population of Sofi, a village on the Atbara River, had permanent enlargement of the spleen 'which could be felt with a slight pressure of the hand, frequently as large as orange, this was called 'Jenna el Wirde' (child of the fever), and was the result of constant attacks of fever in successive rainy seasons' (20). Baker here has unwittingly anticipated the modern-day description of 'tropical splenomegaly; which is well known to occur as a result of recurrent attacks of malaria. He also described how diseases like syphilis (which he remarked is common throughout the country) was treated by getting those affected to eat a specific diet made from slaughtering a sheep. He went further to assert that 'the flesh of the crocodile is eaten greedily, being supposed to promote desire' (21).

About native doctors Baker wrote in some detail, stating that 'The Arabs are wretchedly ignorant of the healing art, and they suffer accordingly' (22). He described in detail the methods they used for healing, which were primarily the same methods of traditional medicine that persisted well beyond the Turco-Egyptian era into modern times. The native doctor, the '*Faky*' (or *Fageer*) used various prescriptions that were centred around writing down a verse from the *Holy Quran*. This could be either a piece of paper that has to be swallowed by the patient or a wooden plate on which the writings (the prescription) was to be washed off by water and that water to be swallowed in perfect faith by the patient. He went on to describe the types of patients who went to those native doctors for consultations for various complaints.

> No 1 arrives, a barren woman who requests some medicine that will promote the blessing of childbirth. No 2, a man who was strong in his youth, but from excessive dissipation has become useless. No 3, a man deformed from his birth, who wishes to become straight as other men. No 4, a blind child.... (23)

He finally elaborated on his observations on the superstitions and relics adopted by the people in that part of the Turco-Egyptian Sudan. He described the method the natives adopt to prevent 'hydrophobia' (rabies), which he was told was prevalent in the area, by making all the dogs pass through a hut set on fire! (24).

Appendix 4

Traditional Sudanese Medical Practices during the Mahdiyya Era

This has already been covered in the section on Medical practices during the Mahdiyya era. the reader is referred to Part III.

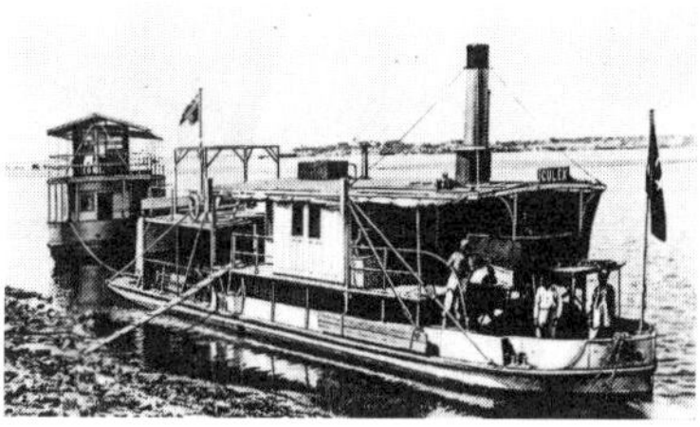

Appendix 5

The Medical Corps Bimbashis

In this section we shall deal with some notable and pioneering doctors from the RAMC and the era of the SMD. The first section will cover the life and times of 'the medical corps Bimbashis'. *Bimbashi* was a Turkish military title equivalent to Major. Those were Dr. Leonard Bousfield, Dr. William Byam, and Dr. Steven Lyle Cummins. They made special contributions to medicine and medical research in their heyday. Further, they have left a rich heritage from their career in the Anglo-Egyptian Sudan and beyond. Two of them; Byam and Cummins, went on to have very distinguished careers in medicine back in Britain. Bousfield, who came to Sudan among the first wave of the RAMC following the Reconquest, effectively spent all his working career in the Sudan, and he made special contributions to earlier research into leishmaniasis, which was a mysterious disease for a good number of years, despite the earlier discovery of its causative parasite by Charles Donovan and William Leishman in the early years of the twentieth century. Bousfield, after he left the RAMC, went on to obtain a public health diploma and to succeed Dr. Balfour as the Medical Officer of Health of Khartoum. Bousfield then became one of the main characters of the 'Central Sanitary Board', which was effectively the main hub of overseeing the public health, not only of Khartoum, but for all of Sudan. Lyle Cummins, a prolific Anglo-Irish and a multi-talented physician and scientist, made special contributions while in Sudan to both research and medical services. He went on after returning to Britain to be one of the pioneers of respiratory medicine and was credited with establishing the diploma of treatment of tuberculosis, a disease he gained much expertise dealing with while in Sudan. That diploma became a useful public health degree for overseas doctors flocking to Cardiff to obtain it well into the dying years of the twentieth century.

Section I: Steven Lyle Cummins, the Irish Pioneer of Tuberculosis

Born in 1873, in Cork, the famous southern Irish coastal town, Stevenson Lyle Cummins belonged to a gifted Irish family by long adoption and he inherited their abilities and the characteristics of his native land. His father, W. J. Cummins, was a doctor. Cummins was educated at St Faughnan's College, Roscarbury, and Queen's College, Cork, whence he graduated in 1896. Soon after graduation he joined the RAMC, in 1897, and his first active involvement in the Sudan was during the Nile Expedition of 1898, and he was involved in the Battle of Omdurman on September 2, 1898. He was then seconded to the EAMC in 1899 and became captain in 1900 (1). He served mostly at Khartoum, where he was Senior Medical Inspector at the Egyptian Army Military Hospital, which later became known as the River Hospital. It was during this period in Sudan that he first developed an interest in tuberculosis, a field in which he would later excel and become a world-renowned expert. In 1908; following observation of Sudanese troops he treated from tuberculosis, Cummins came up with the 'Virgin Soil' theory, which had a significant impact on the thinking in the field of tuberculosis for generations to come (2). Cummins realised that those Sudanese troops who were generally drawn from the Sudanese hinterlands, showed evidence of a more acute form, with a tendency for dissemination and more fulminant disease with higher morbidity and mortality than their Fellaheen counterparts, who were drawn from the Nile Delta of Egypt. This latter group had features of the disease as seen in the Europeans, with disease locality and fibrosis. The concept broadly encompassed the interaction of race, immunity, and migration. Referring to Pearson's work on heredity and tuberculosis, Cummins came up with the 'Virgin Soil' theory, claiming that the Sudanese had no innate immunity stemming from previous exposure; hence, they were more vulnerable from lack of resistance which is witnessed in the Europeans and Egyptians. The tenets of the 'Virgin Soil' theory were that 'primitive tribes' are highly susceptible to infection by the tubercle bacillus and that 'civilised' people are highly protected against it. In a subsequent paper, 'The "Virgin Soil" Theory in Cummins' Concept', was synonymous with absence of acquired immunity (1912 paper) (3). Here he seems to have been influenced by his work in London, where he was appointed to the Vaccine Department in the Royal Army Medical College as pathologist after he left Sudan in 1909. It was in that department that he became involved in the work of developing a vaccine for typhoid. It was possibly here that much of his later expertise and ideas in the field of tuberculosis and immunity were planted. According to Mark Harrison and Michael Worboys, he was influenced by the ideas of his mentor and teacher; Almroth Wright at Netly. Wright had earlier developed the theory and practice of the protective inoculation that Cummins was applying and practicing daily (4). Cummins' 'Virgin Soil' theory had shaped the discussion in medical circles involved in tackling the rising incidence of tuberculosis in the imperial peripheries. However, although the observations made in the field of tuberculosis among 'primitive' and 'civilised' peoples during the First World War cast doubt on the practical application of Cummins' theory, the concept continued to influence much of the thinking in the field of tuberculosis in the subsequent era.

During the War he became Assistant Director of Medical Services, 16 Division, British Armies in France and then in Germany. After the war he succeeded the famous Sir William Leishman as Professor of Pathology, Royal Army Medical College, in July of 1919. Cummins retired from the army in 1921 and was then appointed as David Davies Professor of Tuberculosis, Welsh National School of Medicine, where he served in this capacity for seventeen years (1921-1938). Around this time Cummins had moved the concept of his theory into a new domain, from 'primitive' peoples to British children, drawing an analogy in immunological terms. In his inaugural lecture he stressed that 'Nature is gradually getting rid of tuberculosis by a process of unconscious vaccination, then we should, in our efforts in defending children and susceptible persons from massive doses, and we should concentrate research on efforts to discover a safe and effective vaccine' (5). It was at Cardiff that he helped develop the tuberculosis department, and later was very devoted to developing postgraduate teaching in tuberculosis; indeed, it was to his credit that he was the one who initiated and founded the Tuberculosis Diseases diploma at University of Wales in Cardiff, and the course leading to its diploma. Cummins led clinical research in the pre-antimicrobial era. In Cardiff, Lyle Cummins was involved in all aspects of treating tuberculosis. He did experimental work to investigate the use of urea as an antibacterial agent against the tubercle bacilli. Interestingly, he was drawn into this investigation after he received correspondence from Dr. Roy Humphreys, the Senior Physician of Khartoum Civil Hospital, and his Sudanese assistant, Dr. Halim Mohamed. It is interesting to note that the latter went on to be the first Sudanese physician, and he himself had suffered from tuberculosis as a child and underwent total unilateral pneumonectomy and lived past 100 years of age with a single lung. Drs Humphreys and Halim wrote to Lyle Cummins stating that they had the experience of treating a patient with a tuberculous ulcer on the chest with urea powder (6). The research interests of Lyle Cummins in tuberculosis were diverse. Starting earlier with interest in using sanocrysin, he then developed a special interest in the silico-tuberculosis of South Wales coal miners (7). He held the belief that silicon exposure among those men was protective against tuberculosis and he did several experimental works in support of his ideas (8). In 1926 he was to be involved in an exhaustive investigation of tuberculosis among South African natives, especially those working in the mines around Witwatersrand. He was also involved in another investigation on tuberculosis in Burma in 1937.

Cummins became a world expert on tuberculosis. He was credited with being one of the leading clinicians to conduct research that gave rise to many ideas that helped to understand the development of immunity to tuberculosis. He advanced the notion of relative immunity developing after exposure to the tubercle bacillus, whereby the body's resistance would prevail against infection. Cummins reached this conclusion after he conducted research on the tuberculin skin test in Welsh patients who had become infected with tuberculosis. However, it was his original 'Virgin Soil' theory, despite the intense debate it generated and the controversy around some of its concepts, that gained him his greatest fame. Cummins repeated the mantra that tuberculosis is a disease of civilization, and if the process of civilizing the 'primitive' was to be managed appropriately, there was no reason those populations, experiencing tuberculosis for the first time in the wake of the European colonial enterprises, could not be spared the excess of the tubercular mortality they were suffering. He argued that the 'civilizing mission' should be slowed down, keeping the native population out of the unhealthy urban areas unless they were working there and sending them back home to recuperate if they become ill. In those days, the major remedy for tuberculosis was nursing and 'healthy outdoors' living. Cummins' 'Virgin Soil' theory greatly shaped contemporary thinking. However, it was criticised by modern scholars as being flawed and fraught with misconceptions (9) (10). Further, it was also described as being a reflection of the heyday colonial thinking of 'other primitive races that were out there to be civilised'. Even some modern scholars felt that the theory was 'intersected with Nazi racial excesses' and that it shaped attitudes and policies elsewhere (11). Some also felt that the 'Virgin Soil' theory and its concept invited an apathetic response to the sick of the 'primitive races', blaming poor resistance on 'racial inferiority' rather than on poor working conditions, as in the case of the Rand workers of the South African gold-mines. Furthermore, Black African Americans would not be approved for health insurance policies by leading health insurance companies like the Prudential of New Jersey (ibid.) (12). Nonetheless, Cummins, despite the fact that his main focus of 'racial inferiority' and 'race immunological weakness' was scientifically flawed, his advocacy for more active rule for colonial powers and medical workers to do more to control the spread of tuberculosis ought to give him a pardoning credit.

Lyle Cummins wrote a book titled *Primitive Tuberculosis*, published in 1939 (13), and shortly before his death in 1949 his second book, *Tuberculosis in History,* was published (14). He also authored the section on tuberculosis and tetanus in *The Official History of the War*. Lyle Cummins had other interests in the medical field; e.g., he won the Parker Memorial Prize in 1913 for his essays on enteric fever. He also published in journals and textbooks on other diseases, such as Kala-azar, tetanus, and influenza. In addition to his general medical and surgical ventures in the Anglo-Egyptian Sudan, he discovered a new species of *Culex fatigans* in Sudan that was named after him by the British authority on entomology in the early twentieth century as *C. cumminsii*. Cummins first brought this new species from Bahr el-Ghazal and it was later found in other places, including Khartoum, by Dr. Andrew Balfour, and in Uganda by Drs Low and Moffat (15). Lyle Cummins held many key posts and professional chairmanships of several associations and organizations, including vice-president of the section of tuberculosis at the annual meeting of the British Medical Association in Glasgow in 1922, and then at Winnipeg, Canada in 1930. He conducted many surveys on tuberculosis in several countries, including Burma and South Africa. He was knighted and held several medals and honours, including the Order of Osmanieh in 1907, a Medal with Clasp after the Nile Expedition of 1898, the Legion of Honour (Officer); Couronne de Belgique (Officer), Croix de Guerre (Belgian) in 1918. Lyle Cummins died on May 26, 1949, at 75 years of age, at Oxford. He left three daughters and a son.

Back to his earlier work in Sudan, where the 'Virgin Soil' theory had its beginning, the River Hospital in the 1920s and until the 1950s was the main hospital to treat tuberculosis cases in the Sudan. Further, several Sudanese doctors, who graduated from Khartoum, the first of them Drs Mamoun Hussein Sherif and Abdeen Sharraf, were to come to Cardiff and receive training and obtain the very diploma established by Cummins in tuberculosis management, and then go back to fight the menace of tuberculosis in their native Sudan. One of his friends and acquaintances wrote in his obituary:

> It is perhaps impossible to for any one person to form a complete appreciation of Lyle Cummins. His talents and interests were so diverse, and his facility of impromptu thought and expression so great, that whatever he was doing or discussing seems of first importance. His unfailing courtesy and tolerance, formal or informal, might suggest to the unwary some artificiality, but he

> was genuinely absorbed in everything he did, even when dealing with essentially uncongenial persons or affairs.

He went on to affirm that:

> He was perhaps too diverse for radical scientific research, but he grasped, developed and pronounced ideas about tuberculosis which bore more fruits with others.... He might have made a larger place for himself in literature than in medicine had he devoted himself entirely to it. (16)

Section II:

'Sudan Doctor': Leonard Bousfield, the Isle of Wight Aristocrat

Dr. Leonard Bousfield was amongst the first wave of recruits following the foundation of the military hospitals in Sudan in 1904. Born at St Leonards, Sussex, in 1874, in an English family from Isle of Wight, he was christened in the name of the village, as the youngest of five children to a leisured and aristocratic father of Pulpit Rock, Bonchurch, Isle of Wight. Young Leonard enjoyed a prestigious upbringing and education during the golden years of the Victorian era. When seventeen, he was enrolled in Pembroke College, Cambridge, as an exhibitioner. After winning several prizes, he went on to complete his medical studies at the London Hospital in 1898 (now Royal London Hospital), Whitechapel, qualifying as MBBCh (Cantab.) in 1903 (17). Leonard Bousfield, during his training at the London Hospital, was privileged to be the house physician of a famous London physician, Dr. Percy Kidd, and to one of the British pioneers of neurology and physiology, Dr. (later Sir) Henry Head. He was also house surgeon to Mr (later Sir) Hugh Rigby, the famous Royal Surgeon who saved the life of George V by an operation in 1928. After finishing his basic training at the London Hospital, attracted by the idea of travel overseas and for other private reasons, he decided to join the Royal Army Medical Corps in 1904, gaining the Herbert Scholarship and Pathology Prize at the entry exam.

In his book, *Sudan Doctor*, which he wrote well into his retirement, at age 77, and published in 1954 (only three years before his demise), he reflected on his experience and his life and times in the Sudan. His accounts also shed light on the working life of doctors in Whitechapel and London Hospital in Victorian Britain. Later, Bousfield was to set forth to join another prominent physician, Sir William Boog Leishman, the distinguished pathologist, and one of the early pioneers of tropical medicine. The experience he gained under Leishman's mentorship proved invaluable to him in his later career in the Sudan, when he was set to diagnose and treat many cases of visceral leishmaniasis (Kala-azar), the very parasite that was discovered by Colonel Leishman and named after him. Following two years of work under Colonel Leishman, Bousfield was posted to Malta in 1905 to investigate an outbreak of Malta Fever, in what is known as 'The Malta Fever Commission'. In 1906, Bousfield was attracted to work for the Egyptian Army and, after a short stay in Cairo, he moved up the Nile to Khartoum. Following a short stay in Khartoum, Bousfiled was then posted to Kassala, the main town in eastern Sudan, as Senior Medical Officer. His personal qualities and his noble upbringing added further to his professional dimensions. He was set to practice in an alien country, in a remote spot, away from European civilization. He would practice in every field of medicine: he would be a physician, a surgeon, an obstetrician, an epidemiologist, a public health physician, a pathologist, even a dentist, and he would excel in them all. Further, he would also carry out administrative duties in a conquered country where the pacification of the natives was still in its infancy. Bousfield combined wisdom with science, and courage with sensible thinking. It did not take him long to gain the hearts and minds of his Sudanese patients and his subordinates.

Bousfield made sound observations of protean medical problems he encountered amongst his Sudanese patients. One of the main accomplishments of this *'Fringi*[1] *Hakim Pasha'* was his assigned role as an 'epidemiologist' to map out visceral leishmanisis (Kala-azar) in the eastern and southeastern corner of Sudan (Fourth Report, Wellcome Tropical Research Laboratories, 1911) (18). Leishmaniasis had emerged as a devastating disease in that part of the Sudan. Following advice from Dr. Andrew Balfour, the Government decided to send what came to be known as the 'Kala Azar Commission'. Bousfiled led a team that was assigned to survey the Kassala and Blue Nile regions. They trekked through the Atbara, Rahad, Dinder, and Blue Nile rivers close to the Abyssinian border. Their work helped to estimate the prevalence of disease in that part of the Sudan and added much to the current understanding of leishmaniasis in Sudan. The disease was first described in Sudan by the Wellcome Tropical Resarch Laboratory's 'Travelling Pathologist', Dr. Sheffeild Neave, after he diagnosed the condition in a young Sudanese boy in Omdurman following a splenic puncture (19). Stemming from a personal experience during that Commission, Bousfield cleverly made the observation that there is a vector/intermediate host for the Kala-azar parasite, but he never published it. Many years later, just such a vector was proven to be the sandfly, *Phlebotomus papatasi*. Bousfield during the work of the Commission took a splenic puncture from a woman with suspected Kala-azar and, while handing the needle to one of his subordinates, he accidentally pricked one of his fingers. After Bousfield fixed the slide and examined it under the microscope, he was horrified to see that the slide was full of Leishman-Donovan bodies. Naturally alarmed, concerned, and dreading the worst, he took a scalpel and cut the area of his inoculated finger. Fortunately, to his great relief, he did not contract that lethal disease and this prompted him to make the observation that there must definitely be an intermediate host for the parasite (20).

Bousfield also wrote on 'native medicine and remedies' as practiced by the inhabitants of the Kassala area and its surroundings. In that article, he described surgical instruments, methods of treating surgical conditions like wounds, abscesses, and fractures, as well as various medical conditions, including pneumonia, leprosy, and syphilis. He was particularly intrigued to find out that a finely divided brownish black earth called *'turaba'*, which was used by the natives to treat syphilis, was found on analysis at the Chemical Section of the Wellcome Laboratory in Khartoum to contain mercury (21). Mercury at the time was the agent used in contemporary Western medicine to treat syphilis. According to Bousfield, the earth could only be found in a particular village on the Atbara River in eastern Sudan. A similar observation was made by his RAMC contemporary in the Sudan, Colonel R. G. Anderson, who also published similar findings on traditional medicine used by people of Kordofan region in the western part of Sudan (22). The name described by Anderson as *'tureba'* is slightly different in spelling from the one used by Bousfield, and it reflects the different dialects of the Sudanese natives in different parts of the Sudan. Ahmed Alsafi, in his work, *Traditional Sudanese Medicine,* (23) described the same substance by a not dissimilar name to that of Colonel Anderson (*Turaiba = pterocar puslucens*) for the same substance still used by Sudanese people especially in the rural areas to treat syphilis nearly a century after the observation published by Bousfield and Anderson.

Bousfield also wrote excellent accounts of some of the medical problems he encountered during his extensive career in the Sudan. He wrote on his experience of operating on Sudanese patients, quoting the occasion while he was in the Nuba Mountains, in western Sudan. One of his patients (injured during a military excursion) insisted 'not only to have the amputation without anaesthesia, but he would even assist him in holding the severed limb by the sound arm!' (24). He commented on the paradox of his experience with some of his European subjects who happened to have milder ailments. He also wrote in detail on his experience in dealing with smallpox epidemics he encountered, and how he would start the campaign of mass vaccination by vaccinating himself and his wife in the presence of his domestic servants, so that they can distribute the news in the *suk* (Arabic: market) (25). He wanted his Sudanese patients to know that the '*Fringi Hakim Pasha*' had already vaccinated himself and his family, in an act akin to a campaign of raising public awareness in modern terms and lead by example. Bousfeild did this time and time again, despite his having had vaccination against smallpox in Britain before his arrival in Sudan. He also described his moving experience with a leper family during a visit to Gallabat, a small town on the Sudanese-Abyssinian border, when he spent some time trying to convince a couple with the disease to send away their only son so that he wouldn't get the infection. Bousfield passionately wrote:

> The little lad jumped up crying bitterly and nestled up to his mother, begging not to be sent away. At once the parents also broke into tears and it was so heart-rending that I found myself joining in. It would have been a curious spectacle for any outlooker (sic): a white doctor sitting down with a black man, woman and child, all weeping profusely.... I am not ashamed of my emotion. It would have been a callous man indeed who did not appreciate the noble pathos of the scene. (26)

During his earlier days in the Sudan, there were no dentists in the whole of the Sudan. Bousfield approached his dentist back home in Britain during one of his leaves to give him some 'elementary instructions on dentistry' (27). Back in Sudan, Bousfield used what he learned to ease the sufferings of those who happened to come his way with dental problems. He later wrote about his amazing dental ventures: 'This sideline of mine earned more gratitude than I ever received for my medical care' (28). On the other hand, Bousfield's time in Sudan was not spent only in medical enterprises, but he also documented a lot of other areas dealing with animal and plant life and those accounts are quite valuable to researchers in these areas (29). He also made excellent observations on the customs, traditions, and superstitions of the natives in various regions he worked and visited in the Sudan. Bousfield had excelled not only in medicine, but as an excellent observer who interacted with his environment with the attitude of a true scientific man. Despite that, Bousfield was criticized for some of his views about his Sudanese patients and subordinates, which many felt were outdated by the standards of the day; but one has to remember that some of his views were not uncommon in his heyday. Further, Bousfield also made several commending remarks about the Sudanese and he praised their personal qualities, their courage, endurance of illness, as well as their bravery, personal hygiene, and cleanliness (30). He even put them ahead of his fellow native Europeans.

Leonard Bousfield spent his first few years in Kassala Province, and then he moved to Khartoum Military Hospital till 1910; the year that his first contract with the Sudan Government ended. He left for England to marry his cousin, Miss Jenny M. Emerson, daughter of Sir Emerson. Thereafter, he resumed his duties with the Royal Army Medical Corps in Britain, and he was promoted to Major General in 1911. Following the resignation of Andrew Balfour, Bousfield was contacted by the Sudan Government to be his successor as Medical Officer of Health of Khartoum. The offer was made on the condition that he should obtain the Diploma of Public Health (DPH), which he did, from the Irish Royal Colleges from Dublin, with distinction. He was later appointed Medical Officer of Health for Khartoum District which covered Khartoum, Omdurman, and Khartoum North. With the increasing inhabitants and expansion of the 'three cities', the task of dealing with the increasing demands of keeping mosquito breeding and malaria at bay was challenging. He succeeded in maintaining a high standard of public health in his domain. In 1920, he was appointed Chief Sanitary Officer of the Sudan Government, a post he held till 1925, the year when he retired from his service in the Sudan. He received the Order of Majideah (4th Class) from the Sultan of Turkey, and the Order of the Nile from the King of Egypt. Bousfeild never practiced medicine after he left Sudan. He lived in his home at Shacklin, Isle of Wight. His first wife died and he married the formerly Mrs Agnes D. Galsworthy. He died on February 25, 1956. Paul (Herbert) Squires, one of his contemporaries and friends during his service in Sudan, wrote: 'Sir Andrew Balfour had laid the foundation of a highly efficient sanitary service, and Bousfield faithfully carried on the tradition' (31).

Section III:

The Moth Doctor: Bimbashi Byam 'Bey' & his Sudan Adventures

A descendant of a long line of 'William Byams', who were all very adventurous, William Byam was to follow in the footsteps of his ancestors in a military career. His father, a Taunton and Somerset man, was a Major-General in the British Army. He served in New Zealand during the Maori War and then moved to India, where his son William Byam was born in 1882 (the year the British bombarded Alexandria and took over control of Egypt). It was an irony that William Byam's encounter with the Sudan began when he was only a few years old, in 1885, when his father, on board the military ship *'Serapis'* in the Red Sea; received orders to join the expedition dispatched to rescue Charles Gordon, who was besieged in Khartoum. Landed in the Trinikitat 'a small harbour south of Suakin', his father and his men joined the troops of Sir Gerald Graham in the battles of El Teb and Tamai, where the Mahdist Emir, Osman Digna, broke the 'British square' and set Rudyard Kipling to nominate the 'Fuzzy Wuzzy' as the 'first class of fighting men':

> We 've fought with many men acrost the seas
> An' some of 'em was brave an' some was not
> The Paythan an' the Zulu an' Burmese
> But the Fuzzy was the finest o' the lot
> We never got a ha 'porth's change of 'im
> 'E squatted in the scrub an' 'ocked our 'orses
> 'E cut our sentries up at Suakim
> An' 'e played the cat an' banjo with our forces
> .So 'ere's to you, Fuzzy-Wuzzy, at your 'ome in the Soudan;
> *You big black boundin' beggar—for you broke a British square*!

Little Byam was left at the shore as the 'drum boy'. Later, Byam was to write in his autobiography that that drum remained with him as a souvenir till it was lost when his house in London was bombarded in World War Two. Back in England, the family spent a spell in Pontefract, Yorkshire, and later moved to settle at South-sea, Cosham, near Portsmouth. His father, 'a man of strong likes and dislikes' (as Byam describes him) (32), wants his little feeble son to join the army as an officer, as both parents were from a 'military stock'. Nicknamed by his mother as 'Mr Why-Why'(33), little Byam was noted to be an imaginative and thoughtful child, always craving knowledge and questioning things. Byam was to receive earlier education at Scarborough, then went on to be enrolled at Wellington College at Berkshire. Here, Byam felt he wanted to be a doctor, and became enrolled at St Georges'. He was to write later that he was proud to be a 'St Georges' Man', and follow the track of his grandfather, who also trained at St George's earlier in the 1800s, and his Uncle Sam Byam who was a doctor and anatomy demonstrator in the mid-1800s. Byam, a brilliant student of his generation, went on to win several prizes, including the Thompson Medal in Fifth Year, and graduated in 1904. He declined an offer to join a group of 'City Men', who were keen on a business enterprise in the southern Atlantic, but he could not see himself 'agreeing to be a mate in a game of bridges, and smoke a pipe'. Byam decided to join the Royal Army Medical Corps, especially as he was keen to please his father. He wrote:

> I fondly hoped I might please my father by entering the army, even as a non-combatant. In this I was gravely mistaken, for he informed me in no uncertain terms that he had even less use for a doctor in the army than for his civilian counterparts. (34)

Byam passed the entrance exam of the RAMC, scoring the top mark. The famous British ophthalmologist at the time, Jonathan Hutchinson, Jr. made a remark to one of Byam's mentors that he never before gave the full mark in surgery to any candidate except to Byam (35). Byam, in his first few months in the RAMC, became more fascinated with Sir Patrick Manson:

> ...few lectures were devoted to tropical medicine, a subject I become very much interested in under the guidance of Sir Patrick Manson, who richly deserved his unofficial title of the father of Tropical Medicine. At St Georges he lectured mainly about malaria, but he brought home to us the importance of the insect world to the dwellers of hot climates. My career owes him a great

debt. (36).

After a few assignments to Aldershot and Netley Hospital, he was posted to Egypt in 1906. About the latter, Byam wrote that it was there that he was introduced to the horrors of syphilis (37). He was appointed as an 'Eye Specialist' and was stationed at 'The Citadel', the famous group of palaces build by Mohamed Ali. There he looked after a full ward destined for 'Infectious Diseases'. In summer of 1908, he was approached by Dr. S. Lyle Cummins, Senior Medical Officer of the Egyptian Army (whom Byam describes as being a fine and a cultured man), to join the Egyptian Army Medical Corps with the title of Bimbashi (Major). Such a position at that time was considered an honour and a prestige, with significant financial incentive (38). Byam took the opportunity and he left for England for a month, and there he went to consult Dr. William Leishman on malaria and other tropical diseases. Leishman advised him to use whatever was at his disposal as means of treatment and also to use his common sense, advice that Byam would certainly make use of in his future career (39). He had earlier received his first commission in the Sudan, when he was assigned by Captain Lyle Cummins to the task of vacating the Deputy Governor of Kassala, who was seriously ill, and bringing him to Cairo for treatment. Byam gave a fascinating account of that venture, which involved travelling down the Atbara River, well down stream during the flood season, and then on foot from 'Goz Rajab' to Kassala (40). On arrival back at Cairo after he brought his patient, whom Byam diagnosed as suffering from typhoid, he was immediately appointed as Senior Medical Officer for Kassala Province, succeeding Leonard Bousfield. Byam travelled again to Atbara, and from there he didn't take a boat downstream, but instead learned to ride a camel down the bank of the Atbara River, and he was to take his first '*camel shid*'(short march) on his way to 'Goz Rajab' and then across the semi-arid lands to Kassala.

Byam's *'Kassala Days & Ways'*

Byam described Kassala as a 'town of much interest', with a population of 15,000, and the old town fortified by a wall built in the days of Turco-Egyptian rule (41). The two years Byam spent at Kassala were full of achievement in public health as well as the routine medical and surgical work he did. The public health work was covered earlier in Part V (*vide supra*). Two interesting incidents from his routine medical and surgical work were mentioned by Byam in the first volume of his autobiography, *The Road to Harley Street*. Although Byam was significantly handicapped in terms of resources, especially for surgical emergencies, lack of x-ray apparatus, etc, he managed to make the best of his clinical abilities and his excellent common sense to diffuse hectic situations. The first such situation was an incident with Syed Ali el-Mirghani, the Chief of the Khatmyyia religious Muslim Sect in Sudan, who had symptoms diagnosed by Byam as being due to renal stones. Byam gave the appropriate advice, however, some 'clergymen' felt that the holy man should be treated by a recipe of half a melon after each one of them spat on it. The pain of the renal colic followed the natural history and it eased off spontaneously. The Sudanese notable was very grateful to Dr. Byam's kind review and care and he gave the doctor a nice white camel, which Byam was in desperate need of. Byam called his future journeys invaluable companion, Snodgrass (42). The other incident was when the wife of one Egyptian officer (the woman was morbidly obese) presented with symptoms of acute abdomen, and Byam found a very large abdominal mass. As the patient was chronically constipated, Byam thought of easing off her constipation before he embarked on a major surgery. The enema given twice resulted in the expulsion of large rounded worms, with Medusa's head and complete resolution of symptoms! (43).

The Benevolent Enterprise of Byam: The Leper Colony at Gallabat

Byam did an inspection tour of his province in 1909, travelling southward on his 'Snodgrass', trekking down the valley of the Atbara River and its tributary, Settit. He later wrote about this adventure: 'I marched up the valley of Settit as far as the boundary and found few scattered settlements but not enough to disturb the game which Sir Samuel Baker had recorded as considerable' (44). Byam detected cases of Kala-azar and ordered their transfer to Gedaref

Hospital for treatment. He then crossed the Tacazzy Valley (Takazzy being the name used by the Abyssinians for the River Atbara). Nearly fifty years later, in 1952, Byam revisited the same area in a tour of Ethiopia and crossed from the Abyssinian side of the Tacazzy River, where he met some dwellers and conversed with them in Arabic and he wrote in his autobiography 'they were friendly and took me for an American, having never heard of the English' (45). Reaching Gedaref, he described the military hospital as having been built comparatively recently, on a large mound which is shared with the British Officers Mess. They were situated over a little hill that was cleared of bushes and overlies the town. He described the town as follows:

> '...I left the River and marched westwards for Gedaref over a featureless plain, among stunted trees and bushes of mimosa. On arrival, I found a town which would be hard to beat for drabness, with nothing of interest to be seen, even in the distance.' (46)

He also described the Civil Hospital as composed of four circular thatched huts and one mud-brick building that served as an office, dispensary, and surgical suite. Byam was critical of the Syrian Medical Officer who was in charge of both the military and Civil Hospitals. He also made comments about the poor state of the slaughterhouse. He then left Gedaref, pressing the officials at Khartoum to build a new hospital and improve the slaughterhouse and other public health facilities. (The new hospital, part of which is still existing today, was built in 1911.)

Inspecting Galabat, Byam described the town as the eastern-most frontier post, suffering repetitively from raiding and plundering by the Abyssinians, a *de facto* irony persisting even in modern times. Byam's description of Gallabat is no different from that of British explorer James Bruce, who traversed the town in 1772, when it was still called Ras El Fil (47). He set off to find the whereabouts of the lepers. The sufferers of this dreaded disease during Byam's day were usually evicted from their homes by their neighbours and were abandoned to live in remote spots in the middle of nowhere. In his quest to find and locate these poor souls, Byam was left alone, as his assistants, his cook, and his and *sais* (Arabic, horse-keeper) abandoned him, being scared to death of coming in contact with the lepers, making bizarre excuses and concealing their fear. Eventually, after he succeeded in locating the lepers, Byam had the daunting task of gaining their trust and to setting forth a plan to house them in a decent 'leper colony'. Byam wrote to the PMO at Khartoum, asking for funds and permission to delegate Dr. Hannah (his Syrian subordinate) to oversee the colony, emphasising that he had heard that 'two helpless lepers had recently been carried off by leopards'. The reply he received from one of the PMO's assistants baffled him: 'What a pity the leopard don't finish off your beastly lepers' (48). In an act of benevolence, Byam explored every avenue to establish the colony. He made arrangements with the Inspector of Galabat to impose a levy on the villages that had evicted the lepers, and he even wrote to his mother appealing for funds and asking her to collect all the money she could from her friends and acquaintances. He wrote: 'This she did most successfully' (49). The colony was successfully built, the patients were well stationed in it, and each one of them had his own '*tuckle*' (Sudanese [slang], hut)—despite their grumbling and protesting that they had been 'men of properties…each owning two or more houses, and …they were offered only one tuckl' (50). Byam also made arrangements for each of them to have a little surrounding area where some crops could be cultivated and some animals could be kept. Before Byam left Kassala to take up his post in Khartoum, he paid a visit to inspect the colony and was pleased to see that progress been made; he was satisfied that it was all a splendid venture. He had earlier placed his subordinate medical officer, the Syrian, Dr. Anton Hanna, in charge of the settlement.

Byam's benevolent leper enterprise was the first 'leper colony' to be established in the Sudan. Unfortunately, little additional information has survived in the available record to trace its further developments or its eventual fate. From subsequent reports of the Director of the SMD, it happened that the 'colony' was later transferred to Gedaref, the main town in the region (51). The exact date could not traced. Worth mentioning is that the first 'leper colony', i the capital, Khartoum, known as the 'Leper's *hush*' (Arabic and Sudanese [slang], house-yard), was not established until many years later, at Omdurman. Dr. Alexander Cruickshank, one of the doctors who joined the medical service in the Sudan in the mid-1920s, established a large 'leper colony' in Mongalla Province, southern Sudan, which had the highest prevalence of leprosy in Sudan in those days.

'Dr. Byam Bey': Khartoum Days & 'The Anuak Patrol'

In the spring of 1911, Byam was transferred to Khartoum as Senior Medical Officer, Khartoum District. He wrote: 'this means promotion, and I would be a Bey and service at Headquarters' (52). The most vivid experience of his 'Khartoum Days' was his assignment in the 'Anuak Patrol', a thrilling adventure, of which he wrote and reflected upon in his first book, *The Road to Harley Street*. Byam was commissioned as the Medical Officer to accompany a group of over a thousand men who were given the task of dealing with the Anuak, a tribe in the eastern part of southern Sudan. The Anuak were then famous as 'slave raiders' rather than 'slave traders'. Byam joined the patrol as the Medical Inspector and he had an assistant junior medical officer, the Syrian Ibrahim Abu Haider. The objective of the patrol was to liberate the men, women, and children captured by the Anuak. The second objective was to find the legendary Boma Plateau and to ascertain whether there was gold there, and whether it belonged to Sudan or to Abyssinia. On reaching the junction of the Akobo and Pibor tributaries of the Sobat River, the patrol established a fort, later to become 'Akobo Post', which was the earliest foundation of today's 'Akobo town' in Southern Sudan. After many weeks of wandering in those southern hinterlands, the mission achieved none of its objectives. It neither succeeded in 'hunting the hunters' nor did it have any success in finding any gold or silver in Poma Plateau. After a few skirmishes with and various ambushes by the Anuaks, who turned out to be 'elusive outlaws', playing 'hide and seek' with the expedition, Byam built a hospital to nurse the few members of the patrol who had been wounded during those skirmishes. He himself was struck down by several bouts of malaria and thus handed over the care of the hospital to his Syrian assistant, Ibrahim Abu Haider. He later became very unwell with pneumonia and he was lucky to survive after his close friend, Dr. Robert Archibald, the pathologist at the Wellcome Laboratories in Khartoum, came to his rescue on a special personal 'finding mission' (53). Byam later was to write in his tribute, *'Greater Love Hath No Man'* (54), that he was lucky to survive his illness and was subsequently sick-listed for many months, so that he had to go on a convalescent trip to Asia Minor, the Balkans, Austria, and France before ending up in England. The love of Sudan and Egypt had already taken a toll on his heart, as he later wrote: 'In Budapest I was interested in the organization of the markets as I thought they might well serve as a model for those I hoped some day to see in the Sudan' (55). Thereafter, Byam was involved in the first ever medical evacuation mission by airplane ever attempted in Sudan. When the Frenchman, Marc Pourpe, completed the first intrepid flying mission from Cairo to Khartoum in 1914, he was subsequently involved with Byam in the mission of evacuating a British army officer who was injured by a lion two hundred miles south of Khartoum. The mission was not completed as the plane failed to operate (56).

Trench Fever Research & Discovery: The Moth Doctor Comes True'

Back in Egypt in 1913, Byam was commissioned to file a report on the training of doctors at the American and the French Medical Schools in Beirut on behalf of the Turkish authorities. His companion was his former 'aide', Dr. Asad Malouf, from his Kassala days (57). The Byams finally left Africa and went back to England. Byam continued to suffer from repeated bouts of malaria, which weakened him despite having to go with his Scottish wife to the Scottish Highlands for convalescence. He was listed as sick and invalid for military service. He had earlier received an invitation from Sir Ronald Ross to join a panel of experts on a mission to tackle the menace of malaria which inflicted the British and allied troops in Greece (58). Instead, Byam was instructed by the War Office to join the Heart Hospital at Hampstead, where he worked with a group of physicians headed by Sir William Osler[2] (59). It was there that Byam developed his interest in conducting research to investigate the mystery of Trench Fever. Following a 'brainstorming' discussion with Sir William, Byam was assigned six patients to observe (60). Byam's zest for research flourished, his lifelong love for insects and moths eventually came to pioneering frontiers. Sound clinical observations made by Byam enabled him to start his initial research on patients with Trench Fever. At that time, many cases were seen in Britain, especially from British troops stationed in France. Byam argued that Trench Fever was possibly the cause of many cases admitted to 'Nerve Hospitals' as cases of neuro-asthenia. The War Office became interested and an expert panel headed by the Tropical Medicine pioneer, Sir David Bruce[3], was formed to oversee Byam's research (61). Byam's ventures included basic science research involving inoculating experimental animals with blood from infected patients. Then he realized that it was difficult to reproduce the *acute* stage of Trench Fever by simply injecting blood from *chronically* ill patients. At the time, a hypothetical link was proposed involving the transmission of Trench Fever via biting by body lice, '*cimex leticularis*'. Byam made the observation that there were many officers who got infected who had never been bitten by lice. After several sets of experiments involving human volunteers, Byam and his colleagues finally proved that the disease was actually transmitted from the infected droppings of lice, 'lice excreta'. Skin breaks resulting from inoculation proved to be the usual portal of entry of the organism (62). At a later stage, Byam and his colleagues proved this organism to be a spirochaete (63). Byam first published his work in 1918. In 1923, Byam and Robert Archibald co-edited one the most revered textbooks on tropical medicine at the time, *The Practice of Medicine in the Tropics*. Byam would later write in his autobiography: 'for the second time in my life, entomology moulded my career. Moth and butterflies had led me to make medicine my career, and lice, I might almost say, introduced me to Harley Street' (64).

Byam's Moral Stand over 'Importing' Bilharziasis to Sudan

Byam at some stage decided to settle in British Columbia, Canada, when in 1911 he took an extended leave from work in Khartoum. However, he was destined for other new ventures elsewhere. He was set up as a successful physician running a busy practice in Harley Street. Years later in London, and in the early 1920s, Byam had some discussions with his old Khartoum mess-mates, Drs Archibald and Balfour, concerning the plan of the British administration in Sudan for construction of a dam up the Blue Nile near Makkwar. The aim was to establish one of the largest irrigation schemes in the world at that time, to exploit the Gezira plain for growing cotton. He recollected that his friends had been concerned that such project might not be without health risks to the population, especially as it was obvious that the labour needed to construct the dam had to be imported from Egypt. His years in Cairo, early in his career, had given him the knowledge of the spectrum of health problems of the 'Falaheen'. With this in mind, he could map out the possible health risks associated with 'importing the endemic diseases of Egypt' into the Sudan. Tuberculosis, bilharziasis, hookworm infestations—all were not prevalent at that time in the Sudan but were highly prevalent in Egypt. One day, at his practice at Harley Street, he read that there would be no quarantine at the borders between Sudan and Egypt when the 'Falaheen' labourers would be transported to Sudan. He asserted that:

> It was impossible for me to sit a side indifferent to the future of the country where I have lived and worked for so many years. Besides, how could we be guilty of such crass jolly and expect postgraduate students of medicine to come to our schools for instructions and guidance, knowing we neglected the very rules of hygiene we set ourselves up to teach? (65).

He then came to know that Dr. Edward Crispin (then Director of SMD) was in London on leave. Byam decided to go and speak to him about the health risks of 'importing bilharzia to the Sudan'. He became shocked again to know that no precautions were set in place against such risks, simply because Crispin, who was aware of those risks, did not win against the engineer appointed to oversee the building of the dam. The engineer argued that such measures would jeopardize the labour recruitment process. Sir Lee Stack, the Governor General, took the side of the engineer, and Crispin lost.

Byam immediately became involved in a long and rigorous process of lobbying and counter-lobbying to avert the matter and secure the establishment of a quarantine at the port of entry to Sudan from Egypt. He wrote:

> The Governor General, Sir Lee Stack, had concurred and Crispin had supinely washed his hands of the whole problem. He had proceeded on leave hoping to forget his worries.....instead, after my visit, he found himself precariously poised between the devil and the deep Blue Nile' (ibid., page 115). (66)

Byam decided to go ahead and write a letter to the 'Times':

> My next step was to pen a letter for publication, in 'The Times'.... I described the disease which would inevitably be introduced from Egypt unless proper precautions were taken, and I added that up to the date of my letter apathy reigned and disaster loomed large on the horizon. (ibid, p.115). (67)

Byam passed a copy to Crispin for comment before posting the original. Crispin grimaced and shouted: 'For God's sake Byam, don't publish this letter or I shall be broken' (68). Byam then asserted to Crispin that he would give him one more chance by placing the matter with Sir Walter Morley Fletcher, of the MRC in London.

> Fletcher read my letter with care, mingled with amusement and spasms of horror.... he then told me that his knowledge of tropical medicine is insufficient to allow him to place the matter to the President of the MRC, Sir A J Balfour.... He asked to provide 'supporters of standing'. Byam would rush to seek the help of Andrew Balfour & Lyle Cummins who amicably provided the strongest support. ...with two such supporters, Fletcher agreed he had no option but to place my views before Balfour and His Majesty Privy Council. He insisted however, that I rewrite my letter, which he alluded to as 'scurrilous journalese'. (69)

A flurry of activity was then to follow. Sir Lee Stack was instructed to establish quarantine at Wadi Halfa, and Crispin was to cancel his leave and return to supervise this arrangement. Byam later received an invitation to dine with Sir Lee Stack and two of his senior staff. He wrote:

> ...after hospitality when we had reached the stage of coffee and cigars, the true purpose of the luncheon was revealed. They said:

> why have you made this damaging attack on the Sudan; what would you need to keep your mouth shut in the future? Would you be content with a knighthood?

Byam would assert in few words his stand and his motives, highlighting that advice was made in moral grounds stemming out from medical knowledge of disease prevention. He went on to add:

> ...Crispin far from bearing my ill-will, seemed relieved by the turn of the events and returned to Sudan to carry out what he knew full well should have been done before. Twelve month later, I received a copy of his report on the first year working of the Quarantine at Wadi Halfa. The illustrations included photographs of glass dishes filled with worms removed from Egyptians who had subsequently been allowed to continue their journey to the Blue Nile, rejoicing on their improved health and vigour and, no doubt, more useful members of the society.... (70)

Away from medicine, in 1923 Byam developed a special interest in philately, mentioned as a way of dealing with the stress of a successful private practice in Harley Street (Wikepedia) (71) (see Appendix 2). Following a long and successful career in Harley Street, Byam died at 81 years of age in Guernsey.

Footnotes

1 Fringi or Frankish is a word commonly used in the past in several Arab countries to refer to people of European origin. It probably dates back to the time of the Crusades.

2 Sir William Osler (1849-1919), a reputable Canadian physician, now an icon of medicine, is one of the forefathers of modern clinical medicine and education. He was the son of Featherstone Lake Osler, who was descended from a Cornish family in England that emigrated to Canada in the mid-nineteenth century.

3 Sir David Bruce, the famous discoverer of the trypanosomiasis parasite (named after him, *trypanosome bruceii*) is a descendant of the traveler/explorer, Scotsman James Bruce.

Bibliographic Information

Primary Sources

A. Archival materials

1. Sudan Archive at Durham (SAD)

https://www.dur.ac.uk/library/asc/collection_information/cld-load/?collno=135

Cruickshank A. & Bloss, J. F. E. The Sudan: A medical history (unpublished manuscript), SAD 704/4/1-107.

Christopherson, John Brian. Catalogue of papers, Sudan Archives Durham, GB-0033. http://reed.dur.ac.uk/xtf/view?docId=ead/sad/christoj.xml. (accessed May 15, 2014).

Christopherson, J. B. Description of Sudanese native remedies in the Mahdi's and Khalifa's time in Omdurman, SAD 497/6/1-28.

Atiya Family, SAD 2/20/2.

2. Cambridge University Library Archives

a. Royal Commonwealth Society Section (RCMS)

Military Intelligence Reports, Sudan Government Annual Reports, 1898-1919.

R. Kirk, RCMS 122/3/5.

M. H. Satti, RCMS 122/2/11.

b. Special Reading Room

Crawford, O. G. S. *The Fung Kingdom of Sennar with a Geographical Account of the Middle Nile Region*. John Bellows Ltd, 1951 (first edition).

James Howard Thornton. *Memories of Seven Campaigns: A Record of Thirty-Five Years' Service in the Indian Medical Department in India, China, Egypt, and the Sudan*. London, A. Constable, 1895.

3. Other archival sources

a. Sudan Despatches, Nile Expedition, http://www.northeastmedals.co.uk/britishguide/sudan/despatches_index.htm

b. Kings College London, Liddell Hart Centre for Military Archives, www.kcl.ac.uk/ihcma/summary/cu05-001.shtml.

publishing.eur.nl/ir/repub/asset/8151/HOOFDSTUK3.PDF.

Published Sources

Abu Salim, Mohamed Ibrahim. *History of Khartoum*. Irshad House Publications, Khartoum, 1970 (in Arabic).

Abu Shouk, A. I. *Heritage & Power in Sudan*. Abdelkariem Mirghani Cultural Centre Publications, 2008 (in Arabic).

Ahmed Bin Ali. *Kattib Al-Shouna' Manuscript on History of Sennar Sultanate & the Turco-Egyptian Administration of the Sudan*. Al Dar All Soudania for Books, Khartoum, 2009 (In Arabic),

Al-Gaddal, Mohamed Saeed. *Mohammed Ahmed el-Mahdi (The Mahdi); a Portrait of a Sudanese Rebel*. Khartoum University Press, 1st edition, 1985 (in Arabic).

al-Jindi & Tagher. *Ismail* (in Arabic) (Publisher unknown).

Alsafi, A. *Traditional Sudanese Medicine*. Sudan Currency Printing Press, 2006.

Atiyah, Edward. *An Arab Tells His Story: A Study in Loyalties*. London, Murray, 1946.

Atiyah, Edward. *The Black Vanguard.* Peter Davies, London 1952

Baker W. S. *The Abyssinian Tributaries of the Blue Nile & the Sword Hunters of Hamran Arabs*. London, MacMillan Press, 1868.

Baker, S. W. *Ismailia: A Narrative of the Expedition to Central Africa for the Suppression of the Slave Trade*. London, Macmillan & Co., 1874.

Baker, S. W. *The Albert Ny'anza Great Basin of the Nile and Exploration of the Nile Sources*. London, MacMillan & Co. Ltd., 1866.

Bayoumi, A. *The History of Sudan Health Services*. Kenya Literature Bureau, 1979.

Bell, H. *Frontiers of Medicine in the Anglo-Egyptian Sudan*. Oxford University Press,1999.

Beveridge, C. E. G. *Allah Laughed.* Melbourne, The National Press, PTY, Ltd, 1949.

Bjorkelo, Andres. *Prelude to the Mahdiyya: Peasants and Traders in Shendi's region, 1821-1885*. Cambridge University Press, 1989.

Boddy J. Barbaric Customs & Colonial Science: teaching the female body in the Anglo-Egyptian Sudan. In: Michael Lambek & Paul Antz. *Illness & Irony: On the Ambiguity of Suffering in Culture*. Berghahn Books 2003.

Bousfiled, L. *Sudan Doctor*. C Johnson, London, 1954.

Boyd, Alexander. *From The Niger to the Nile*. Edward Arnold, London 1907.

Burckhardt, John Lewis. *Travels in Nubia*. London, John Murray, Albermarle Street, 1819.

Browne, W. G. *Travels in Africa, Egypt and Syria from the Year 1792 to 1798*. London, 1806.

James Bruce. *Travels to Discover the Source of the Nile, in the Years 1768, 1769, 1770, 1771, 1772 and 1773*. Five volumes. G.G.J. and J. Robinson, London, 1790.

Byam, W. *The Road to Harley Street*. London, Geoffrey Bles, 1963.

Byam, W. *Dr. Byam in Harley Street*. London, Geoffrey Bles, 1963.

Byam, W. *Trench Fever. Lice and their Menace to Man*. London, Oxford University Press, 1919.

Cain, P. J, Hopkins, A. J. *British Imperialism*. London, Longman, 1993.

Churchill W. S. *The River War: An Account of the Reconquest of the Soudan*. New York, Award Books, 1965.

Clot Bey, A. B. *Memoires de A. B. Clot Bey*. Le Caire institute Francias 1949, Apercu general sur L'Egypte.

Crawford, O. G. S: *The Fung Kingdom of Sennar with a Geographical Account of the Middle Nile Region*. John Bellows Ltd, 1951 (first edition).

Crichton-Harris, A. *Poison in Small Measures. Dr. Christopherson and the cure for Bilharzia*. Amsterdam, Brill, 2009.

Cromer, Earl of. *Modern Egypt*. New York, Macmillan, 1916.

Cruickshank A. *Itchy Feet: A Doctor's Tale*. Elms Court, Ifracombe, Devon, Arthur H Stockwell Ltd, 1991.

Daly, W. M. *Empire on the Nile, the Anglo-Egyptian Sudan, 1898-1934*. Cambridge University Press, 1986.

D'Arcy, P. W. *Laboratory on the Nile*. London, CRC Press, 1999.

Elnur, Ibrahim. *Contested Sudan: The Political Economy of War and Reconstruction*. London, Routledge, 2009.

English, George B. *A Narrative of the Expedition to Dongola and Sennar*. London, John Murray, 1822.

Ewald, Janet. *Soldiers, Traders and Slaves: State Formation in the Greater Nile Valley, 1700-1885*. Madison, University of Wisconsin, 1990, p.126.

Fahmy, Khalid. *All the Pasha's Men. Mehmed Ali, His Army and the Making of Modern Egypt*. Cambridge University Press, 1997.

Ferguson, Niall. *Empire: How Britain Made the Modern World*. New York, Penguin Books, 2004.

Fothergil, E. *Five Years in the Sudan*. London, John Ashworth, 1911.

Gaetano Casati. *Dieceanni in Equatoria*. Milan, 1891. [*Ten years in Equatoria*. Translated from the Italian manuscript by J Randolph Clay & Walter Savage Landor. London, Fredrick Warne and Co., 1898.]

George Waddington, Barnard Hanbury. *A Journal of a Visit to Some Parts of Ethiopia*. London, John Murray, 1822.

Gray, Richard. *A History of the Southern Sudan 1839-1889*. London, Oxford University Press, 1961

Hamid, Musa Abdalla & Salih, Kamal. *Omdurman Teaching Hospital: Past, Present and Future* (in Arabic). 1986. Publisher unknown.

Hassan, Yusuf Fadul. *An Introduction to the History of the Eastern Sudanese Islamic Kingdoms of the Sudan* (in Arabic). Fifth edition, 2012.

Hill, R. L. *The Sudan Memoirs of Carl Christian Giegler Pasha, 1873-1883*. Translated from the German by Thirza Kupper. London, 1984.

Hill, R. L. *Egypt in the Sudan*. Oxford, 1959.

Hill, R. L. *Biographical Dictionary of the Anglo-Egyptian Sudan*. Oxford, 1951.

Holroyd, A. T. *Suakim and the Country of Soudan*. Sydney, Thomas Richards, Govt Printer, 1885.

Holt, P. M. and Daly, W M. *History of the Sudan, from the Coming of Islam to the Present Day*. London, Longman, 1988.

Holt, P. M. *The Mahdist State in the Sudan 1881-1898. A Study of its Origin, Development and Overthrow*. Oxford, Clarendon Press, 1958.

James, R. *Henry S. Wellcome*. London, John Curtis Books, 1996.

Kramer, R. S. *Holy City on the Nile: Omdurman during the Mahdiyya 1885-1898*. Princeton, New Jersey, Markus Wiener Publishing, 2010.

Krump, Theodoro. *Hoher und Fruchtbarer Palm-Baum des Heiligen Evangelij*. Augsburg, Georg Schulter & Martin Happach, 1710.

Lamothe, R. M. *Slaves of Fortune, Sudanese Soldiers in the River War 1896-1989*. Suffolk, UK, Boydell & Brewer, 2011.

MacMichael, H. A. *The Sudan*. London, Ernest Benn, 1954.

Melly, George. *Khartoum and the Blue and White Niles*. London, Colburn & Co., 1852.

Mohamed Abdel-Rahim. *'Alindaa fi-Daffie el-Iftraa* (in Arabic), Cairo, Parliament Press, 1952.

Abu Shouk, A. I. *Yusuf Michaeil Memoirs on Turco-Egyptian, Mahdist, and Anglo-Egyptian Sudan* (in Arabic). Khartoum, Abdelkariem Mirghani Cultural Centre Publications, 2004.

Moore-Harell, Alice. The Turco-Egyptian Army on the eve of the Mahdiyya, 1877-1880. *Int J Middle East Stud* 31(1999), pp. 19-37.

Moore-Harrel, A. *Gordon and the Sudan. Prologue to the Mahdiyya 1877-1880*. Oxford, Routlege, 2013.

Moorehead, Alan. *The Blue Nile*. London, The Reprint Society, 1963, pp.166-184.

Moorehead, A. *The White Nile*. Harper & Brothers, 1960.

Mowafi, Reda. *Slavery, Slave Trade and Abolition Attempts in Egypt and the Sudan 1820-1882*. Lund Studies in International History. Scandanavian Universities Books, 1981.

Monsieur Poncet, M. D. *A Voyage to Ethiopia in the Years 1698, 1699, 1700*. Covent Garden, W. Lewis, London, 1709.

Mukherjee, R. *Ancient Inhabitants of Jebel Moya Sudan*. Cambridge University Press, 2010.

Nachtigal G. *Sahara & Sudan: Wadai and Darfur*. Vol. 4. 1877.

Nicoll, F. *The Sword of the Prophet. The Mahdi of the Sudan and the Death of General Gordon*. Gloucestershire, Sutton Publishing Ltd, 2004.

O'Fahey, R. S. *The Darfur Sultanate: A History*. Columbia Hurst, 2008.

Ohrwalder, Fr. Joseph. *Ten Years of captivity in the Mahdi's Camp 1882-1892*. Translated from the German by F. R. Wingate. 10th edition. London, Sampson Low, Marston & Co., 1893.

Pallme, Ignatius. *Travels in Kordofan: Embracing a Description of thatProvince of Egypt, and of Some of the Bordering Countries, with a Review of the Present State of Place under the Government of Mehemed Ali*. London, Unknown Binding, 1844.

Parke, Thomas Hazel. *My Personal Experiences in Equatorial Africa as a Medical Officer of the Emin Pasha Relief Expedition*. London, William Clowers & Sons, 1891.

Parkyns, Mansfield. *Life in Abyssinia. Being Notes Collected during Three Years*. Albemarle Street, John Murray, 1853.

Pelligrini, Mattucci. *Sudan e Gallas*. Milan, Fratelli Treves, 1879.

Reid, J. W. *Traveller Extraordinary. The life of James Bruce of Kinnaird*. London, Eyre and Spottiswoode, 1968.

Santi, P. and Hill R. *The Europeans in the Sudan 1834-1878*. Oxford, 1980.

Seligman, C. G., and Seligman, B. Z. *The Pagan Tribes of the Nilotic Sudan*. London, George Routledge & Son, 1932.

Selim. *Voyage aux sources du Nil Blanc*. Ed., E. F. Jomard. *Memoires Soc. Geog. de Paris*, vol. xviii, 1842.

Shebieka, M. *'Al-Sudan abr algroon'* (in Arabic). Beirut, 1963.

Shugair, N. *Tareekh wa geograhiet al-Sudan* (in Arabic). Revised by Fadwa Abdel Rahman Ali Taha. Cairo, 1907.

Sonbol, Amira El-Azhari. *The Creation of a Medical Profession in Egypt 1800-1922*. New York, Syracuse University Press, 1991.

Slatin, R von. *Fire and Sword in the Sudan*. Translated by Colonel F. R. Wingate. London, Popular Edition, 1897.

Squires, H. C. *Sudan Medical Service, An Experiment in Social Medicine*. London, Heineman, 1958.

Stanley, H. M. *How I Found Livingstone*. Dover Publications, 2002 (first published, 1872).

Taylor, Bayard. *A Journey to Central Africa, or Life and Landscapes from Egypt to the Negro Kingdoms of the White Nile, with a Map and Illustrations by the Author*. New York, G. P. Putman & Co., circa 1854.

Theobald, A. B. *The Mahdiya. A History of the Anglo-Egyptian Sudan 1881-1899*. London, Longmans, Green and Co., Ltd., 1951.

Toniolo, Elias & Hill, Richard. *The Opening of the Nile Basin. Writings by Members of the Catholic Mission to Central Africa on the Geography and Ethnography of the Sudan, 1842-1881*. New York, Barnes & Noble Books, 1975.

Wallis Budge, E. A. *The Egyptian Soudan: Its History and Monuments*. London, 1907.

Wingate, F. R. *Mahdiism and the Egyptian Sudan: Being an Account of the Rise and Progress of Mahdiism and of Subsequent Events in the Sudan Up to the Present Time*. Macmillan and Company, 1891.

Warburg, G. *Islam, Sectarianism and Politics in Sudan since the Mahdiyya*. London, Hurst & Co., 2003

Wellcome H. S., Addison, F. *Jebel Moya*. Oxford University Press, 1949.

Wenyon, Charles Morley. *Protozoology; A Manual for Medical Men, Veterinarians and Zoologists*. Baillieri Tindall & Cox, 1926.

Werne, F. *Expedition to Discover the Sources of the White Nile in the Years 1840, 1841*. Translated by C. W. O'Reilly. London, 1849.

Wilson, Rev C. T. & Felkin, Rev R. W. *Uganda and the Egyptian Soudan*. Stuttgart, 1883.

Endnotes

Part I, Chapter 1: Sources

Abu Salim, Mohamed Ibrahim. *History of Khartoum.*

AlGaddal, Mohamed Saeed. *Mohammed Ahmed el-Mahdi (The Mahdi).*

Crawford, O. G. S. *The Fung Kingdom of Sennar*. Gloucester, 1951.

Hassan, Yusuf Fadul. *An Introduction to the History of Islamic Kingdoms of the Eastern Sudan 1450-1821.*

Holt, P. M. & Daly, M. W. *History of the Sudan, from the Coming of Islam to the Present Day*. 6th Edition. 2011.

MacMichael, H. *The Sudan*. London, Ernest Benn, 1954.

Nachtigal, G. *Sahara & Sudan: Wadai and Darfur*. Vol. 4. 1877.

O'Fahey, R. *The Darfur Sultanate: A History*. Columbia Hurst, 2008.

Wallis Budge, E. A. *The Egyptian Soudan: Its History and Monuments*. London, 1907.

www.thefreedictionary.com

Part I, Chapter 2: Endnotes

1. James Bruce, *Travels to Discover the Source of the Nile*, London, 1790.
2. W.G. Browne, *Travels in Africa, Egypt and Syria from the Year 1792 to 1798.*
3. Trade & Plantations Committee Report of 1789, Part VI (Trade in the interior of Parts of Africa).
4. John Lewis Burkhardt, *Travels in Nubia*, London, John Murray, Albermarle Street, 1819.
5. Mansfield Parkyns, *Life in Abyssinia, Being Notes Collected during Three Years Residence and Travels in that Country*, London, 1853.
6. George Melly, *Khartoum and the Blue and White Nile*, London, 1851.
7. A. Moorhead, *The Blue Nile*, pp.166-184.

8. George B. English, *A Narrative of the Expedition to Dongola and Sennar*.
9. F. Caillaud, *Voyage à Meroë: au fleuve Blanc,* 4 volumes, Paris (1823–1827).
10. Moorhead, op. cit., p.176.
11. Waddington & Hanbury, p.54.
12. A. E. Robinson, The Mamelouks in the Sudan, *Sudan Notes & Records*, Vol. 5, 1922, pp.88-94.
13. R. L. Hill, *Egypt in the Sudan*, op. cit., p.157.
14. Moorhead, *The Blue Nile*, p.184.
15. Andres Bjorkelo, *Prelude to the Mahdiyya*, p.35.
16. Ibid., pp.83-84.
17. Ibid., p.76.
18. N. Shugair, *Tareekh wa geograhiet al-Sudan* (in Arabic), Cairo, 1907.
19. Bjerkelo, op. cit., p.52.
20. R. L. Hill, The Period of the Egyptian Occupation, 1820-1881, *Sudan Notes & Records*, 1959, Vol. 40, pp.101-106.
21. Ahmed bin elHaj Ali, *'Katib Alshuna', History of Sinnar Kings and the Turco-Egyptian Rule, 1504-1872* (in Arabic), p.22.
22. Cailliaud, op. cit., pp.309-318.
23. Ahmed bin Ali, op. cit., p.23.
24. Mohamed Abdel-Rahim, *'Alindaa fi Radd el-Iftraa* (in Arabic), p.104.
25. B. E. Babiker, *Khartoum: Past, Present and the Prospects for the Future*, Durham Middle East Papers, Sir William Luce Publications Series, p.9, Dro.dur.ac.uk/89/1/Babiker.pdf.DDD35.
26. Ahmed bin Ali, op. cit.
27. Melly, op. cit.
28. Richard Gray, *A History of the Southern Sudan 1839-1889*, London, Oxford University Press, 1961.
29. Ibid., pp.58-69.
30. Ibid., p.42.
31. Stafford Poole, Notable Vincentians {7}: Luigi Montouri. *Vincentian Heritage J* 4-1-1995.
32. E. Toniolo, The First Centenary of the Roman Catholic Mission to Central Africa, 1846-1946, *Sudan Notes & Records*, Vol. 27, 1946, pp.99+.
33. Brun Rollet diary, *Le Nil Blanc et le Soudan*, 1855, pp.193-194.
34. Gray, op. cit., p.48.
35. Ibid., pp.51-58.

36. Ibid., p.47.
37. John Udal, John Petherick, the First British Resident, *Sudan Studies*, No 17, 1995, pp.2-22.
38. Ibid., p.5.
39. Gray, op. cit., pp.58-69.
40. A. B. Theobald, *The Mahdiya. A History of the Anglo-Egyptian Sudan 1881-1899*, London, Longmans, Green and Co. Ltd., 1951.
41. Nial Ferguson, op. cit.
42. Ibid., p.13.
43. Ibid., p.12.
44. Ibid.
45. H. M. Stanley, *How I Found Livingstone*, Dover Publications, 2002 (first published 1872).
46. Hill, *Egypt in the Sudan*, op. cit., p.68.
47. Ibid.
48. Anniversary address of Mr W. R. Hamilton, President of the RGS, The J of R G Society, London, 9th vol., 1839, London, Albemarle Street, John Murray, p.xxxiii
49. Hill, op cit., p.69.
50. F Werne, *Expedition to Discover the Sources of the White Nile*, 1849, 2 vols.
51. Selim, *Voyage aux sources du Nil Blanc*, ed. E. F. Jomard, *Memoires Soc. Geog. de Par*is, vol. xviii, 1842.
52. https://en.wikipedia.org/wiki/Richard_Francis_Burton
53. https://global.britannica.com/biography/John-Hanning-Speke
54. Gray, op. cit., p.52.
55. Baker, *Ismailia.*
56. Baker, *Albert Nyanza.*
57. P. M. Holt, *The Mahdist State in the Sudan 1881-1898*, Oxford, Clarendon Press, 1958, pp.26-27.
58. Stanley, op. cit.
59. Holt, op. cit., pp.39-40.
60. Gaetano Casati, *Ten Years in Equatoria*, London, Fredrick Warne & Co., 1898, p.23.
61. Ibid., p.23.
62. Holt, op. cit., p.57.
63. Ohrwalder, *Ten Years of Captivity in the Mahdi's Camp*, op. cit.
64. Fergus Nicoll, *The Sword of the Prophet: The Mahdi of the Sudan and the Death of General Gordon*, Gloucestershire, Sutton Publishing Ltd., 2004. p.159.
65. Holt, op. cit., pp.71-72.

66. Ibid., p.79.
67. Ibid., pp.79-80.
68. Ibid, p.80.
69. Earl of Cromer, *Modern Egypt* (in two volumes), London, MacMillan Press, 1908.
70. Holt, op. cit., pp.88-90.
71. Cromer, op. cit., pp.487-488.
72. Holt, op. cit., p.89.
73. Theobald, *Mahdiyya*, op. cit., pp.167-168.
74. Ohrwalder, op. cit.
75. R. Slatin, *Fire and Sword in the Sudan*, op. cit.
76. F. R. Wingate, *Mahdiism and the Egyptian Soudan.*
77. Abu Shouk, *Heritage & Power in Sudan* (in Arabic).
78. Holt, op. cit., p.209.
79. M. S. Yusuf Mikha'il (1); f. 96, {quoted by Holt, op. cit., p. 209})
80. W. S. Churchill, *The River War.*

Part II, Chapters I & 2: Endnotes

1. S. Hillelson, David 'ha' Reubeni an early visitor to Sennar, *Sudan Notes & Records*, 1933, Vol. 16, Part I, pp.55-66.
2. M. D. Poncet, *A Voyage to Ethiopia in the years 1698, 1699, 1700*, London, Covent Garden, W. Lewis, 1709.
3. Theodoro Krump, *Hoher und Fruchtbarer Palm-Baum des HeiligenEvangelij,* Augsburg, Georg Schulter& Martin Happach, 1710.
4. Jay Spalding, 1974.The Sudanese Travels of Theodoro Krump, 1700-1702. www.kean.edu/~jspauldi/krump2home.html
5. Krump, op. cit., p.291.
6. Ibid.
7. Ibid., p.290.
8. Ibid., pp.291-292.
9. Ibid., p.319.
10. Krump, op. cit., p.320.
11. Ibid., pp.319-320.
12. Ibid., p.320.
13. Ibid., p.315.
14. Ibid., pp.301-319.
15. Cruickhsahnk & Bloss, SAD, op. cit.
16. E. A. Wallis Budge, *The Egyptian Sudan*, pp.4-11.
17. J. W. Reid, *Traveller Extraordinary. The Life of James Bruce of Kinnaird*, London, Eyre and Spottiswoode, 1968.

18. Ibid., p.53.
19. James Bruce, *Travels to Discover the Source of the Nile, In the Years 1768, 1769, 1770, 1771, 1772 and 1773*, Five volumes, London, G.G.J. and J. Robinson, 1790.
20. Reid, *Traveller Extraordinary*, op. cit., p.172.
21. Ibid., p.225.
22. Cruickshank & Bloss, op. cit.
23. O. G. S. Crawford, *The Fung Kingdom of Sennar with a Geographical Account of the Middle Nile Region*, John Bellows Ltd., 1951 (first edition).
24. James Bruce, *Travels to Discover the Nile*, p.129.
25. Ibid., pp.128-129.
26. Ibid., p.129.
27. Ibid., pp.126-127.
28. Ibid., pp.130-131.
29. Cruicksahnk & Bloss, op. cit.
30. Bruce, *Travels*, op. cit., p.133.
31. F. Nigel Hepper, On the Botany of James Bruce's Expedition to the Source of the Blue Nile, *J. Soc. Biophys. Nat. Hist.*, 1980, 9(4), 527-537.
32. W. G. Browne, *Travels in Africa, Egypt & Syria 1792-1798*, Londres, 1799.
33. Browne, Ibid., p.190.
34. Ibid., p.312.
35. Ibid., p.325.
36. Ibid., p.326.
37. Ibid., p.327.
38. Autobiography, Diaries, Recollections, Berberian11.tripod.com/stambolski memoirs.htm
39. Browne, op. cit., p. 332.
40. Browne, ibid., p.334.
41. Browne, ibid., pp.332-333.
42. *Brucea Anti-dysenterica*; see *Encyclopedia Britannica, A Dictionary of Arts & Sciences*, vol. 2.
43. Browne, op. cit., p.337.
44. Ibid., p.338.
45. Ibid., p.339.
46. Ibid., p.346.
47. Ibid., p.350.
48. John Lewis Burckhardt, *Travels in Nubia.*
49. Ibid., pp.viii-ix.

50. Ibid., p.xxix.
51. Ibid., p.212.
52. Ibid.
53. Ibid., pp.211-212.
54. Ibid.
55. Ibid.
56. Ibid., p.290.
57. Ibid., p.212.
58. Ibid., p.213.
59. Ibid., p.295.
60. Ibid., pp.295-296.
61. Ibid., pp.296-297.
62. Ibid., p.304.
63. Ibid.
64. Ibid., p.261.
65. Ibid., p.263.
66. Hill, *Biographical*, op. cit., p.xii..
67. Wallis Budge, *The Egyptian Sudan*, op. cit.
68. Amira El-Azhari Sonbol, *The Creation of a Medical Profession in Egypt 1800-1922*, New York, Syracuse University Press, 1991.
69. Ibid., p.36.
70. Gerard N. Burrows, Clot Bey: The Founder of Modern Western Medicine in Egypt, *The Yale Journal of Biology and Medicine*, 1975, 48, pp.251-257.
71. Ibid.
72. Ibid.
73. Sonbol, op. cit.
74. K. Fahmy, *All the Pasha's Men*, 1991.
75. A, B, Clot Bey, *Memoires de A. B. Clot Bey*, 1949.
76. Cailliaud, op. cit.
77. Ahmed bin Ali Katib al-Shouna, op. cit., p.23.
78. Mohamed Abdel Rahim, *Alnidaa fi- dafi el-Iftraa* (in Arabic), p.104.
79. Ibid.
80. S. I. Khalil, The First Hospital in Sudan, 1826-1959: A Historical perspective, *Sudan Medical Journal*, 2014, 50(1), pp.48-52.
81. Ahmed Ahmed Sid Ahmed, op. cit., p.109.
82. I. Pallme, *Travels in Kordofan*, 1844.
83. Ibid., p.211.
84. Ibid., p.214.
85. P. Santi and R. Hill, *The Europeans in the Sudan 1834-1878*.

86. A. Cruickshank & J. F. E. Bloss, The Sudan: A Medical History (unpublished manuscript), SAD 704/4/1-107.
87. G. Waddington & B. Hanbury, *A Journal of a Visit to Some Parts of Ethiopia*, 1822.
88. Hill, *Biographical Dictionary*, 1967, op. cit., p.334.
89. Ibid., p.117.
90. Extracts from Private Memorandum Kept by Lord Prudhoe on a Journey from Cairo to Sennar in 1829, *Journal of the Royal Geographical Society of London*, 1835, vol. 5, pp.38-58.
91. Hill, op. cit., p.126.
92. Santi & Hill, op. cit.
93. Ibid.
94. Prudhoe, op. cit.
95. Ibid., p.47.
96. Pallme, op. cit., p.258.
97. Ibid., p.212.
98. Ibid., p.196.
99. Ibid., p.197.
100. Mansfield Parkyns, *Life in Abyssinia*, 1853.
101. Hill, *Biographical Dictionary*, 1967, op. cit., p.131.
102. F. Werne, *Expedition to Discover the Sources of the White Nile*, 1849, p.5.
103. Stafford Poole, Notable Vincentians (7): Luigi Montuori, *Vincetian Heritage Journal*, Vol. 16, Issue 1, 1995.
104. A. Alsafi, *Traditional Sudanese Medicine*, 2006, op. cit., p.449.
105. Ibid., p.454.
106. Hill, *Biographical Dictionary*, 1967, op. cit., p.305.
107. G. O. Whitehead, Andre Melly's Visit to Khartoum, 1850, *Sudan Notes & Records*, 1938, 21, pp.291-306.
108. Dr.. A. Peney, Memoires sur l'ethnograpie du Soudan Egyptien, *Rev. Ethnographie* I, II, III.
109. Santi & Hill, *Letters to Adolfo Antognoli*.
110. Hill, op. cit.
111. Santi & Hill, op. cit.
112. E. Rossi, *La Nubia edil Sudan*, Constantinople, 1858.
113. Hill, *Biographical Dictionary*, 1967, op. cit., p.299.
114. Hill, ibid., p.114.
115. Cruickshank & Bloss, op. cit.
116. *Voyage au Darfour, traduit de l'Arabe par le Dr.. Ferron public par les soins de M. Jomard*, Paris, 1845.
117. Ahmed Ahmed Sid Ahmed, op. cit., p.275.

118. Hill, *Egypt in Sudan*, 1959, p.128.
119. File 47, M.S; No 874, encl 1,22 March 1871 (quoted in R. L. Hill, *Egypt in Sudan*, 1958).
120. S. W. Baker, *The Albert Ny'anza Great Basin of the Nile and Exploration of the Nile Sources*, London, MacMillan & Co., Ltd., 1866.
121. Ibid., p.461-493.
122. al-Jindi & Tagher, *Ismail*, p.165.
123. Hill, *Egypt in the Sudan*, 1959; p.128 .
124. Hill, *Biographical Dictionary*, 1967, op. cit., p.54.
125. Dr.. W. Junker, *Travels in Africa, 1875-1878*, p.21.
126. Bayoumi, op. cit., 1974.
127. Sir Aly Tewfik Shousha Pasha, Cholera Epidemic in Egypt (1947): A Preliminary Report, *WHO Bulletin, 1948, 1(2), pp.353-381.*
128. George C. Kohn, MacNamara, A History of Asiatic Cholera, In: *Encyclopaedia of Plague & Pestilence.*
129. Whitehead, 1938, op. cit.
130. R. L. Hill, Unpublished Fragments of a Manuscript Concerning Events in the Sudan 1843-1848, *Sudan Notes & Records*, 1955, Vol. 36(2), pp.112-122.
131. Katib Al Shona, *The History of the Fung and the Turco-Egyptian Administration*, pp.133-134.
132. Cruickshank & Bloss, op. cit.
133. Ibid.
134. Hill, *Biographical Dictionary*, 1967, op. cit., p.133.
135. Samuel W Baker, *Ismailia: A Narrative of the Expedition to Central Africa for the Suppression of the Slave Trade*, London, Macmillan & Co., 1874.
136. Ibid., p.385.
137. Ibid.
138. Dr. Richard Pankhurst, The Pankhurst History Library, the History of Epidemics in Ethiopia, 6.
139. Gaetano Casati, *Dieceanni in Equatoria*, Milan, 1891 [*Ten years in Equatoria*, translated from the Italian manuscript by J. Randolph Clay & Walter Savage Landor, London ,Fredrick Warne and Co., 1898.]
140. Ibid., pp.17-18.
141. Ibid., p.15.
142. Baker, *Albert N'yanza*, op. cit., p.11.
143. Bayard Taylor, *A Journey to Central Africa*, 1856.
144. Ibid., pp.269-278.
145. Ibid.

146. Luigi Montouri to Vincenzo Spaccapietra, 3 September 1843, quoted in Pane, Il Beato Guistino de Jacobis, pp.839-848, and Bano, 'Lazzaristi,' p.291.
147. Rev C. T. Wilson & Rev R. W. Felkin, *Uganda and the Egyptian Soudan*, Stuttgart, 1883.
148. Mattucci Pelligrini, *Sudan e Gallas*, Milan, Fratelli Treves, 1879.
149. Alice Moore-Harell, The Turco-Egyptian Army on the eve of the Mahdiyya, 1877-1880, *International Journal of Middle East Studies*, 31, 1999, pp.19-37.
150. Gordon to Cabinet Secretariat 25th April 1877, 11 Rabi Awal 1294H, DW box 19,24/4 (Quoted in A. Moore-Harrel Gordon).
151. R. L. Hill, *The Sudan memoirs of Carl Christian Giegler Pasha, 1873-1883*, London, 1984.
152. Casati, op. cit., p.12.
153. Elias Toniolo, Richard Hill, *The Opening of the Nile Basin: Writings by Members of the Catholic Mission to Central Africa on the Geography and Ethnography of the Sudan, 1842-1881*, New York, Barnes & Noble Books, 1975.
154. Alice Moore-Harel, *Gordon*, p.167.
155. The Khediev Council Papers, Dar Al-Wathaig al-Qawmia, Cairo, box 20.
156. Hill, *Biographical Dictionary*, p.347.
157. Thomas Hazel Parke, *My Personal Experiences in Equatorial Africa as a Medical Officer of the Emin Pasha Relief Expedition*, 1896.
158. A. T. Holroyd, Notes on a Journey to Kordofan in 1836-7, *The Journal of the Royal Geographical Society*, 1839, Vol. 9, pp.166-191.
159. Reda Mowafi, *Slavery, Slave Trade and Abolition Attempts in Egypt and the Sudan 1820-1882*, Lund Studies in International history, Scandanavian Universities Books, 1981.
160. Arthur T. Holroyd, *Suakim and the Country of Soudan*, Sydney, Thomas Richards, Govt Printer, 1885.
161. Thornton, *Memories of Seven Campaign 1895.*
162. Holroyd, 1839, op. cit.
163. Ibid.
164. Hill, 1967, op. cit., p.282.
165. J. F. E. Bloss, Notes on the Health of the Sudan Prior to this Government, *Sudan Notes & Records*, 1941, 24, pp.131-143.
166. Cruickshank & Bloss, op. cit.
167. Ibid.

Part II, Chapter 3: Endnotes

1. Francis R. Wingate, *Mahdiism and the Egyptian Sudan: Being an Account of the Rise and Progress of Mahdiism and of Subsequent Events in the Sudan Up to the Present Time*, Macmillan and Company, 1891.
2. Fr .Joseph Ohrwalder& R. F. Wingate, *Ten Years of Captivity in the Mahdi's Camp*, 1893.
3. R. von Slatin, *Fire and Sword in the Sudan*, 1897.
4. Slatin, op. cit.
5. Ohrwalder, op. cit.
6. Robert S. Kramer, *Holy City on the Nile*, 2010.
7. J. B. Christopherson, Description of Sudanese Native Remedies in the Mahdi's and Khalifa's Time in Omdurman, SAD 497/6/1-28.
8. Musa Abdalla Hamid & Kamal Salih, Omdurman Teaching Hospital, 1986.
9. Ibid.
10. A. Bayoumi, *The History of Sudan Health Services*, Kenya Litreature Bureau, 1979.
11. P. M. Holt, *The Mahdist State in the Sudan 1881-1898. A Study of Its Origin, Development and Overthrow*, Oxford, Clarendon Press, 1958.
12. Kraemer, op. cit.
13. Ibid., p.69.
14. Ibid., p.70.
15. Ibid.
16. Kraemer, op. cit., p.73.
17. Abu Salim AI: Al-Bulis fi'l Mahdiyya', 'Majalat Al-Bulis, July 1966. (In Arabic)
18. Kraemer, op. cit., p.74.
19. Ibid., p.78.
20. Ibid., p.75.
21. Third Wellcome Report, 1908, The Healing Act as Practised by the Dervishes in the Sudan during the Rule of the Mahdi and of the Khalifa, by El Bimbashi Hassan Effendi Zaki, Sudan Medical department, Medical Officer, Gordon Memorial College (translated from Arabic).
22. Third Wellcome Report, 1908, Additional Notes Contributed by Sir Rudolph Baron von Slatin Pasha, Inspector General, Sudan Government.
23. Hill, *Egypt in Sudan*, 1959, p.128.

24. Zaki, op. cit., p.269.
25. Ibid.
26. Ibid.
27. Ibid., p.270.
28. Ibid.
29. Ibid., p.277.
30. Ibid., p.278.
31. Ibid., p.277.
32. A. Alsafi, *Traditional Sudanese Medicine*, 2006.
33. Slatin, op. cit., pp.278-279.
34. Zaki, op. cit., p.271.
35. Ibid., p.270.
36. Alsafi, op. cit.
37. R. G. Anderson, Medical Practices and Superstitions amongst the People of Kordofan: Their Treatment of Diseases and Chief Drugs, Instruments and Appliances in Common Use, Third Wellcome Report, 1908, pp.281-322.
38. L. Bousfield, The Native Methods of Treatment of Diseases in Kassala and Neighbourhood, Third Wellcome Report, 1908, pp.273-275.
39. M. Shebieka, *'Al-Sudan abr algroon'* (in Arabic), Beirut, 1963.
40. Slatin, op. cit.
41. Ohrwalder, op. cit.
42. Yusuf Michaeil, Memoirs (in Arabic; revised and authenticated by Ahmed Ibrahim Abu Shouk).
43. R. Lamothe, *Slaves of Fortune, Sudanese Soldiers in the River War 1896-1989*, Suffolk, UK, Boydell & Brewer, 2011, p.92.
44. G. Ayoub Balamoan, *Migration Policies in the Anglo-Egyptian Sudan, 1884-1956*, Cambridge, Mass., Harvard University Centre for Population Studies, 1976, p.26.
45. Lamothe, op. cit., p.93.
46. N. H. Hunter, Historical Records of the Xth Sudanese, 1886-1910, National Army Museum 1968-07-330-1.
47. Zaki, op. cit., p.271.
48. Ohrwalder, p.176.
49. Janet Ewald, *Soldiers, Traders and Slaves: State Formation in the Greater Nile Valley, 1700-1885*, Madison, University of Wisconsin, 1990, p.126.
50. G. Warburg, *Islam, Sectarianism and Politics in Sudan since the Mahdiyya*, London, Hurst & Co., 2003, p.47.
51. Musa & Salih, op. cit.

52. MIR 1904, RCSM, Cambridge University Library.
53. S. I. Khalil, The First Hospital in Sudan 1826-1959, a Historical Perspective, *Sudan Medical Journal*, 2014, 50(1), pp.48-52.
54. MIR 1899, RCMS, Cambridge University Library.

Part III, Chapter I: Endnotes

1. James Howard Thornton, *Memories of Seven Campaigns*, 1895.
2. Ibid., p.215.
3. Ibid., p.228.
4. Ibid., p.222.
5. Ibid., p.228.
6. Ibid., pp.244-247.
7. Ibid., p.248.
8. Cruickshank & Bloss, SAD.
9. Walter H. Wallis, *Anglo-African Who's Who and Biographical Sketchbook 1907*, Jeppestown Press, 2006, p.281.
10. James Baird, Sir Alexander Ogston & the Royal Army Medical Corps. Repub.euro.nl/pub/8151/HOOFDST1JK.3.PDF
11. Cruickshank and Bloss, op. cit.
12. Ohrwalder, 1892, op. cit.
13. Cruickshank and Bloss, op. cit.
14. Sudan Despatches, Nile Expedition. http://www.northeastmedals.co.uk/britishguide/sudan/despatches_index.htm
15. Military Intelligence Reports, Sudan Government Annual Reports, Years 1898-1899, Royal Commonwealth Society Section, (RCMS), Cambridge University Library.
16. Ibid., p.22.
17. Ibid., p.24.
18. Cruickshank and Bloss, op. cit.
19. MIR 1898-1899, op. cit. p.26.
20. Ibid., p.32.
21. Military Intelligence Reports, Sudan Government Annual Reports 1900, RCMS, Cambridge University Library.
22. Ibid., p.25.
23. Military Intelligence Reports, Sudan Government Annual Reports 1901, RCMS, Cambridge University Library.
24. Ibid.
25. Ibid., p.77.
26. MIR 1901 & 1902.

27. Medical & Sanitary Dept, Military Intelligence Reports, Sudan Government Annual Reports 1903, RCMS, Cambridge University Library.
28. Ibid.
29. Military Intelligence Reports, Sudan Government Annual Reports 1905, RCMS, pp.83-84.
30. Military Intelligence Reports, Sudan Government Annual Reports 1904, RCMS, Cambridge University Library.
31. Ibid.
32. MIR 1905, op. cit.
33. Squires, Sudan Health Services, 1958, p.xxx (Syrian Medical Colleges).
34. H. Bell, *Frontiers of Medicine in the Anglo-Egyptian Sudan*, 1999.
35. MIR 1905, op. cit.
36. Squires, op. cit., p.3.
37. Ibid., p.14.
38. MIR 1905, op. cit.
39. R Kirk, unpublished papers, RCMS 122/3/5, Cambridge University Library.
40. Byam, *The Road*, op. cit., p.62.
41. Ibid., pp.76-77..
42. W. Byam, *The Road to Harley Street*, London, Geoffrey Bles, 1963.
43. Squires, op. cit., p.8.
44. Squires, op. cit., pp.23-28.
45. Annual Report SMD, RCSM.
46. Byam, op. cit., p.175.
47. Atiyah, *An Arab Tells His Story*.
48. Atiyah, *The Black Vanguard*.
49. Atiya Family, SAD 2/20/2.
50. Michael Atiyah.
51. Ann Crichton-Harris, *Poisons in Small Measures: Bilharzia Drug Discovery & Dr. Christopherson*, Amsterdam, Brill, 2009 (George Morhig).
52. Ibid., Alfred Morhig.
53. Hadi Stambolia, personal communication.
54. Dr. Musa Abdalla Hamid & Dr. Kamal Salih, 'Omdurman Teaching Hospital: Past, Present and Future 1986 (in Arabic) (publisher unknown).
55. SAD 407/2/1-79.
56. Ibid.
57. Byam, *The Road*, p.62.

58. Ibid., p.82.
59. Ibid., p.135.
60. Ibid., p.149.

Part III, Chapter 2: Endnotes

1. M. W. Daly, *Empire on the Nile, the Anglo-Egyptian Sudan, 1898-1934*, Cambridge University Press, 1986, pp.259-265.
2. A. Cruickshank, *Golden Age of Tropical Medicine: Essays in Honour of Richard Hill*, 1985.
3. H. Bell, Frontiers of Medicine, p.31.
4. H. C. Squires, Sudan Medical Service, An Experiment in Social Medicine, London Heineman, 1958, p.5.
5. Crichton-Harris, *Poisons in Small Measures*, 2009, p.122.
6. A. Crichton-Harris, Undercurrent on the Nile, *Journal of Medical Biography*, 2006, 14(1), pp.8-16.
7. Crichton-Harris, *Poisons*, op. cit., p.119.
8. Squires, op. cit., p.8.
9. Daly, op. cit., p.260.
10. Squires, op. cit., p.4.
11. R Kirk, Doctors in the Sudan Medical Service: A List for the Years 1901-1950, RCMS 122, Cambridge University Library.
12. Squires, op. cit., p.109.
13. Ibid.
14. Ibid.
15. Crichton Harris, *Undercurrent on the Nile*, 2006, op. cit.
16. P. W. D'Arcy, *Laboratory on the Nile*, 1999, pp.39-40.
17. Sudan Medical Service, Annual Report, 1928.
18. A. A. Abdel Hameed, Wellcome Tropical Res Laboratory, Medical History, 1997.
19. L. Bousfield, *Sudan Doctor*, p.64.
20. Squires, op. cit., p.15.
21. J. B. Christorpherson, Letter to the Editor, *St. Bartholomew Medical Journal*, 1928.
22. Squires, op. cit., p.8.
23. Atiyah Family, SAD, 2/20/2.
24. MIR 1906, RCS 122/3/4.
25. MIR 1904, RCS 122/3/4.
26. MIR 1905, Public Health, RCS 122/3/4.
27. Bousfield, *Sudan Doctor*, op. cit., p.70.
28. MIR 1905, op. cit.

29. Crichton-Harris, *Poison*, op. cit., p.129.
30. SAD 406/5/28.
31. Squires, op. cit., p.16.
32. MIR 1906, op. cit.
33. MIR 1908.
34. Squires, op. cit., p.16.
35. Crichton-Harris, *Poisons*, op. cit., p.172.
36. Phipps to Wingate, SAD.
37. Byam, *The Road*, p.5.
38. Cruickshank, *Itchy Feet*, op. cit., p.32..
39. P. J. Cain & A. J. Hopkins, *British Imperialism*, London, Longman, 1993.
40. S. Mollan, Recruitment to the Sudan Medical Service 1898-1938: Some Speculations Based on the Use of Social Ntwork Analysis, SSSUK, 29 (June 2002), pp.35-54.
41. K. Owen, Sudan Interlude, *Retired Fellows Journal, Royal Society of Medicine*, 2006.
42. Mullan, op. cit.
43. Ibid.
44. Byam, *The Road*, op. cit., p.71.
45. Ibid., p.73.
46. *Sudan Gazette*, No. 29, November 1901.
47. *Sudan Gazette*, No. 71, February 1905.
48. MIR, Sudan Government, 1910, Royal Common Wealth Society, Cambridge University Library.
49. MIR, 1911.
50. MIR, 1912.
51. Squires, op. cit., p.79.
52. MIR, 1913.
53. MIR, 1914.
54. *Sudan Gazette*, No. 285, 11 September 1915.
55. *Sudan Gazette*, No. 310, 7 December 1916.
56. MIR, 1915-1919.
57. MacMichael, *The Sudan*, p.168.
58. MIR, 1915-1919, op. cit.
59. Ibid.
60. Ibid.
61. Ibid.
62. MacMichael, *The Sudan*, op. cit., p.168.
63. Squires, op. cit., p. 79.
64. MIR, 1915-1919, op. cit.

65. Ibid.
66. Public Health Reports, Governor General Annual Report, Sudan Government, 1920, Royal Commonwealth Society, Cambridge University Library.
67. Ibid.
68. Ibid.
69. Ibid.
70. Ibid.
71. Ibid.
72. Public Health Reports, Governor General Annual Report, Sudan Government, 1921, Royal Commonwealth Society, Cambridge University Library.
73. Squires, op. cit., p.49.
74. Public Health Report, 1921, op. cit.
75. Ibid.
76. Ibid.
77. Ibid.
78. Ibid.
79. Ibid.
80. Ibid,
81. Ibid.
82. Ibid.
83. Squires, op. cit., p.50.
84. Sudan Medical Department, Annual Report, 1922.
85. Ibid.
86. Ibid.
87. Ibid.
88. Ibid.
89. Ibid.
90. Ibid.
91. Annual Report, Sudan Medical Department, 1923.
92. Ibid.
93. Ibid.
94. Ibid.
95. Ibid.
96. Ibid.
97. Cruickshank, *Itchy Feet*, op. cit., p.46.
98. Annual Report, 1923, op. cit.
99. Ibid.
100. Ibid.
101. Squires, op. cit., p.50.

102. Squires, op. cit., p.51.
103. Annual Report, Sudan Medical Department, 1922, op. cit.
104. Ibid.
105. Ibid.
106. Ibid.
107. Ibid.
108. Ibid.
109. Ibid.
110. Ibid.
111. Ibid.
112. Ibid.
113. Ibid.

Part III, Chapter 3: Endnotes

1. Sudan Medical Department Annual Report, 1922, 1923.
2. D. A. Messinezy, Notes on the Health Personnel Training Programme of the Anglo-Egyptian Sudan, *Bulletin of the World Health Organization*, 1949, 2, 289-298.
3. Ibid.
4. Ibrahim Elnur, *Contested Sudan: The Political Economy of War and Reconstruction*, London, Routledge, 2009, p.174.
5. Daly, *Imperial Sudan*, p.122. {ref 124}
6. Ibid., p.123.
7. K. Owen, *Sudan Interlude*, 2006.
8. S. Neave, *Leishmania donovani* in the Soudan, *British Medical Journal*, 1904, 1252.
9. Bousfield, *Sudan Doctor*, pp.76-78.
10. Bousfield, Third Wellcome Report, pp.107-119.
11. S. L. Cummins, Third Wellcome Report, 1908, pp.100-106.
12. D. S. B. Thomson, Fourth Wellcome Report, 1911, pp.142-156.
13. W. E. Marshall, Fourth Wellcome Report, pp.157-172.
14. R. W. Stephenson, Leishmaniasis among Dinka Tribe in Melut, Southern Sudan, *Annals of Tropical Medicine & Parasitology*, 1940, 34, p.176.
15. MH Satti, RCMS 122/2/11, Cambridge University Library.
16. R. G. Archibald & M. A. Haseeb. Some Observation on the Epidemiology of Kala azar in the Sudan. *Transactions of the Royal Society of Tropical Medicine and Hygiene*, 1937, Vol. XXX, No. 4, pp.895-400.
17. Report of the Royal Soc. of Sleeping Sickness, 1903; pp.213-214.

18. A. Castellani, Presence of Trypanosomes in Sleeping Sickness, In: Reports of the Sleeping Sickness Commission of the Royal Society, 1903, 1, 3-10,
19. D. Bruce et al., Further Report on Sleeping Sickness in Uganda, In: Reports of the Sleeping Sickness Commission of the Royal Society, 1903; 4, pp.2-87.
20. J. F. E. Bloss, The History of Sleeping Sickness in the Sudan, *Royal Society of Medicine, Proceedings*, 1960, 53, 421, pp.7-12.
21. S. Neave, Second Wellcome Report, 1906.
22. Ibid.
23. A. J. Balfour, Trypansomiasis in the Sudan, Report of the Sleeping Sickness Commission. Second WellcomeReport, 1906.
24. Fourth Wellcome Report, 1911, p.SSC.
25. The Anglo-Egyptian Sudan & Sleeping Sickness, *Bulletin of the Sleeping Sickness Bureau*, 9 (1909), pp.347ff.
26. H. Ensor, Report on the Investigation Carried Out in Bahr el-Ghazal Province on Behalf of the Sudan Sleeping Sickness Commission 1907-1908, *Journal of the Royal Army Medical Corps*, 1909, 12, pp.376-401.
27. A. B. Mathias, Sleeping Sickness in the Anglo-Egyptian Sudan, Report of the Sleeping Sickness Commission, Fourth Wellcome Report, 1911, Volume A: Medical, pp.31-40.
28. Bloss, op. cit.
29. Ibid.
30. Ibid.
31. B. H. H. Spence, Annual Report on Tuberculosis & Sleeping Sickness in Equatorial Africa, Geneva, League of Nations, 1923.
32. P. H. Abbott, Observation on the Control of Sleeping Sickness among the Azande Tribe of Southern Sudan, *East African Medical Journal*, 1952, 29(8), pp.298-308.
33. G. K. Maurice, Bulletin of the Sleeping Sickness Bureau, *Journal of the Royal Army Medical Corps*, 1930, 55, pp.161-241.
34. Bloss, op. cit.
35. A. Bayoumi, 1970, op. cit.
36. MIR 1903.
37. MIR 1901.
38. MIR 1902.
39. Crichton-Harris, *Poisons*, 2009, p.97.
40. MIR 1903, op. cit.
41. MIR 1904.
42. Annual Report of Sudan Medical Department, 1920.

43. Annual Report of Sudan Medical Department, 1921.
44. H. Ensor, A Case of Cerebro-spinal Meningitis, *Journal of the Royal Army Medical Corps*, 1904.
45. R. B. U. Somers, M & B 693 in Cerebrospinal Fever, *The Lancet*, 1, 921-922, 1939.
46. MIR 1900.
47. Squires, *Sudan Medical Service*, op. cit. p. 38.
48. J. Bryant & H. D. Fairman, Chemotherapy for Cerebrospinal Fever in the field, *The Lancet*, 1, 923-926, 1939.
49. N. L. Corkhill, Vitamin A in Cerebrospinal Fever, *Journal of Tropical Medicine (Hygiene)* 1936.
50. M. E. Wolff, Some Notes on the Sudan, SAD 582/10/16.
51. H. Bell, Frontiers of Medicine in the Anglo-Egyptian Sudan, 1999, Oxford University Press.
52. MIR 1908.
53. MIR 1911.
54. MIR 1908, op. cit.
55. Bell, op. cit.
56. Cruickshank, *Itchy Feet: A Doctor's Tale*, London, 1991, p.144.
57. J. Boddy, Barbaric Customs & Colonial Science: Teaching the Female Body in the Anglo-Egyptian Sudan, In: Michael Lambek & Paul Antz, *Illness & Irony: On the Ambiguity of Suffering in Culture*, Berghahn Books, 2003.
58. Annual Report SMD, 1922.
59. E. M. Kendall, A Short History of the Training of Midwives in the Sudan, *Sudan Notes & Records*, 1953, 33, pp.42-53.
60. Ibid.
61. Ibid.
62. Messinzy, op. cit.
63. Kendall, op. cit.
64. M. E. Wolff, Elementary Practical Lessons for Midwives, Sudan Archives of Durham, 581/5/7.
65. Squires, op. cit., p.xxx.
66. Kendall, op. cit.
67. Annual Report SMD 1922, op. cit.
68. Annual Report SMD 1923.
69. Annual Report SMS 1925.
70. Annual Report SMS 1926.
71. Cruickshank, op. cit., p.144.
72. S. I. Khalil, The First Hospital in the Sudan 1826-1959, *Sudan Medical Journal*, 2014, vol. 50(1), 48-52.

73. Crichton-Harris, *Poisons*, p.xxx.
74. Dr. Christopherson Papers, SAD 400/5.
75. W. F. Sanders, *The Royal Engineers in Egypt and the Sudan.*
76. Squires, 1958, op. cit., p.83.
77. Khalil, op. cit.
78. Bousfield, *Sudan Doctor*, op. cit., pp.160-175.
79. Squires, op. cit, p.14.
80. Ibid.
81. Beveridge, *Allah Laughed*, p.102.
82. Squires, op. cit., p.48.
83. Ibid., pp.48-49.
84. SMD Annual Report, 1923.
85. Squires, op. cit., p.49.

Part IV: Endnotes

1. Robert James, Henry S Wellcome, 1996, John Curtis Books, London (The Plight of the Sioux Indians, pp.7-33).
2. Ibid., p.134.
3. Ibid., p.49.
4. H. S. Wellcome, miscellaneous letters, Wellcome Archives.
5. Wellcome to Kitchener, miscellaneous correspondence, 1899, Wellcome Archives.
6. R. James, op. cit., p.250.
7. F. W. Sandes, The Royal Engineers in Egypt and the Sudan, Chatham, 1937.
8. James, op. cit., p.50.
9. Wellcome to Wingate, miscellaneous correspondence, 1899, Wellcome Archives.
10. Wellcome to Currie, miscellaneous correspondence, Wellcome Archives GWGA; 171-2, Hb62.
11. First Wellcome Report, 1904, p.11.
12. *Sudan Gazette*, No. 60, March 1904.
13. E. Fothergil, *Five Years in the Sudan*, 1910.
14. Talbot to Wingate, 21/05/1903, SAD 273/5/27-29.
15. A. Balfour, Mosquito Work in Khartoum and in the Anglo-Egyptian Sudan Generally, First Wellcome Report, 1904, pp.14-36.
16. Ibid., p.14-18.
17. Ibid., p.18.
18. Ibid., p. 20

19. P. F. D'Arcy, *Laboratory on the Nile: A History of the Wellcome Tropical Research Laboratories*, CRC Press, 1999.
20. A. Balfour. Mosquito Work in the Anglo-Egyptian Sudan and in the Anglo-Egyptian Sudan Generally, Second WellcomeReport, 1906, pp.15-28.
21. D'Arcy, op. cit., p.71.
22. Second Wellcome Report, 1906, op. cit., p.25.
23. Ibid., p.18 .
24. Ibid., p.23.
25. Ibid., p.19.
26. Ibid., p.17.
27. MIR1903, RCMS 122/3/4.
28. Colonel Bray, Work in Kassala.
29. Byam, *The Road*; 1964, p.63.
30. Ibid., p.62.
31. A. Balfour, Sanitary Notes, Khartoum, Third WellcomeReport, 1908, pp.60-92.
32. Ibid., p.17.
33. D'Arcy, op. cit.
34. S. Neave, Obituary, *British Medical Journal*, Nov. 7, 1936 vol. 2 (3957) 951.
35. www.encyclopedia.com
36. S. Neave, *Leishman donovani* in the Soudan, *British Medical Journal*, May 28, 1904; p. 1252.
37. Second Wellcome Report, p.183.
38. S. Neave, Report of the Travelling Pathologist and Naturalist, Second Wellcome Report, 1906, pp.183-204.
39. Ibid.
40. D'Arcy Laboratory, op. cit., pp.115-116.
41. Second Wellcome Report, 1906, pp.12-13.
42. D'Arcy, Laboratory, op. cit., p.117.
43. C. M. Wenyon, Report of the Travelling Pathologist and Protozoolgist, Third Wellcome Report, 1908, pp.121-168..
44. Charles Morley Wenyon, *Protozoology: A Manual for Medical Men, Veterinarians and Zoologists*, Baillieri Tindall & Cox, 1926.
45. D'Arcy, op. cit.
46. First Wellcome Report, 1904, op. cit., p.14.
47. A. Balfour, Biting and Noxious Insects Other than Mosquitoes, First Wellcome Report, 1904, pp.38-40.
48. A. Balfour, Biting and Noxious Insects Other than Mosquitoes, Second Wellcome Report, 1906, pp.29-50.

49. First Wellcome Report, 1904, op. cit., p.38.
50. A. Balfour, Insects and Vegetable Parasites Injurious to Crops, First Wellcome Report, pp.46-47.
51. Ernest E. Austen, Some Blood Sucking Diptera from the Anglo-Egyptian Sudan Collected during 1905 with Description of Some New Insects, Second Wellcome Report, pp.51-66.
52. F. V. Theobald, The Mosquitoes of Egypt, The Sudan & Abyssinia, First Wellcome Report, 1904, pp.51-66.
53. Ibid.
54. F. V. Theobald, Report on Economic Entomology, Second Wellcome Report, 1906, pp. 67-96.
55. Balfour A. Haemogregarine of Mammals, Second Wellcome Report, 1906, pp.97-112.
56. Laveran, Comptesrendus des seaness de L'Aead des Sciences, Vol. CXLI. p.295, 1905.
57. Balfour, Second Wellcome Report, p. 111.
58. David Waterston, Report upon the Physical Characters of Some of the Nilotic Negroid Tribes, Third Wellcome Report, 1908, pp.325-376.
59. Ibid., p.325.
60. Ibid., p.328.
61. Ibid., p.338.
62. Ibid., p.356.
63. Ibid., p.346.
64. Ibid., p.350.
65. D. J. Vallance, Notes on Ethnographical Specimens Collected by Dr. A. MacTier Pirrie, Third Wellcome Report, 1908, pp.377-380.
66. Ibid., pp.377-384.
67. Ibid., pp.378.
68. Alexander Boyd, *From the Niger to the Nile*, London, Edward Arnold, 1907.
69. Vallance, op. cit., p.380..
70. C. G. Seligman & B. Z. Seligman, *The Pagan Tribes of the Nilotic Sudan*, London, George Routledge & Son, 1932.
71. Fourth Wellcome Report, 1911, p.26.
72. D'Arcy, 1999, op. cit., p.209.
73. Ibid., p.213.
74. First Wellcome Report, 1904, op. cit., p.9.
75. Ibid..
76. Ibid., p.13.
77. Second Wellcome Report, 1906, p.9.

78. Ibid., p.11.
79. Third Wellcome Report, 1908, op. cit., p.16.
80. Ibid., p.16.
81. Ibid., p.17.
82. Third Wellcome Report, 1908, op. cit., p.16.
83. Ibid., p.23.
84. Ibid., p.22.
85. Ibid., p.59.
86. Fourth Wellcome Report, 1911, op. cit., p.19.
87. Ibid., p.20.
88. Ibid.
89. Ibid.
90. Ibid., pp.21-22.
91. Ibid., p.25.
92. Ibid., p.26.
93. Ibid.
94. Third Wellcome Report, Supplement, 1908, op. cit., p.6.
95. Ibid., pp.25-27.
96. Ibid., p.26.
97. Wellcome Fourth Report, Supplement, 1911.
98. Ibid., p.6.
99. Ibid., p.141.
100. Ibid., p.15.
101. A. A. Abdel Hameed, *Medical History*, 1997, 41, pp.30-58.
102. J. B. Christopherson, *Lancet*, 1919, op. cit.
103. Abdel Hameed, op. cit.
104. Archibald & Haseeb, *Proceedings of the Royal Society of Medicine*, 1937.
105. T. A. Elhadd, *Journal of the Royal College of Physicians of Edinburgh*, 2015.
106. Udal to Wellcome, Wellcome Archives, 1930.
107. A. Ibrahim , Government Analyst, Robert Kirk Papers, RCSM 122/2/1; The Wellcome Chemical Laboratories, A Contribution to the 8th Annual Conference of the Philosophical Society of the Sudan, January 1960.
108. D'Arcy, 1999, op. cit., p.252.
109. Sir Andrew Balfour, Obituary, *British Medical Journal*, Feb. 7, 1931, 1(3657):245-6.

Endnotes to Appendix I

1. Obituary, J. B. Christopherson, *British Medical Journal*, July 1955, p.327.
2. The Annual Presidential Address of the Royal College of Physicians of London, Monday, March 26, 1956.
3. A. Crichton-Harris, Undercurrent on the Nile, *Journal of Medical Biography*, 2006, 14(1), pp.8-16..
4. Crichton-Harris, *Poison*, pp.71-201.
5. John Brian Christopherson, Catalogue of papers, Sudan Archives Durham, GB-0033. http://reed.dur.ac.uk/xtf/view?docId=ead/sad/christoj.xml. (accessed May 15, 2014)+
6. Crichton-Harris, *Poison*, op. cit., pp.171-201.
7. Crichton-Harris, *Poison*, op. cit., pp.119-138.
8. Squires, *The Sudan Medical Services*, p.6.
9. Ibid., p.11.
10. Crichton-Harris, *Poison*, p.147.
11. Squires, op. cit., p.5 .
12. Crichton-Harris, *Poison*, op. cit.. p.147.
12. Ibid., pp.148-151.
13. Ibid., pp.149-164.
14. SAD 407/2/1-79.
15. SAD 407/6/1-14.
16. Crichton-Harris, *Poison*, op. cit., pp.159-164.
17. Ibid., p.161.
18. Bousfield, *Sudan Doctor*, op. cit.
19. Byam, *The Road*, op. cit., pp.114-116.
20. J. B. Christopherson & A. J. Chalmers, A Sudanese Actinomycosis, *Annals of Tropical Med*icine (Section Parasitology), 1916-17, x.223-282.
21. SAD 407/6/27.
22. J. B. Christopherson, The Successful Use of Antimony in Bilharziosis, *The Lancet*, 7 Sept 1919, pp.325-327.-
23. Crichton-Harris, pp.269-292.
24. 15. SAD 407/2/1-25.
25. SAD 407/6/27.
26. *The London Gazzette*, 14 March 1916, pp.2782.
27. *The Sudan Diocesan Review*, Autumn 1956, 50/1/248.

Endnotes to Appendix 2

1. William Byam (2016, September 3) In; *Wikipedia, The Free Encyclopedia*. Retrieved 01:10, September 3, 2016, https://en.wikipedia.org/w/index.php?title=William_Byam&oldid=737471644
2. Who Is Who in Br. Philately, Association of British Philatelic Societies, 2014.
3. Dr. W. Byam, *The London Philatelist*, Vol. 72, No. 852, Dec 1963.
4. *The Canadian Philatelist*, Vol. XV, No. 1, Jan-Feb 1964, pp.32-34.
5. William Byam, *Dr. Byam in Harley Street*, Geoffrey Bles, 1963.

Endnotes to Appendix 3

1. Robert James, Wellcome, 1996, p.14.
2. John Symons, The Benevolent Autocrat, *The Wellcome Journal*, Vol. 6, 1991.
3. H. S. Wellcome & F. Addison, *Jebel Moya*, Oxford University Press, 1949.
4. R. Mukherjee, *Ancient Inhabitants of Jebel Moya Sudan*, Cambridge University Press, 2010.
5. Towards an archaeology of social organization at Jebel Moya, 5th – 1st millennium BC, *Sudan & Nubia,* 2009, 13, pp.120-125 .
6. Rudolf Gerharz, 1994. Jebel Moya in Neuer Interpretation (Institut fuer Sudan archaeologie und Aegyptologie der Humboldt-Universitaet zu Berlin - Meroitica).

Endnotes to Appendix 4

1. Poncet, *A Voyage to Ethiopia*, 1709.
2. Jay Spalding, op. cit., p.358.
3. J. Bruce, *Travels*, op. cit.
4. Ibid., pp.728-729 .
5. Ibid., pp.402-403.
6. W. G. Browne, *Travels*, op. cit.
7. W. G. Browne, *Travels*, ibid., p.346.
8. Burckhardt, *Travels in Nubia*, pp.211-212.
9. Ibid., p.261.
10. Ibid., p.263.

11, Pallme, *Travels in Kordofan*, op. cit., pp.194-195.

12. Ibid., p.195.
13. Ibid.
14. Ibid., p.196.

15. Holroyd, *Suakim and the Soudan*, 1885, pp.14-15.
16. S. W. Baker, *The Nile Tributaries*, op. cit., p.96.
17. Ibid., p.91.
18. Ibid., p.96.
19. Ibid., p.91.
20. Ibid.
21. Ibid., p.97.
22. Ibid., p.92.
23. Ibid.
24. Ibid., p.96.

Endnotes to Appendix 5

1. Kings College London, Liddell Hart Centre for Military Archives, www.kcl.ac.uk/ihcma/summary/cu05-001.shtml.: *publishing.eur.nl/ir/repub/asset/8151/HOOFDSTUK3.PDF).*
   (Kings College London, Liddell Hart Centre for Military Archives, www.kcl.ac.uk/ihcma/summary/cu05-001.shtml
2. S. L. Cummins, Tuberculosis in the Egyptian Army, *British Journal of Tuberculosis*, 1908, 2/1, pp.35-46.
3. S. L. Cummins, 1912 paper.
4. Michael Worboys, Tuberculosis and Race in Britain and its Empire 1900-1950, In: Ernst Waltraud & Bernard Harris, *Race, Science & Medicine 1700-1960*, Routledge, 1999, p.84.
5. S. L. Cummins, Tuberculosis in Wales, *British Medical Journal*, 1922, 1, Pp.340.
6. S Lyle Cummins, Tubercle Bacilli and Urea, *British Medical Journal*, June 16, 1945, p.841.
7. S. L. Cummins, Pneumoconiosis with Special Reference to the Silico-anthracosis of Coal Miners, *British Medical Journal*, 17 Aug. 1935, pp.287-289.
8. S. L. Cummins, The Pneumoconiosis in South Wales, *Journal of Hygiene*, 1937, XXXVI, No. 4, pp.547-568.
9. Michael Worboys, *Migrants, Minorities & Health*, 1997.
10. Michael Worboys, *Tuberculosis and Race*, 1999, pp.93-124.
11. Helen Bynum, *Spitting Blood*, p.185.
12. Ibid., p.188.
13. Ibid., p.186 .
14. S. L. Cummins, *Primitive Tuberculosis*, London, John Bale Medical Books, 1939.

15. S. L. Cummins, *Tuberculosis in History*, London, Ballierie Tindal & Cox, 1949, p.15.
16. Obituary, *British Medical Journal*, June 11, 1949, p.1054.
17. Leonard Bosfield, *Sudan Doctor*, London, 1957.
18. Leonard Bousfield, Observation on Kalaz azar in the Kassala Province, Third Report of Wellcome TRL, Khartoum, 1908, pp.107-119.
19. S. Neave, *Leishmania donovani* in the Soudan, *British Medical Journal,* 1904, 1, p.1252.
20. *Sudan Doctor*, op. cit., pp.76-78.
21. Bousfield, Third Wellcome Report, op. cit., pp.270-275.
22. R. G. Anderson, Medical Practices and Superstitions as Practiced by the Natives in Kordofan, Third Report of Wellcome TRL, Khartoum, 1908, pp.280-322.
23. Ahmed Alsafi, *Traditional Sudanese Medicine*, op. cit., pp.233-234.
24. Bousfied, *Sudan Doctor*, op. cit., p.83.
25. Ibid., p.89.
26. Ibid., pp.91-92.
27. Ibid., p.100.
28. Ibid., p.101.
29. Ibid.
30. Ibid., pp.86-95.
31. L. Bousfield, Obituary, *British Medical Journal*, 1956, March 10, H. C. Squires et al., pp.577-578.
32. Byam, *The Road*, p.5.
33. Ibid., p.1.
34. Ibid., p.28.
35. Ibid.
36. Ibid., p.36.
37. Ibid., p.38.
38. Ibid., pp.50-51.
39. Ibid., p.58.
40. Ibid., pp.51-55.
41. Ibid., p.61.
42. Ibid., pp.69-70.
43. Ibid., pp.70-71.
44. Ibid., p.73.
45. Ibid., p.74.
46. Ibid., p.76.
47. James Bruce, *Travels in Abyssinia*, op. cit.
48. Byam, *The Road*, op. cit., p.81.
49. Ibid., p.82.

50. Ibid.
51. SMD, Annual Report, 1920.
52. Byam, *The Road*, op. cit., p.97.
53. Ibid., pp.118-148.
54. Ibid., p.149.
55. Ibid., p.155.
56. Ibid., p.178.
57. Ibid., pp.170-175.
58. Ibid., p.210.
59. Ibid., p.211.
60. Ibid.
61. Ibid., p.221.
62. Ibid., pp.217-226.
63. W. Byam, *Trench Fever. Lice and their Menace to Man*, London, Oxford University Press, 1919, pp.120-130.
64. Byam, *The Road*, op. cit., p.227.
65. Ibid., p.114.
66. Ibid., p.115.
67. Ibid.
68. Ibid.
69. Ibid., p.116.
70. Ibid., pp.112-117.
71. William Byam (2016, September 3). In: *Wikipedia, The Free Encyclopedia*. Retrieved 01:10, September 3, 2016, https://en.wikipedia.org/w/index.php?title=William_Byam&oldid=737471644

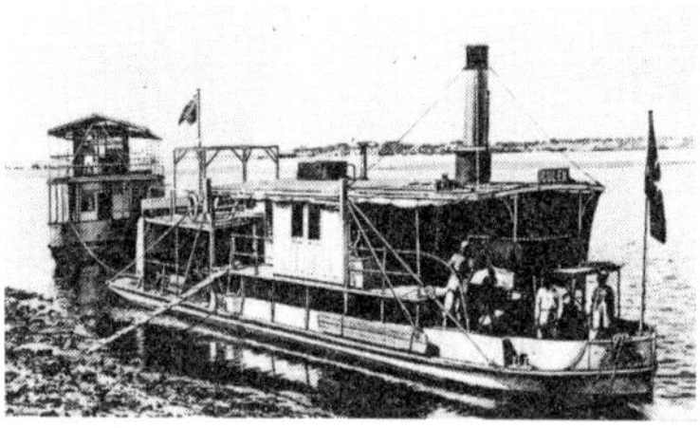

Index

B

D

E

H

K

M

N

O

P

Q

R

S

T

Y

Z